Board Review Series

GROSS ANATOMY

Board Review Series

GROSS ANATOMY

KYUNG WON CHUNG, Ph.D.

Professor
Department of Anatomical Sciences
University of Oklahoma College of Medicine
Oklahoma City, Oklahoma

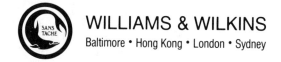

WILLIAMS & WILKINS
Baltimore • Hong Kong • London • Sydney

Editor: Kim Kist
Associate Editor: Victoria M. Vaughn
Copy Editor: Deborah Tourtlotte
Design: Norman W. Och
Illustration Planning: Wayne Hubbel
Production: Raymond E. Reter
Cover Design: Betsy Bayley

Copyright © 1988
Williams & Wilkins
428 East Preston Street
Baltimore, MD 21202, U.S.A.

Printed in the United States of America

Library of Congress Cataloging-in-Publication Data

Chung, Kyung Won.
  Gross anatomy.

  Includes bibliographies and index.
    1. Anatomy, Human—Outlines, syllabi, etc.
2. Anatomy, Human—Examinations, questions, etc.
I. Title. [DNLM: 1. Anatomy—examination questions.
2. Anatomy—programmed instruction. QS 18 C559g]
QM31.C54 1988   611   87-15948
ISBN 0-683-01564-8

88 89 90 91 92   10 9 8 7 6 5 4 3 2 1

To My Wife, Young Hee,
and
My Sons, Harold and John

PREFACE

This book is designed for medical and dental students, presenting the essentials of human anatomy in the form of condensed descriptions and simple diagrams. The text is organized in a review format with related test questions following each section. This makes the study of human anatomy pleasant, more interesting, and understandable. It is the wish of the author to include all of the information without introducing a vast amount of material or entangling students in a web of details. However, because the book is in summary form, students are encouarged to consult a standard textbook for a comprehensive study of difficult concepts and fundamentals.

The book begins with a brief introduction to the skeletal, muscular, nervous, and circulatory systems. Following are chapters on regional anatomy, which include the upper limb, lower limb, thorax, abdomen, perineum and pelvis, back, and head and neck.

It is the author's belief that anatomy is a visual science of the configuration of the body, and thus the success of learning and understanding it depends largely on the quality of dissection and illustrations of human structure. Many of the illustrations are simple schematic drawings to help the reader to understand the descriptive text; they often beneficially replace the written word. A few of the illustrations are quite complex, attempting to exhibit important anatomical relationships. A considerable number of tables of muscles may prove to be useful as a summary and review. In addition, several summary charts for muscle innervation and action, cranial nerves, autonomic ganglia, and foramina of the skull are included in hopes that these will highlight and summarize pertinent aspects of the system.

Test questions at the end of each chapter can be studied in a relatively short time. The test questions are designed to emphasize important points, leading to a better understanding of the essential material. These are also intended for self-evaluation of one's progress in learning, to make students aware of any areas of weakness, and to enable them to correct deficiencies in their knowledge of anatomy. Answers and explanations are provided immediately after the review questions. If the answer comes directly from the question, no explanation is provided. It is hoped that this book will fill any obvious gaps in anatomical knowledge and serve as a useful guide for the review of regular human anatomy as well as for the National Board Examination.

I am deeply indebted to Mrs. Mary Barr for her tireless typing efforts and skilled word processing which brought the work to speedy completion. I am particularly grateful to Ms. Nancy Giger and Mr. John L'Ecuyer for their proofreading during the preparation of this manuscript. I wish to express my appreciation to Ms. Diane Abeloff, Medical Illustrator, for her book, *Medical Art, Graphics for Use*, which was used for illustrations with a little modification in some cases. I would like to express my special thanks to Mr. Shawn C. Schlinke for his excellent illustrations and full cooperation. Special thanks are extended to Mrs. Sherrie Brandt for her splendid schematic drawings. My very special thanks also to Mr. Ben Han for his outstanding photographic preparation of illustrations. I greatly appreciate and enjoy the privilege of working with Mr. John Gardner, Vice President and Editor-in-Chief, Ms. Kimberly Kist, Senior Editor, Ms. Victoria M. Vaughn, Associate Editor, and other staff members of William & Wilkins for their invaluable efforts in the production of this book.

Kyung Won Chung

CONTENTS

1

Introduction

Skeleton and Joints

I. Bones

–are calcified connective tissue consisting of cells (osteocytes) in a matrix of ground substance and collagen fibers.

–act as levers on which muscles act to produce the movements permitted by joints.

–serve as a reservoir for calcium and phosphorus.

–their internal soft tissue, the marrow, forms blood cells.

–are classified, according to shape, into long, short, flat, irregular, and sesamoid bones.

A. Long Bones

–their length is greater than their breadth and include the clavicle, humerus, radius, ulna, femur, tibia, fibula, metacarpals, metatarsals, phalanges, etc.

–have a shaft (diaphysis) and two ends (epiphyses).

–their shaft is the central region and composed of a thick collar of compact bone, surrounded by a connective tissue sheath, the periosteum.

–their shaft also has the marrow cavity and the metaphysis, which is the more recently developed part adjacent to an epiphysial disc.

–their ends (epiphyses) are composed of a trabecular bony meshwork, surrounded by a thin layer of compact bone.

–their articular surfaces (i.e., the ends) are covered by hyaline cartilage.

–develop by replacement of hyaline cartilage plate.

B. Short Bones

–are found only in the wrist and ankle.

–are approximately cuboidal in shape.

–are composed of spongy bone and marrow surrounded by a thin outer layer of dense compact bone.

C. Flat Bones

–include the ribs, sternum, scapulae, and bones in the vault of the skull.

–consist of two layers of compact bone, separated by spongy bone and marrow space (diploë).

–their articular surfaces are covered with cartilage or fibrous tissue.

–grow by replacement of connective tissue.

1

D. Irregular Bones

—include bones of mixed shapes, such as bones of the skull, vertebrae, and coxal bones.

—comprise mostly spongy bone enveloped by a thin outer layer of dense compact bone.

E. Sesamoid Bones

—develop in certain tendons.

—serve to reduce friction on the tendon, and thus protect the tendon from excessive wear.

—are commonly found where tendons cross the ends of long bones in the limbs and the wrist.

II. Joints

—are places of union between two or more bones of the skeleton.

—are classified on the basis of their structural features into fibrous, cartilaginous, and synovial types.

A. Fibrous Joints (Two Types)

1. Sutures

—are connected by several fibrous connective tissues.

—are found between the flat bones of the skull.

2. Syndesmoses

—are joined by fibrous connective tissue.

—occur as the inferior tibiofibular and tympanostapedial syndesmoses.

B. Cartilaginous Joints

1. Synchondroses (Primary Cartilaginous Joints)

—are united by hyaline cartilage.

—permit no movement but growth in the length of the bone.

—include epiphysial cartilage plates (the union between the epiphysis and the diaphysis of a growing bone) and spheno-occipital and manubriosternal synchondroses.

2. Symphyses (Secondary Cartilaginous Joints)

—are joined by a plate of fibrocartilage and are slightly movable joints.

—include the pubic symphysis (symphysis means "grown together") and the intervertebral discs (unions between the bodies of the vertebrae).

C. Synovial Joints (Diarthrodial Joints)

—permit a great degree of free movement.

—are characterized by four distinguishing features including a joint cavity, an articular cartilage, a synovial membrane (which produces synovial fluid), and an articular capsule.

—are classified according to axes of movement into plane, hinge, pivot, ellipsoidal, saddle, and ball-and-socket joints.

1. Plane Joints

—their movement is limited by the articular capsule.

—permit simple gliding or sliding movement between two flat surfaces.

—exist in the intercarpal, intermetacarpal, carpometacarpal, and acromioclavicular joints.

2. **Hinge (Ginglymus) Joints**
   —allow movement around one axis (uniaxial) at right angles to the bones (have one degree of freedom).
   —allow movements of flexion and extension only.
   —are found in the elbow joint and interphalangeal joint.

3. **Pivot (Trochoid) Joints (trochoid means "resembling a wheel")**
   —allow movement around one axis (uniaxial), but around a longitudinal axis. A central bony pivot rotates within a bony ring.
   —allow rotation only and have one degree of freedom.
   —occur in the superior radioulnar joint and in the joint between the first and second cervical vertebrae.

4. **Ellipsoidal (Condyloid) Joints**
   —allow movement in two directions (biaxial) at right angles to each other (i.e., they have two degrees of freedom).
   —allow flexion-extension and abduction-adduction, but no rotation.
   —occur in the wrist (radiocarpal) and metacarpophalangeal joints.

5. **Saddle (Sellar) Joints**
   —permit movement around two horizontal axes (biaxial) at right angles to each other (i.e., they have two degrees of freedom).
   —allow movement in several directions but less free movements of flexion-extension, abduction-adduction, and rotation than do the ball-and-socket type.
   —occur in the carpometacarpal joint of the thumb.

6. **Ball-and-Socket (Spheroidal) Joints**
   —allow movement in many directions (multiaxial) (i.e., they have three degrees of freedom or greatest "freedom of motion").
   —allow flexion and extension, abduction and adduction, medial and lateral rotations, and circumduction.
   —are seen at the shoulder and hip joints.

Muscular System

I. Muscle

—consists predominantly of contractile cells.
—has three types, including skeletal, cardiac, and smooth muscles.
—produces the movements of various parts of the body by contraction.

A. Skeletal Muscle

—is distinguished as striated and voluntary.
—comprises about 40% of the body mass in man.
—has two attachments, an origin and an insertion. (The origin is the more fixed and proximal attachment, the insertion the more movable and distal attachment.)
—is enclosed by **epimysium,** a thin layer of connective tissue. Smaller bundles of muscle fibers are surrounded by **perimysium.** Each muscle fiber is enclosed by **endomysium.**
—the longest one is the sartorius muscle of the thigh, which is about 24 inches long.

B. Cardiac Muscle

–is known as myocardium and forms the middle layer of the heart.

–is innervated by the autonomic nervous system.

–contracts spontaneously without any nerve supply.

–responds to increased demands by increasing the size of its fiber, which is known as compensatory hypertrophy.

–can have a necrosis, called myocardial infarction, as a result of occlusion of a coronary artery.

C. Smooth Muscle

–is generally arranged in two layers, circular and longitudinal, in the walls of many visceral organs.

–is innervated by the autonomic nervous system, regulating the size of the lumen of a tubular structure.

–undergoes rhythmic contractions called peristaltic waves in the walls of the gastrointestinal tract, uterine tubes, ureters, and other organs.

D. Muscles are Named by their shapes, positions, sizes, attachments, and actions—singly or in combination. For example:

–by their shapes (trapezius, rhomboid, deltoid).

–by their positions (interossei, supraspinatus, infraspinatus).

–by their shapes and positions (biceps brachii, quadriceps femoris).

–by their positions and sizes (latissimus dorsi).

–by their attachments (coracobrachialis).

–by their actions (levator scapulae, supinator).

–by their actions and shapes (pronator teres, pronator quadratus).

–by their actions and positions (flexor digitorum profundus and superficialis).

–by their actions and sizes (adductor brevis, longus, and magnus).

–by their shapes and sizes (teres major and minor).

–by their origins and insertions (sternocleidomastoid, stylohyoid).

II. Structures Associated with Muscles

A. Tendons

–are fibrous bands of dense connective tissue that attach muscles to other structures.

–always have one end attached to muscle and the other end blending with the fibrous connective tissue of the structure to which they attach (usually bone).

–may continue into the muscle as septa.

–are supplied by sensory fibers extending from muscle nerves.

B. A Bursa

–is a flattened sac of synovial membrane, containing a film of fluid to moisten its wall.

–is found where a tendon passes over a bone.

–occurs between muscles, bones, tendons, and ligaments or between two muscles.

–facilitates movement by minimizing friction.

–is prone to fill with fluid when infected or injured (e.g., swelling of the bursa below the patella, known as housemaid's knee).

C. Synovial Tendon Sheaths

—are tubular sacs wrapped around the tendons; they are similar to bursae in their fundamental structure and are filled with synovial fluid.
—occur where tendons pass under ligaments, retinacula, and through osseofibrous tunnels.
—facilitate movement by reducing the friction.
—respond to infection by forming more fluid and proliferating more cells, causing adhesions and thus restriction of movement of the tendon.

D. An Aponeurosis

—is a flat fibrous sheet or expanded broad tendon, giving attachment to muscles and serving as the means of origin or insertion of a flat muscle.

E. A Ligament

—is a fibrous band or sheet connecting two or more bones, cartilages, or visceral structures.

F. Fascia

—is a fibrous sheet or band that covers the body under the skin and invests the muscles and certain organs.
—may limit the spread of pus.

1. Superficial Fascia

—is composed of connective tissue between the dermis and the deep (investing) fascia.
—contains medium-sized vessels, nerves, and skin muscles such as platysma.
—its superficial layer is fatty and its deep layer is membranous.

2. Deep Fascia

—is a sheet of fibrous tissue that invests the muscles and helps to support them by serving as an elastic sheath or stocking.
—forms potential pathways for infection or extravasation of fluids.

Nervous System

I. Nervous System

—may be divided anatomically into the central nervous system, consisting of the brain and spinal cord, and the peripheral nervous system, consisting of 12 pairs of cranial nerves and 31 pairs of spinal nerves.
—is divided functionally into the somatic nervous system, which controls primarily voluntary activities, and the visceral (autonomic) nervous system, which controls primarily involuntary activities.
—is composed of neurons (nerve cells), which typically have two types of processes: axon and dendrites.
—controls and integrates the activity of the various parts of the body.

II. Neurons

—are the structural and functional unit of the nervous system (neuron doctrine).
—consist of cell bodies together with their processes, dendrites and axons.
—their dendrites (dendron means tree) are usually short, highly branched, and carry impulses to the cell body.

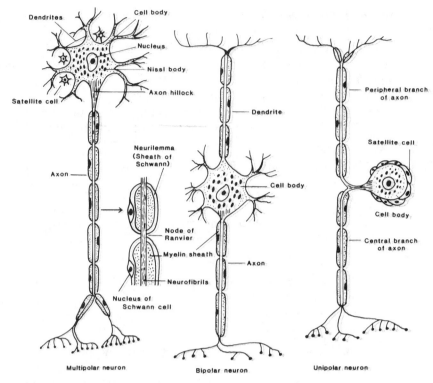

Figure 1.1. Three types of neurons.

—their axons are usually single and long, have fewer branches (collaterals), and carry impulses from the cell body.

—are unipolar, bipolar, or multipolar in shape.

—are specialized for the reception, integration, transformation, and transmission of information.

A. Classification

1. Unipolar Neurons

—have only one process, which divides into a central branch that functions as an axon, and a peripheral branch that serves as a dendrite.

—are sensory neurons of the peripheral nerve (i.e., cerebrospinal ganglion cells).

2. Bipolar Neurons

—have two processes, one dendrite and one axon.

—are found in the olfactory epithelium, in the retina of the eye, and in the inner ear.

3. Multipolar Neurons

—have several dendrites and one axon.

—are most common in the central nervous system (i.e., motor cells in anterior and lateral horns of the spinal cord, autonomic ganglion cells).

B. The Cells Supporting Neurons

–include Schwann cells and satellite cells in the peripheral nervous system.
–are called neuroglia in the central nervous system and are composed mainly of three types: oligodendrocytes, astrocytes, and microglia.

1. Myelin

–is the fat-like substance forming a sheath around certain nerve fibers.
–is formed by **Schwann cells** in the peripheral nervous system and **oligodendrocytes** in the central nervous system.

III. Central Nervous System

A. Brain

–is enclosed within the cranium or brain case.
–its cortex is the outer part of the hemispheres and composed of gray matter that consists largely of the nerve cell bodies.
–its interior part is composed of white matter that consists largely of axons forming tracts or pathways.
–its interior also contains ventricles that are filled with cerebrospinal fluid.

B. Spinal Cord

–is cylindrical in shape and occupies approximately the upper two-thirds of the vertebral canal.
–has cervical and lumbar enlargements for nerve supply of upper and lower limbs, respectively.
–its gray matter lies centrally, in contrast to the cerebral hemispheres, and white matter is located in the periphery.
–has a conical end known as the conus medullaris.
–grows much more slowly than the bony vertebral column during the intrauterine development, and thus its terminal end gradually shifts to a higher level.
–ends at the level of L2 in the adult and at the level of L3 in the newborn.
–is enveloped and protected by the meninges.

C. Meninges

–consist of three layers of connective tissue membranes that surround and protect the brain and spinal cord.

1. Pia Mater

–is closely applied to the surface of the brain and spinal cord.
–has lateral extensions between the dorsal and ventral roots of spinal nerves, known as denticulate (dentate) ligaments.
–enmeshes blood vessels on the surfaces of the brain and spinal cord. (The spinal pia mater is less vascular than the cerebral pia mater.)

2. Arachnoid

–is a filmy, transparent, spidery layer and is connected to the pia mater by web-like trabeculations.
–has the subarachnoid space, which is the interval between the arachnoid and pia mater that is filled with cerebrospinal fluid. It also contains blood on hemorrhage of a cerebral artery.

—may have the arachnoid granulations, which are tuft-like collections of highly folded arachnoid that project through the dura mater.

3. **Dura Mater**

—is the tough, fibrous, outermost layer of the meninges.

—has the **subdural space** internal to it (between the arachnoid and dura).

—has the **epidural space** external to it, which contains the vertebral venous plexus, and the middle meningeal arteries in the cranial cavity.

—is a two-layered structure in the cranium, having meningeal and periosteal layers.

—forms the dural venous sinuses, which are spaces between the periosteal and meningeal layers or between duplications of the meningeal layers.

4. **Cerebrospinal Fluid**

—is contained in the subarachnoid space between the arachnoid and pia mater.

—is formed by vascular choroid plexuses in the ventricles of the brain.

—circulates through the ventricles, enters the subarachnoid space, and eventually filters into the venous system.

IV. Peripheral Nervous System

A. Cranial Nerves

—consist of 12 pairs which, along with 31 pairs of spinal nerves, comprise most of the peripheral nervous system.

—are connected to the brain rather than to the spinal cord.

—have motor fibers whose cell bodies are located within the central nervous system, and sensory fibers whose cell bodies form sensory ganglia that are located in the nerve outside the central nervous system.

—ermerge from the ventral aspect of the brain except the trochlear nerve (fourth cranial nerve).

—contain all of the functional components of spinal nerves.

—are described individually in the chapter on the head and neck.

B. Spinal Nerves

—have 31 pairs including 8 cervical, 12 thoracic, 5 lumbar, 5 sacral, and 1 coccygeal nerves.

—are divided into the ventral and dorsal primary rami.

—are connected with the sympathetic chain ganglia by rami communicantes.

—are mixed nerves, containing motor fibers and sensory fibers.

—contain sensory fibers whose cell bodies are in the dorsal root ganglion (general somatic afferent and general visceral afferent).

—contain motor fibers whose cell bodies are in the anterior horn of the spinal cord (general somatic efferent).

—contain motor fibers (general visceral efferent) whose cell bodies are in the lateral horn of the spinal cord (only segments between T1-L2).

1. Ventral Primary Rami

—contain somatic sensory fibers (general somatic afferent) whose cell bodies are in the dorsal root ganglia.

—contain somatic motor fibers (general somatic efferent) whose cell bodies are in the anterior horn of the spinal cord.

—contain visceral motor fibers (general visceral efferent) whose cell bodies are in the sympathetic chain ganglia.

—is also called intercostal nerves in the thoracic area (T12 is a subcostal nerve).

2. Dorsal Primary Rami

—innervate the skin and deep muscles of the back.

C. Nerve Components in Peripheral Nerves

1. General Somatic Afferent (GSA) Nerves

—transmit pain, temperature, touch, and proprioception from the body to the central nervous system (CNS).

2. (General) Somatic Efferent (GSE) Nerves

—carry motor impulses to skeletal muscles of the body; they arise from myotomes of the embryonic somites.

3. Special Somatic Afferent Nerves

—convey special senses of vision, hearing, and equilibration to the CNS.

4. General Visceral Afferent (GVA) Nerves

—convey sensory impulses from the visceral organs to the CNS.

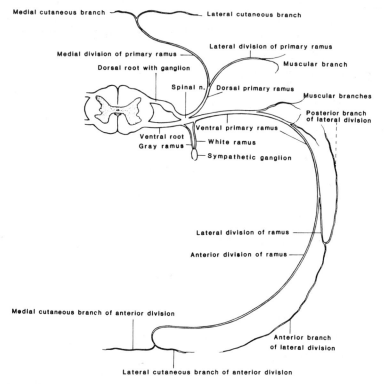

Figure 1.2. Typical spinal nerve.

5. General Visceral Efferent (GVE) Nerves (Autonomic Nerves)
   –transmit motor impulses to smooth muscle, cardiac muscle, and glandular tissues.

6. Special Visceral Afferent (SVA) Nerves
   –transmit smell and taste sensations to the CNS.

7. Special Visceral Efferent (SVE) Nerves
   –conduct motor impulses to the muscles of the head and neck; they arise from branchiomeric structures, such as muscles for mastication, muscles for facial expression, and muscles for elevation of pharynx and movement of larynx.

V. Autonomic Nervous System

–is divided into the sympathetic (thoracolumbar outflow) and parasympathetic (craniosacral outflow) systems.
–is composed of general visceral efferent neurons.
–regulates the activity of cardiac muscle, smooth muscle, and glands.
–is composed of two neurons: preganglionic and postganglionic.

A. Sympathetic Nerve

–has preganglionic nerve cell bodies that are located in the lateral horn of the thoracic and upper lumbar levels of the spinal cord.
–has preganglionic fibers that pass through ventral roots, spinal nerves, white rami communicantes and enter adjacent sympathetic chain ganglia where they synapse or run farther through the splanchnic nerves to reach collateral ganglia located along the major abdominal blood vessels.
–has postganglionic fibers from the chain ganglia that return to spinal nerves by way of gray rami communicantes and supply the skin with

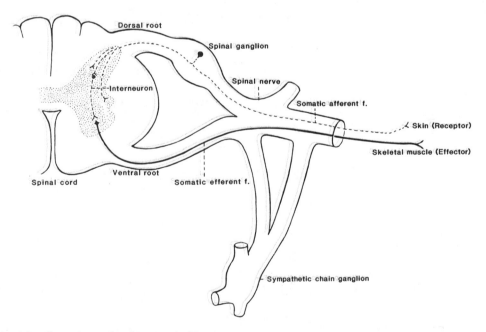

Figure 1.3. General somatic afferent and efferent nerves.

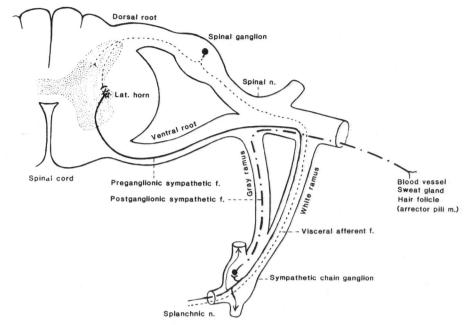

Figure 1.4. General visceral efferent (autonomic) and afferent nerves.

(*a*) secretory fibers to sweat glands, (*b*) motor fibers to smooth muscles (arrector pili muscles) of the hair follicles, and (*c*) vasomotor fibers to the blood vessels.

–functions primarily in emergencies, preparing individuals for fight or flight.

–increases heart rate, inhibits gastrointestinal motility and secretion, dilates pupil and bronchial lumen, etc.

–has widespread effects.

B. Parasympathetic Nerve

–comprises the preganglionic fibers that arise from the brain stem (cranial nerves, 3, 7, 9, and 10) and sacral part of the spinal cord (second, third, and fourth sacral segments).

–is characterized by long preganglionic fibers and short postganglionic fibers.

–decreases heart rate, increases peristalsis, and stimulates secretory activity.

–functions primarily in homeostasis, tending to promote quiet and orderly processes of the body.

–has specific, discrete, and local effects.

Circulatory System

I. Vascular System

–functions to transport vital materials between the external environment and the internal fluid environment of the body.

–consists of the heart and vessels (arteries, capillaries, veins) that transport the blood through all parts of the body.

–has two circulatory loops:

1. Pulmonary circulation

–pumps blood from the right ventricle to the lungs through the pulmonary arteries and returns it to the left atrium of the heart through the pulmonary veins.

2. Systemic circulation

–pumps blood from the left ventricle through the aorta to all parts of the body and returns it to the right atrium through the superior and inferior vena cavae and the cardiac veins.

–also includes the lymphatic vessels, a set of channels that begins in the tissue spaces and returns excess tissue fluid to the bloodstream.

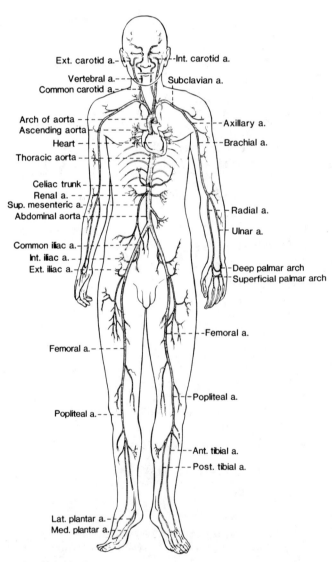

Figure 1.5. Major arteries of the body.

A. Heart

—begins as a contractile tube during embryological development.

—is a hollow, muscular organ that pumps blood through the pulmonary and systemic circulations.

—receives the venous blood from the body in the right atrium and then passes it into the right ventricle, which pumps it to the lungs for oxygenation.

—receives the oxygenated blood from the lungs in the left atrium whence it passes to the left ventricle, which forces it through the arteries to supply the tissues of the body.

—is regulated in its pumping rate and strength by the autonomic nervous system, which controls a pacemaker (the sinoatrial node).

B. Fetal Circulation

1. **In the fetus, oxygenation of the blood occurs in the placenta, rather than in the lungs.**

2. **Before birth three shunts exist partially bypassing the lungs and liver.**

   a. *Foramen Ovale*

   —shunts blood from the right atrium to the left atrium, without passing through the lungs (pulmonary circulation).

   b. *Ductus Arteriosus*

   —shunts blood from the pulmonary trunk to the aorta, without passing through the lungs (pulmonary circulation).

   c. *Ductus Venosus*

   —shunts oxygenated blood from the umbilical vein (returning from the placenta) to the inferior vena cava, without passing through the liver.

C. Blood Vessels

—carry blood to the lungs, where carbon dioxide is exchanged for oxygen.

—carry blood to the intestine, where nutritive materials in fluid form are absorbed, and to the endocrine glands, where hormones pass through their walls, distributing hormones from the glands to target cells.

—transport the waste products of tissue fluid to the kidneys, intestines, lungs, and skin, where they are excreted.

—are of three types: arteries, veins, and capillaries.

1. **Arteries**

   —carry blood away from the heart and distribute it to all parts of the body.

   —have thicker and stronger walls than those of veins.

   —have three main types:

   a. *Elastic Arteries*

   —are the largest arteries in the body and their walls consist chiefly of elastic fibers, which tend to smooth the pressure and lessen the velocity of the blood.

—include the aorta, pulmonary artery, brachiocephalic trunk, common carotid artery, subclavian arteries, etc.

b. *Muscular Arteries*

—are the medium-sized arteries, whose wall consists chiefly of smooth muscle fibers.
—are controlled by the autonomic nervous system.

c. *Arterioles*

Thick Muscular wall

—are the smallest arteries.
—have a relatively narrow lumen and thick muscular walls.
—their pressure is mainly regulated by the degree of tonus in the smooth muscle in their walls.

2. Veins

—return the blood to the heart.
—have thinner walls than arteries.
—carry dark venous blood, except the pulmonary vein.
—may be distended and tortuous as varicose veins, which are most commonly seen in the lower extremities, probably as a result of congenitally incomplete valves. Varicose veins are also commonly seen among persons in occupations requiring long periods of standing and in pregnant women.
—closely accompany an artery as a pair or more that are known as venae comitantes.

3. Capillaries

—comprise anastomosing networks called capillary beds.
—are distributed throughout the body to bring the blood into close contact with the cells of the tissues.
—are composed of endothelium and its basement membrane, and connect the arterioles to the venules.
—are the exchange site where oxygen and nutritive materials from oxygenated blood diffuse across the endothelial wall of the arteriolar end of the capillary into the tissue space, whereas metabolic waste products and carbon dioxide diffuse from the tissue spaces into the blood through the wall of the venous end.
—are absent in the cornea, epidermis, and hyaline cartilage.
—may not present in some area where the arterioles and venules have direct connection. These arteriovenous anastomoses (AV shunts) bypass the capillaries, and are especially numerous in the skin (of the nose, lips, finger, and ears), where they conserve the heat of the body.

4. Sinusoids

—are wider than capillaries and are also more irregular.
—substitute capillaries in the liver, spleen, red bone marrow, carotid body, adenohypophysis, suprarenal cortex, and parathyroid glands.
—have walls that consist largely of phagocytic cells.

antibodies formation

—form a part of the reticuloendothelial system, chiefly concerned with phagocytosis and antibody formation.

II. Lymphatic System

—provides an important immune mechanism for the body. (When foreign proteins are drained from an infected area by the lymphatic capillaries, immunologically competent cells produce a specific antibody to the foreign protein, or lymphocytes are dispatched to the infected area. Lymphocytes have an important role in the development of antibodies and immune reactions.)
—is involved in the metastasis (spread) of cancer cells.

A. Lymphatic Vessels

—serve as a one-way drainage, toward the heart.
—return lymph to the bloodstream through the thoracic duct, the largest lymphatic vessel.
—are not visible in dissections.
—are the major route by which carcinoma metastasizes.
—function to absorb the large protein molecules and transport them to the bloodstream because they cannot pass through the walls of the blood capillaries into the tissue fluid.
—carry lymphocytes from lymphatic tissues to the bloodstream.
—have valves to ensure flow of lymph away from the tissues and toward the venous system.
—are constricted at the sites of valves, showing a knotted or beaded appearance.
—are absent in the brain, spinal cord, eyeball, bone marrow, splenic pulp, hyaline cartilage, nails, and hair.

B. Lymphatic Capillaries

—begin blindly in most tissues, collect tissue fluid, and join to form large collecting vessels that pass to regional lymph nodes.
—are wider than blood capillaries.
—absorb plasma from the tissue spaces and transport it back to the venous system.
—are called lacteals in the villi of the small intestine and absorb emulsified fat.

C. Lymph Nodes

—are organized collections of lymphatic tissue permeated by lymphatic channels.
—have fibroelastic capsules from which connective tissue trabeculae extend into the substance of the organ.
—have the cortex (outer part) that contains collections of lymphatic cells called germinal centers, and the medulla (inner part) that contains cords of lymphatic cells.
—receive afferent vessels through the capsule. (Efferent vessels leave through the hillus, through which blood vessels also enter and leave.)
—produce lymphocytes and plasma cells.
—trap bacteria drained from an infected area and ingest them by the reticuloendothelial cells or phagocytic cells (macrophages).
—are decreased in size during malnutrition and after irradiation.

–serve as filters; thus, the cancer cells in lymph vessels migrate or metastasize to lymph nodes and tend to remain within the nodes, where they proliferate and gradually destroy them.)

D. Lymph

–is a clear, transparent, watery fluid that is collected from the intercellular spaces. It contains no cells until lymphocytes are added in its passage through the lymph nodes.

–contains the similar constituents as blood plasma (e.g., proteins, fats and lymphocytes).

–often contains fat droplets (called chyle).

–is filtered by passing through several lymph nodes before entering the venous system.

REVIEW TEST
INTRODUCTION

DIRECTIONS: For each of the questions or incomplete statements in this section, *one* or *more* of the answers or completions given are correct. Choose answer:
- A. if only **1**, **2**, and **3** are correct.
- B. if only **1** and **3** are correct.
- C. if only **2** and **4** are correct.
- D. if only **4** is correct.
- E. if **all** are correct.

1.1. The saddle joint
1. allows rotation only.
2. allows movements of flexion and extension only.
3. occurs in the joint between the first and second cervical vertebrae.
4. occurs in the carpometacarpal joint of the thumb.

1.2. The cerebrospinal fluid
1. is formed by the arachnoid granulations, which are tuft-like collections of folded arachnoid.
2. is formed by vascular choroid plexuses in the ventricles of the brain.
3. is contained in the subdural space.
4. is contained in the subarachnoid space.

1.3. The spinal cord
1. has a conical end known as the conus medullaris.
2. occupies the whole length of the vertebral canal.
3. is enveloped by the meninges.
4. has gray matter that lies in the periphery as in the brain.

1.4. The special visceral afferent nerves transmit:
1. sense of vision to the central nervous system.
2. smell sensation to the central nervous system.
3. pain sensation to the central nervous system.
4. taste sensation to the central nervous system.

1.5. The lymphatic vessels
1. serve as a one-way drainage.
2. are well shown in dissections.
3. are absent in the brain.
4. have no valves.

DIRECTIONS: Each set of lettered headings below is followed by a list of numbered words or phrases. Choose answer.

A. if the item is associated with **A** only.

B. if the item is associated with **B** only.

C. if the item is associated with both **A** and **B**.

D. if the item is associated with neither **A** nor **B**.

A. Fetal circulation
B. Postnatal circulation
C. Both
D. Neither

1.6. Right atrium receives oxygenated blood.

1.7. Right atrial pressure is higher than left atrial pressure.

1.8. Left ventricle delivers oxygenated blood to the aorta.

1.9. Left atrium receives oxygenated blood from lungs via pulmonary veins.

1.10. Blood flows from pulmonary artery to aorta via the ductus arteriosus.

A. Sympathetic nerve
B. Parasympathetic nerve
C. Both
D. Neither

1.11. Has the preganglionic fibers that arise from the spinal cord.

1.12. Has widespread effects.

1.13. Supplies the sweat glands.

1.14. Functions primarily in homeostasis.

1.15. Regulates the activity of cardiac and skeletal muscles.

A. Cardiac muscle
B. Smooth muscle
C. Both
D. Neither

1.16. Is generally arranged in circular and longitudinal layers in the walls of many visceral organs.

1.17. Is innervated by the autonomic nervous system.

1.18. Is distinguished as striated and voluntary and enclosed by epimysium, a thin layer of connective tissue.

1.19. Contracts spontaneously without any nerve supply.

1.20. Typically has two attachments, an origin and an insertion.

DIRECTIONS: Each of the questions or incomplete statements below is followed by suggested answers or completions. Choose the *one* that is *best* in each case.

1.21. Which of the following structures is a fibrous sheet or band that covers the body under the skin and invests the muscles?

A. tendon.
B. ligament.
C. synovial tendon sheath.
D. aponeurosis.
E. fascia.

1.22. Which one of the following muscles is named by its shape and position?

A. trapezius.
B. levator scapulae.
C. biceps brachii.
D. pronator teres.
E. stylohyoid.

1.23. The cranial nerves
A. consist of 31 pairs.
B. have motor fibers whose cell bodies are located in the nerve outside the central nervous system.
C. are connected to the brain.
D. emerge from the dorsal aspect of the brain except for the trochlear nerve.
E. are connected with the sympathetic chain ganglia by gray rami communicantes.

1.24. The dura mater
A. is closely applied to the surface of the brain and spinal cord.
B. is the fibrous innermost layer of the meninges.
C. has the subdural space external to it, which contains the middle meningeal arteries.
D. has the epidural space external to it, which contains the vertebral venous plexus.
E. forms the filum terminale internus, which extend from the end of the conus medullaris.

1.25. Which one of the following blood vessels returns <u>oxygenated</u> blood to the heart?
A. superior vena cava.
B. pulmonary arteries.
C. pulmonary veins.
D. ascending aorta.
E. cardiac veins.

DIRECTIONS: For each numbered item, select *one* lettered heading that is most closely associated with it. Each lettered heading may be selected once, more than once, or not at all.

A. Long bones
B. Short bones
C. Flat bones
D. Irregular bones
E. Sesamoid bones

A. Syndesmoses
B. Synchondroses
C. Hinge (ginglymus) joints
D. Ellipsoidal (condyloid) joints
E. Ball-and-socket (spheroidal) joints

1.26. Consists of two layers of compact bone, separated by spongy bone and marrow (diploë).

1.27. Serve to reduce friction on the tendon, and thus protect the tendon from excessive wear.

1.28. Are found only in the wrist and ankle.

1.29. Have a shaft (diaphysis) and two ends (epiphyses).

1.30. Are bones of mixed shapes, such as bones of the skull, vertebrae, and coxal bones.

1.31. Occur in the radiocarpal and metacarpophalangeal joints.

1.32. Allow movements of flexion and extension only and occur in the elbow and interphalangeal joints.

1.33. Are fibrous joints and occur at the tympanostapedial joints.

1.34. Allow movement in many directions and occur at the shoulder and hip joints.

1.35. Are primary cartilaginous joints, including epiphysial cartilage plates.

ANSWERS AND EXPLANATIONS

INTRODUCTION

1.1. D. The saddle joint allows movement around two horizontal axes (biaxial) at right angles to each other. It occurs in the carpometacarpal joint of the thumb. The joint between the first and second cervical vertebrae is the pivot (trochoid) joint.

1.2. C. The cerebrospinal fluid is formed by vascular choroid plexuses in the ventricles of the brain and contained in the subarachnoid space between the pia and arachnoid maters. The subdural space is a potential space between the arachnoid and dura mater and contains only a film of fluid to moisten its walls.

1.3. B. The spinal cord ends as the conus medullaris at the level of the second lumbar vertebra. It is enveloped and protected by three layers of the meninges. Its gray matter lies centrally, in contrast to the cerebral hemispheres, and white matter lies in the periphery.

1.4. C. The special visceral afferent nerves transmit smell and taste sensations to the central nervous system, whereas the special somatic afferent nerves convey the special senses of vision, hearing, and equilibrium to the central nervous system. The general somatic afferent nerves transmit pain, temperature, touch, and pressure sensations to the central nervous system.

1.5. B. Lymphatic vessels serve as a one-way drainage and are not visible in dissections. They are constricted at the sites of valves, showing a knotted or beaded appearance. Lymphatic vessels are not present in the central nervous system.

1.6. A. In the fetal circulation, the right atrium receives oxygenated blood from the placenta.

1.7. A. In the fetus, the right atrial pressure is higher than the left; thus, the oxygenated blood from the placenta is delivered to the left atrium through the foramen ovale.

1.8. C. The left ventricle delivers oxygenated blood to the aorta in both the pre- and postnatal circulations.

1.9. B. In postnatal circulation, the left atrium receives oxygenated blood from the lungs by way of the pulmonary veins.

1.10. A. In the fetus, blood flows from the pulmonary artery to the aorta via the ductus arteriosus.

1.11. C. Preganglionic sympathetic fibers arise from the thoracic and upper lumbar part of the spinal cord, whereas preganglionic parasympathetic fibers arise from the brain stem (cranial nerves, 3, 7, 9, and 10) and sacral part of the spinal cord.

1.12. A. The sympathetic nerve has widespread effects, whereas the parasympathetic nerve has specific, discrete, and local effects.

1.13. A. Postganglionic sympathetic fibers innervate the skin with secretory fibers to glands, motor fibers to arrector pili muscles of hair follicles, and vasomotor fibers to blood vessels.

1.14. B. The parasympathetic nerve functions primarily in homeostasis, tending to promote quiet and orderly processes of the body, whereas the sympathetic nerve functions primarily in emergencies, preparing individuals for fight or flight.

1.15. D. The sympathetic nerve increases the heart rate, whereas the parasympathetic nerve decreases the heart rate. The skeletal muscle is not innervated by autonomic nerves.

1.16. B. The smooth muscle is generally arranged in two layers, circular and longitudinal, in the walls of many visceral organs.

1.17. C. The autonomic nervous system consists of motor (or efferent) nerves through which smooth muscle, cardiac muscle, and glandular cells are innervated.

1.18. D. The skeletal muscle is distinguished as striated and voluntary, and enclosed by epimysium, a thin layer of connective tissue.

1.19. A. The cardiac muscle contracts spontaneously without any nerve supply.

1.20. D. The skeletal muscle typically has two attachments, an origin and an insertion.

1.21. E. The fascia is a fibrous sheet or band that covers the body under the skin and invests the muscles.

1.22. C. The biceps brachii muscle is named by its shape and position. The trapezius is named by its shape, the levator scapulae by its function, the pronator teres by its function and shape, and the stylohyoid by its origin and insertion.

1.23. C. The cranial nerves consist of 12 pairs, some of which have sensory fibers whose cell bodies are located in the nerve outside the central nervous system. They emerge from the ventral aspect of the brain except for the trochlear nerve.

1.24. D. The dura mater is the tough, fibrous outermost layer of the meninges and has the subdural space internal to it, which contains a film of fluid to moisten its walls. The dura mater has the epidural space external to it, which contains the vertebral venous plexus and the middle meningeal arteries in the cranial cavity. The pia mater is closely applied to the surface of the brain and spinal cord and forms the filum terminale (internus) by its prolongation from the end of the conus medullaris.

1.25. C. The pulmonary arteries carry deoxygenated blood from the heart to the lungs for oxygen renewal, and the pulmonary veins return the oxygenated blood from the lungs to the heart. The aorta carries oxygenated blood from the left ventricle to all parts of the body.

1.26. C. Flat bones consist of two layers of compact bone, separated by the spongy bone and marrow, and include the ribs, sternum, scapulae, and bones in the vault of the skull.

1.27. E. Semamoid bones serve to reduce friction on the tendon, and thus are commonly found where tendons cross the ends of the long bones in the limbs and the wrist. They protect the tendon from excessive wear.

1.28. B. Short bones are approximately cuboidal in shape and found only in the wrist and ankle.

1.29. A. Long bones have a shaft (diaphysis) and two ends (epiphyses). Their diaphysis also has the marrow cavity, and the metaphysis which is the more recently developed part adjacent to an epiphysial disc. The epiphyses are composed of a trabecular bony meshwork, surrounded by a thinner collar of the compact bone.

1.30. D. Irregular bones are bones of mixed shapes, such as bones of the skull, vertebrae, and coxal bones.

1.31. D. Ellipsoidal (condyloid) joints occur in the wrist (radiocarpal) and metacarpophalangeal joints and allow flexion-extension and abduction-adduction.

1.32. C. Hinge (ginglymus) joints allow movements of flexion and extension only and are found in the elbow and interphalangeal joints.

1.33. A. Syndesmoses are fibrous joints and occur at the tympanostapedial and inferior tibiofibular joints.

1.34. E. Ball-and-socket (spheroidal) joints allow movement in many directions (multiaxial) and are found at the shoulder and hip joints.

1.35. B. Synchondroses are united by hyaline cartilage and include epiphysial cartilage plates.

2
Upper Limb

Cutaneous Nerves, Superficial Veins, and Lymphatics

I. Cutaneous Nerves

A. Supraclavicular Nerve

—arises from the cervical plexus (C3,4) and supplies the skin over the upper pectoral, deltoid, and outer trapezius area.

B. Medial Brachial Cutaneous Nerve

—arises from the medial cord of the brachial plexus and supplies the medial side of the arm.

C. Medial Antebrachial Cutaneous Nerve

—arises from the medial cord of the brachial plexus and supplies the medial side of the forearm.

D. Lateral Brachial Cutaneous Nerve

—arises from the axillary nerve and supplies the lateral side of the arm.

E. Lateral Antebrachial Cutaneous Nerve

—arises from the musculocutaneous nerve and supplies the lateral side of the forearm.

F. Posterior Brachial and Antebrachial Cutaneous Nerves

—arise from the radial nerve and supply the posterior side of the arm and forearm.

G. Intercostobrachial Cutaneous Nerve

—is the lateral cutaneous branch of the second intercostal nerve.

—emerges from the second intercostal space by piercing the intercostal and serratius anterior muscles.

—may communicate with the medial branchial cutaneous nerve.

—provides cutaneous distribution along the medial and posterior surface of the arm from the axilla to the elbow.

—contains somatic sensory fibers (general somatic afferent) whose cell bodies are in the dorsal root ganglia.

—contains the postganglionic sympathetic fibers whose cell bodies are in sympathetic chain ganglia.

23

II. Superficial Veins

A. Cephalic Vein

–begins as a radial continuation of the dorsal venous network.

–lies on the lateral side of the front of the elbow.

–is often connected with the basilic vein by the median cubital vein in front of the elbow.

–ascends along the lateral surface of the biceps, pierces the brachial fascia, and lies in the deltopectoral triangle, along with the deltoid branch of the thoracoacromial trunk.

–pierces the clavipectoral fascia and empties into the axillary vein, but occasionally communicates with the external jugular vein.

B. Basilic Vein

–arises from the dorsum of the hand.

–accompanies the medial antebrachial cutaneous nerve.

–joins the brachial veins to form the axillary vein at the lower border of the teres major.

–ascends on the posteromedial surface of the forearm and passes anterior to the medial epicondyle.

C. Median Cubital Vein

–connects the cephalic to the basilic vein.

–is frequently used for intravenous injections and blood transfusions.

–lies superficial to the bicipital aponeursis, which separates it from the brachial artery.

D. Median Antebrachial Vein

–arises in the palmar venous network and ascends on the front of the forearm.

–terminates in the median cubital or the basilic vein.

III. Superficial Lymphatics

A. Lymphatics of the Fingers

–drain into the plexus on the dorsum and palm of the hand.

B. Medial Group of Lymphatic Vessels

–accompanies the basilic vein, passes through the cubital or supratrochlear nodes, and ascends to enter the lateral axillary nodes.

C. Lateral Group of Lymphatic Vessels

–accompanies the cephalic vein and drains into the lateral axillary nodes and also into the deltopectoral (infraclavicular) nodes. The deltopectoral nodes drain in the apical nodes.

Bones and Joints

I. Bones

A. Clavicle

–forms the girdle of the upper limb along with the scapula.

–is the first bone to begin ossification during the fetal development, but is the last one to complete ossification.

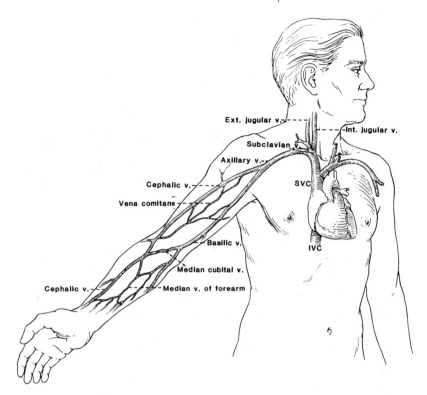

Figure 2.1. Venous drainage of the upper limb.

–has its medial two-thirds convex forward, whereas the lateral one-third is flattened with a marked concavity.

–articulates with the sternum at the sternoclavicular joint and with the scapula at the acromioclavicular joint.

–is a commonly fractured bone. Its **fracture**

–results in upward displacement of the proximal fragment, due to the pull of the sternomastoid muscle, and downward displacement of the distal fragment, due to the pull of the deltoid and the gravity.

–may occur by the hand of the obstetrician in breech (buttocks) presentation or may occur during passage of the child through the birth canal by being pressed against the maternal symphysis pubis.

–may cause an injury of the brachial plexus (lower trunk) and a fatal hemorrhage from the subclavian vein.

–is also responsible for thrombosis of the subclavian vein, causing a pulmonary embolism.

B. Scapula (Shoulder Blade)

–is a flat bone of triangular shape.

1. Spine

–is a triangular process and continues laterally as the acromion.

–divides the dorsal surface into upper supraspinous and lower infraspinous fossae.

–provides an origin for the deltoid and insertion for the trapezius.

2. Acromion

–is the lateral end of the spine.
–articulates with the lateral end of the clavicle.
–provides an origin for the deltoid and an insertion for the trapezius.

3. Coracoid Process

–provides the origin of the coracobrachialis and biceps brachii muscles and the insertion of the pectoralis minor muscle.
–gives attachment for the coracoclavicular ligament (trapezoid portion), coracohumeral ligament, and costocoracoid membrane and ligament.

4. Scapular Notch

–is bridged by the transverse scapular ligament and converted into a foramen that permits passage of the suprascapular nerve.

5. Glenoid Cavity

–articulates with head of the humerus.
–is deepened by a fibrocartilaginous lip or glenoidal labrum.

6. Supraglenoid and Infraglenoid Tubercles

–provide origins for the tendons of the long heads of the biceps and triceps muscles, respectively.

C. Humerus

1. Head

–has the smooth, rounded, articular surface, and articulates with the scapula at the glenohumeral joint.

2. Anatomical Neck

–is an indentation distal to the head for the attachment of the articular capsule.

3. Greater Tubercle

–lies on its lateral side, just lateral to the anatomical neck.
–provides attachments for the following muscles:

  a. *Supraspinatus.*
  b. *Infraspinatus.*
  c. *Teres minor.*

4. Lesser Tubercle

–lies on its medial side of the front, just distal to the anatomical neck.
–provides an insertion for the subscapularis muscle.

5. Intertubercular (Bicipital Groove)

–lies between the greater and lesser tubercles.
–lodges the tendon of the long head of the biceps brachii muscle, which forces the humeral head medially into the joint.
–is connected by the transverse humeral ligament, which restrains the tendon of the biceps long head.
–provides insertions for the pectoralis major on its lateral lip, the teres major on its medial lip and the latissimus dorsi on its floor.

6. Surgical Neck

   −is a narrow area distal to the tubercles and a common site of fracture.
   −is in contact with the axillary nerve and the posterior humeral circumflex artery.

7. Deltoid Tubercle

   −is a V-shaped roughened area on the lateral aspect of the midshaft.
   −marks the insertion of the deltoid muscle.

8. Spiral Groove

   −is a groove for the radial nerve.
   −separates the origin of the lateral head of the triceps above and of the medial head below.

9. Trochlea

   −is shaped like a spool or pulley and has a deep depression between two margins, which articulates the trochlear notch of the ulna.

10. Capitulum

   −is globular in shape and articulates with the head of the radius.

11. Olecranon Fossa

   −is located above the trochlea on the back.
   −houses the olecranon of the ulna in full extension of the forearm.

12. Coronoid Fossa

   −is located above the trochlea on the front.
   −receives the coronoid process of the ulna, upon flexion of the elbow.

13. Radial Fossa

   −is located above the capitulum on the front.
   −is occupied by the head of the radius during full flexion of the elbow joint.

14. Medial Epicondyle

   −projects from the trochlea.

15. Lateral Epicondyle

   −projects from the capitulum.

D. Radius

   −has its head (proximal end) articulating with the capitulum of the humerus and radial notch of the ulna.
   −usually has its distal end articulating with the proximal row of carpal bones including the scaphoid, lunate, and triquetrum, but excluding the pisiform.
   −when fractured at its distal end, called Colles' fracture, is characterized by displacement of the hand backward and outward.
   −is shorter than the ulna.
   −its tuberosity is an oval prominence distal to the neck and gives attachment to the biceps brachii tendon.
   −has, on its distal end, a styloid process that is about 1 cm distal to that of the ulna.

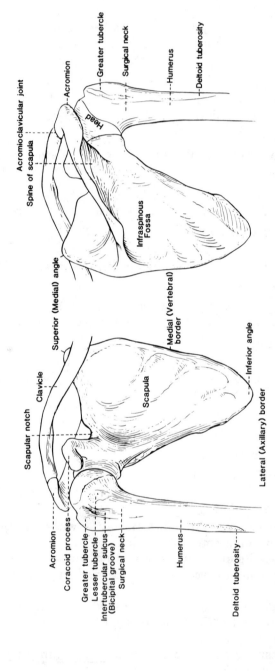

Figure 2.2. Pectoral girdle and humerus.

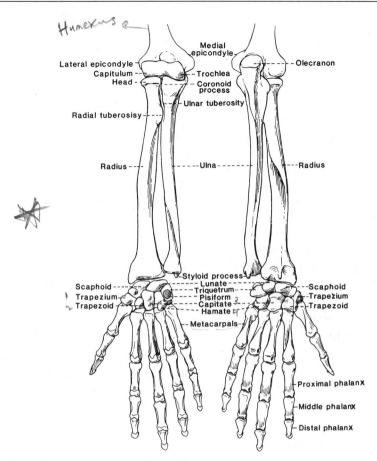

Figure 2.3. Bones of the forearm and hand.

E. Ulna

–has its olecranon, which is the curved projection on the back of the elbow and gives attachment to the triceps tendon.

–has its coronoid process, below the trochlear notch, which gives attachment to the brachialis.

–has its trochlear notch, which receives the trochlea of the humerus.

–has its radial notch for accommodation of the head of the radius.

–has its head (distal end), which articulates with the articular disc of the distal radioulnar joint.

–has a styloid process on its distal end.

F. Carpal Bones

–are eight in number and are arranged in two rows of four.

–Proximal row—scaphoid, lunate, triquetrum, and pisiform (from lateral to medial).

–Distal row—trapezium, trapezoid, capitate, and hamate.

–in the proximal row (except for pisiform), articulates with the radius. (The ulna does not contact with the carpal bones.)

G. Metacarpals

–are miniature long bones, consisting of bases (proximal ends), shafts (bodies), and heads (distal ends).

H. Phalanges

–are miniature long bones, exhibiting bases, shafts, and heads.
–are three in each finger but two in the thumb.
–form the knuckles by their proximal and middle heads.

II. Joints

A. Shoulder (Glenohumeral) Joint

–is a multi-axial ball-and-socket (spheroidal) joint between the glenoid cavity of the scapula and the head of the humerus.
–its articular surface consists of hyaline cartilage.
–its capsule lies deep to the tendon of the musculotendinous cuff.
–its cavity communicates with the subscapular bursa.
–is supplied by the axillary, suprascapular, and lateral pectoral nerves.
–its capsule is attached to the glenoid outside the labrum and to the anatomical neck of the humerus.

B. Elbow Joint

–forms a hinge (ginglymus) joint between the capitulum of the humerus and the head of the radius (humeroradial joint) and between the trochlea of the humerus and the trochlear notch of the ulna (humeroulnar joint).
–also includes the proximal radioulnar joint within a common articular capsule.

C. Proximal Radioulnar Joint

–forms a pivot (trochoid) joint, in which the head of the radius articulates with the radial notch of the ulna.

D. Distal Radioulnar Joint

–is a pivot joint, formed between the head of the ulna and the ulnar notch of the radius.
–has triangular fibrocartilaginous articular disc that unites structure of the joint but excludes the ulna from the wrist (radiocarpal) joint.

E. Wrist (Radiocarpal) Joint

–is an ellipsoid (condyloid) joint formed by the radius, the articular disc, and the proximal row of carpal bones, exclusive of the pisiform. (The ellipsoidal or egg-shaped surface of the carpal bones fits into the concave surface of the radius and articular disc.)
–allows flexion, extension, abduction, adduction, and circumduction.
–its articular capsule is strengthened by radial and ulnar collateral ligaments and dorsal and palmar radiocarpal ligaments.

F. Midcarpal Joint

–is an articulation between the proximal and distal rows of carpal bones.
–forms an ellipsoid joint, by fitting the hamate and the head of the capitate into the concave of the scaphoid, lunate, and triquetrum.
–also forms a plane joint, by joining the scaphoid with the trapezium and trapezoid.

G. **Carpometacarpal Joint**

—forms a saddle (sellar) joint, between the trapezium and the base of the first metacarpal bone.

—also forms plane joints, between the carpal bones and the medial four metacarpal bones.

H. **Metacarpophalangeal Joint**

—is an ellipsoid joint.

—is supported by a palmar ligament and two collateral ligaments.

I. **Interphalangeal Joint**

—is a hinge joint.

—has a strong palmar ligament and two collateral ligaments.

Pectoral Region and Axilla

I. Breast and Mammary Gland

A. **Breast**

—consists of mammary gland tissue, fibrous and adipose tissue, together with blood and lymph vessels and nerves.

—extends from the second to sixth ribs and from the sternum to the midaxillary line.

—has its nipple at the level of the fourth intercostal space. ᵀ4

—has an areola, a ring of pigmented skin around the nipple.

—has glandular tissue, which lies in the superficial fascia.

—is supplied by the anterior perforating branches of the internal thoracic artery and branches of the lateral thoracic artery.

—is innervated by the lateral cutaneous branches of the intercostal nerves and by branches of the supraclavicular nerve.

—has suspensory ligaments (Cooper's), which are numerous, strong fibrous processes that extend from the skin to the underlying deep fascia through the mammary gland.

—has an axillary tail, which is a part of the mammary gland that extends upward and laterally into the axilla because the mammary gland is larger than the breast.

B. **Mammary Gland**

—is a modified sweat gland.

—is located in the superficial fascia (between the superficial and deep layers of the subcutaneous tissue).

—has 15–20 compound alveolar glands or lobes, each of which opens by a lactiferous duct onto the tip of the nipple. Each duct enlarges to form a lactiferous sinus, which serves as a reservoir for milk.

C. **Lymphatic Drainage of Breast or Mammary Gland**

—is of great importance in view of the frequent development of cancer and subsequent dissemination of cancer cells through the lymphatic stream.

—goes mostly (75%) to the axillary nodes, more specifically to the pectoral nodes (including drainage of the nipple).

—follows the perforating vessels through the pectoralis major and the thoracic wall to enter the parasternal (internal thoracic) nodes, lying along the internal thoracic artery.

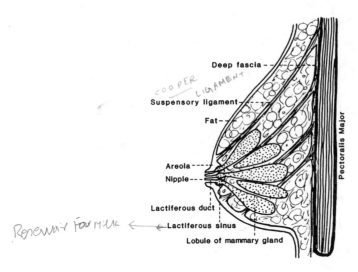

Deep fascia

COOPER LIGAMENT

Suspensory ligament

Fat

Areola

Nipple

Lactiferous duct

Reservoir for Milk ← Lactiferous sinus

Lobule of mammary gland

Pectoralis Major

Figure 2.4. The breast.

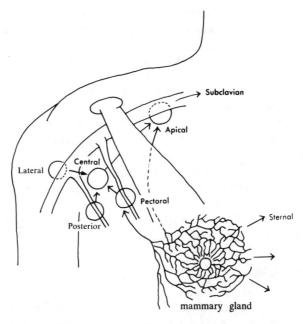

Subclavian

Apical

Lateral

Central

Posterior

Pectoral

Sternal

mammary gland

Figure 2.5. Lymphatic drainage of the breast and axillary lymph nodes.

—also goes to the apical nodes as well as nodes of the opposite breast and of the anterior abdominal wall.

D. Cancer of Breast

—forms a palpable mass in the breast.

—enlarges, attaches to the suspensory ligaments of Cooper, and produces shortening of the ligaments, causing depression or dimpling of the overlying skin.

—may also attach to and shorten the lactiferous ducts, causing the nipple to become retracted or inverted.

—may invade the deep fascia of the pectoralis major muscle; thus contraction of this muscle produces a sudden upward movement of the whole breast.

1. **Radical Mastectomy**

    —is an extensive surgical removal of the breast and its related structures including the pectoralis major and minor, axillary lymph nodes and fascia, and even part of the thoracic wall.

    —may injure the long thoracic and thoracodorsal nerves.

    —may cause postoperative swelling (edema) of the upper limb due to lymphatic obstruction caused by the removal of most of the lymphatic channels that drain the arm, or due to venous obstruction caused by the thrombosis of the axillary vein.

II. Fasciae of Pectoral and Axillary Regions

A. Clavipectoral Fascia

—extends between the coracoid process, the clavicle, and the thoracic wall.

—envelops the subclavius and pectoralis minor muscles.

B. Costocoracoid Membrane

—is a part of the clavipectoral fascia between the first rib and the coracoid process.

—is pierced by the

1. cephalic vein.
2. thoracoacromial artery.
3. lateral pectoral nerve.

C. Pectoral Fascia

—covers the pectoralis major muscle.

—is attached to the sternum and clavicle and is continuous with the axillary fascia.

D. Axillary Fascia

—is continuous anteriorly with the pectoral and clavipectoral fasciae, laterally with the brachial fascia, and posteromedially with the fascia of the latissimus dorsi and serratus anterior muscles.

E. Axillary Sheath

—is a fascial prolongation of the prevertebral layer of the cervical fascia into the axilla.

—encloses the axillary vessels and the brachial plexus.

III. Boundaries of Axilla

A. Medial Wall

—upper ribs and their intercostal muscles and serratus anterior.

B. Lateral Wall

—humerus.

C. Posterior Wall

—subscapularis, teres major and latissimus dorsi.

D. Anterior Wall

–pectoralis major and minor.

E. Base

–axillary fascia.

F. Apex

–interval between clavicle, scapula, and first rib.

IV. Muscles

A. Pectoralis Major

–arises from the medial half of the clavicle, the manubrium and body of the sternum, and the upper six costal cartilages.

–inserts on the lateral lip of the intertubercular groove (the crest of the greater tubercle) of the humerus.

–is supplied by the medial and lateral pectoral nerves.

–adducts and medially rotates the arm; the clavicular part can rotate the arm medially and flex it, whereas the sternocostal part depresses the arm and shoulder.

–has lower fibers that can help to extend the arm.

–receives blood from the pectoral branch of the thoracoacromial artery.

B. Pectoralis Minor

–arises from the external surfaces of the second to the fifth ribs.

–inserts into the coracoid process.

–is innervated by the medial pectoral nerve and by the lateral pectoral nerve.

–depresses the shoulder.

–is invested by the clavipectoral fascia.

–divides the axillary artery into three parts.

–forms part of the anterior wall of the axilla.

–crosses the cord of the brachial plexus.

C. Subclavius

–originates from the junction of the first rib and its cartilage.

–inserts on the lower surface of the clavicle.

–is supplied by the nerve to the subclavius.

–assists in depressing the lateral portion of the clavicle.

D. Serratus Anterior

–arises from the external surfaces of the upper eight ribs.

–is inserted on the whole length of the medial border of the scapula.

–is innervated by the long thoracic nerve.

–rotates the scapula upward so that the inferior angle swings laterally, abducts the arm, and elevates the arm above the horizontal.

–when paralyzed, results in winging of the scapula and inability to elevate the arm above the horizontal.

–forms the medial wall of the axilla.

V. Axillary Artery

–extends from the outer border of the first rib to the inferior border of the teres major muscle, where it becomes the brachial artery.

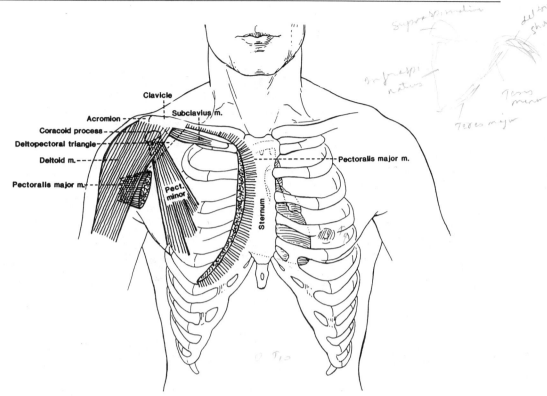

Figure 2.6. Muscles of the pectoral region.

–divides into three parts by the pectoralis minor muscle.
–is considered to be the central structure of the axilla.
–is bordered on its medial side by the axillary vein.

A. Supreme Thoracic Artery

–supplies the first and second intercostal spaces.

B. Thoracoacromial Artery

–is a short trunk from the first or second part of the axillary artery.
–has pectoral, clavicular, acromial, and deltoid branches.
–pierces the costocoracoid membrane (or clavipectoral fascia).

C. Lateral Thoracic Artery

–runs along the lateral border of the pectoralis minor.
–supplies the pectoralis major and minor, serratus anterior, and axillary lymph nodes and gives rise to lateral mammary branches.

D. Subscapular Artery

–is the largest branch of the axillary artery.
–arises at the lower border of the subscapularis muscle and descends along the axillary border of the scapula.
–divides into the thoracodorsal and circumflex scapular arteries.

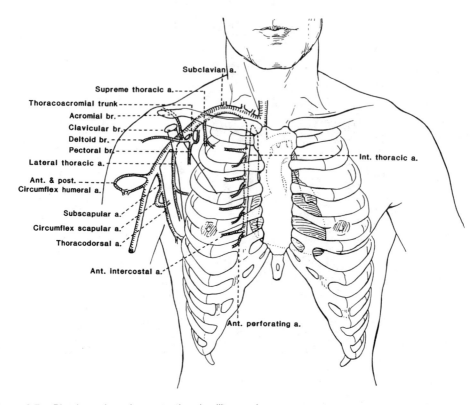

Figure 2.7. Blood supply to the pectoral and axillary regions.

1. Circumflex Scapular Artery

—passes posteriorly into the triangular space bounded by the subscapularis and teres minor above, the teres major below, and the long head of the triceps laterally.

—ramifies in the infraspinous fossa and anastomoses with branches of the dorsal scapular and suprascapular arteries.

2. Thoracodorsal Artery

—accompanies the thoracodorsal nerve.

—supplies the latissimus dorsi and lateral thoracic wall.

E. Anterior Circumflex Humeral Artery

—passes anteriorly around the surgical neck of the humerus.

—anastomoses with the posterior circumflex humeral artery.

F. Posterior Circumflex Humeral Artery

—runs posteriorly with the axillary nerve through the quadrangular space.

—anastomoses in the acromial network and with an ascending branch of the profunda brachii artery.

VI. Veins

A. Axillary Vein

—begins at the lower border of the teres major, as the continuation of the basilic vein.

—ascends along the medial side of the axillary artery.

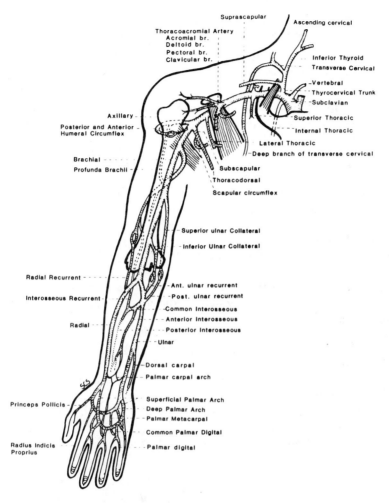

Figure 2.8. Blood supply to the upper limb.

—continues as the subclavian vein at the inferior margin of the first rib.

—commonly receives the thoracoepigastric veins directly or indirectly, and thus provides a collateral circulation if the inferior vena cava becomes obstructed.

—its tributaries are the cephalic vein, brachial veins, and veins that correspond to the branches of the axillary artery with the exception of the thoracoacromial vein.

B. Cephalic Vein

—runs in the deltopectoral triangle, along with the deltoid branch of the thoracoacromial trunk.

—perforates the costocoracoid membrane and terminates in the axillary vein.

VII. Axillary Lymph Nodes

A. The **central** nodes lie near the base of the axilla between the lateral thoracic and subscapular veins. They receive lymph from the lateral, pectoral, and posterior groups of nodes and then drain into apical nodes.

B. The **lateral** nodes lie posteromedial to the axillary veins, receive lymph from the upper limb, and drain into the central nodes.

C. The **subscapular** group lies along the subscapular vein and drains lymph from posterior thoracic wall and posterior aspect of the shoulder to the central group.

D. The **pectoral** nodes lie along the inferolateral border of the pectoralis minor and drains lymph from the anterior and lateral thoracic walls, including the breast.

E. The **apical** nodes lie at the apex of the axilla medial to the axillary vein and above the upper border of the pectoralis minor, receive lymph from all of the other axillary groups (and occasionally from the breast), and drain into the subclavian trunks.

VIII. Brachial Plexus

—is formed by the ventral primary rami of the lower four cervical and first thoracic nerves (C5–T1).
—has roots that pass between the scalenus anterior and medius muscles.
—is enclosed with the axillary artery and vein in the axillary sheath.
—has the following branches from:

A. Roots

1. Dorsal Scapular Nerve (C5)

—pierces the scalenus medius muscle to reach the posterior cervical triangle.
—descends deep to the levator scapulae and the rhomboid minor and major muscles.
—supplies the levator scapulae and rhomboids.

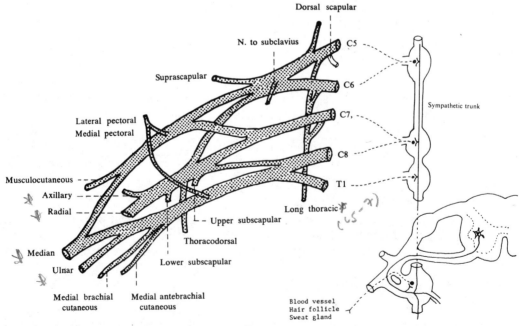

Figure 2.9. The brachial plexus.

2. **Long Thoracic Nerve (C5–7)**

–runs behind the brachial plexus and enters the axilla between the axillary artery and the serratus anterior.

–supplies the serratus anterior muscle.

–when damaged causes "winging of the scapula" and makes elevation of the arm above the horizontal impossible.

winging of the scapula

B. **Upper Trunk**

1. **Suprascapular Nerve (C5)**

–runs laterally across the posterior cervical triangle.

–passes through the scapular notch under the transverse scapular ligament, whereas the suprascapular artery passes over the ligament. So it is said that army (artery) runs over the bridge (ligament) and navy (nerve) runs under the bridge.

–supplies the supraspinatus muscle and the shoulder joint, and then descends through the notch of the scapular neck to end the infraspinatus muscle.

2. **Nerve to Subclavius (C5)**

–descends in front of the brachial plexus and the subclavian artery and behind the clavicle, to reach the subclavius muscle.

–also supplies the sternoclavicular joint.

C. **Lateral Cord**

1. **Lateral Pectoral Nerve (C5–7)**

–arises from the lateral cord of the brachial plexus.

–contains nerve fibers from the fifth, sixth, and seventh cervical nerves.

–supplies primarily the pectoralis major muscle, but also supplies the pectoralis minor muscle.

–sends a branch over the first part of the axillary artery to the medial pectoral nerve and forms a nerve loop through which the lateral pectoral nerve conveys motor fibers to the pectoralis minor muscle.

–pierces the costocoracoid membrane of the clavipectoral fascia.

–is accompanied by the pectoral branch of the thoracoacromial artery.

2. **Musculocutaneous Nerve (C5–7)**

–arises from the lateral cord of the brachial plexus.

–pierces the coracobrachialis muscle and descends between the biceps and brachialis muscles, and innervates these three muscles.

–continues into the forearm as the lateral antebrachial cutaneous nerve.

–contains nerve fibers whose cell bodies are located in the

   a. Dorsal root ganglia (for sensory fibers).

   b. Anterior horn of the spinal cord (for somatic motor fibers).

   c. Sympathetic chain ganglia (for sympathetic postganglionic fibers).

D. **Medial Cord**

1. **Medial Pectoral Nerve (C8–T1)**

–arises from the medial cord of the brachial plexus.

–contains nerve fibers originating from the eighth cervical and first thoracic nerves.

—passes forward between the axillary artery and vein.

—forms a loop in front of the axillary artery with the lateral pectoral nerve.

—enters and supplies the pectoralis minor, and reaches the overlying pectoralis major muscle.

2. **Medial Brachial Cutaneous Nerve (T1)**

—runs the medial side of the axillary vein.

—supplies skin on the medial side of the arm.

—may communicate with the intercostobrachial cutaneous nerve.

—contains nerve fibers whose cell bodies are located in the

a. *dorsal root ganglia (for sensory fibers).*

b. *sympathetic chain ganglia (for sympathetic postganglionic fibers).*

3. **Medial Antebrachial Cutaneous Nerve (C8–T1)**

—runs between the axillary artery and vein and then medial to the brachial artery.

—supplies skin on the medial side of the forearm.

4. **Ulnar Nerve (C7–T1)**

—runs downward the medial aspect of the arm and has no branches in the brachium.

—passes posteriorly to the medial epicondyle in a groove and may be damaged by the fracture of the medial epicondyle, producing funny-bone symptom.

—passes between the two heads of the flexor carpi ulnaris and innervates this muscle and the flexor digitorum profundus.

—crosses the anterior surface of the flexor retinaculum close to the pisiform bone, with the ulnar artery on its lateral side.

—enters the hand deep to the tendon of the flexor carpi ulnaris and palmaris brevis.

—supplies the hypothenar muscle by its deep branch, as well as all the interossei, the third and fourth lumbricals, and the adductor pollicis.

—supplies the palmaris brevis by its superficial branch and divides into a proper digital nerve to the little finger and a common digital nerve to the little and ring fingers.

E. **Medial and Lateral Cords**

1. **Median Nerve (C5–T1)**

—runs down the anteromedial aspect of the arm and has no branches in the brachium.

—enters the forearm between the two heads of the pronator teres muscle.

—passes through the cubital fossa, deep to the bicipital aponeurosis, medial to the brachial artery.

—may be injured by supracondylar fracture of the humerus.

—gives off its largest branch to the forearm, the anterior interosseous nerve.

—passes through the wrist deep to the flexor retinaculum and divides into a muscular branch to thenar muscles and digital branches to the thumb and two and one-half fingers.

F. Posterior Cord

   1. Upper Subscapular Nerve (C5,6)

   –supplies the upper portion of the subscapularis muscle.

   2. Thoracodorsal Nerve (C7,8)

   –runs behind the axillary artery and accompanies the thoracodorsal artery to enter the latissimus dorsi muscle.

   3. Lower Subscapular Nerve (C5,6)

   –arises from the posterior cord of the brachial plexus.
   –innervates the lower part of the subscapularis and teres major muscles.
   –contains nerve fibers from the fifth and sixth cervical spinal nerves.
   –courses downward behind subscapular vessels to the teres major muscle.

   4. Axillary Nerve (C5,6)

   –innervates the deltoid by its anterior and posterior branches and teres minor by its posterior branch.
   –gives rise to the lateral brachial cutaneous nerve.
   –passes posteriorly through the quadrangular space accompanied by the posterior humeral circumflex artery.
   –winds around the surgical neck of the humerus.

   5. Radial Nerve (C5–T1)

   –is the largest branch of the brachial plexus.
   –runs down the posterior aspect of the arm.
   –lies in the musculospiral groove on the back of the humerus with the profunda brachii artery.
   –passes anterior to the medial epicondyle, between the brachialis and brachioradialis muscles, where it divides into superficial and deep branches.
   –may be damaged by the midhumeral fracture, causing paralysis of the extensor muscles of the wrist and hand.
   –gives off the posterior brachial and antebrachial cutaneous nerves.
   –its superficial branch descends in the forearm under cover of the brachioradialis and then passes dorsally around the radius under the tendon of brachioradialis. The nerve runs distally to the dorsum of the hand to distribute the radial side of the hand and radial two and one-half digits.
   –its deep branch enters the supinator muscle, winds laterally around the radius in the substance of the muscle, and continues as the posterior interosseous nerve with the posterior interosseous artery. It supplies muscles of the back of the forearm.

IX. Lesion of Brachial Plexus

A. Upper Trunk Injury (Erb-Duchenne Paralysis)

   –is caused by a violent separation of the head from the shoulder, such as results from a fall from a motorcycle or horse.
   –results in a **"waiter's tip" hand**, in which the arm tends to lie in medial rotation, due to paralysis of lateral rotator muscles.

B. Lower Trunk Injury (Klumpke's Paralysis)

—is caused during a difficult breach delivery (birth palsy or obstetrical paralysis) or by a cervical rib (cervical rib syndrome), or abnormal insertion or spasm of anterior and middle scalene muscles (scalene syndrome).

—results in a "claw hand."

C. Injury to Posterior Cord

—is caused by the pressure of the crosspiece of a crutch, resulting in paralysis of the arm, called **"crutch palsy."**

—results in loss of the extensors of the arm, forearm, wrist, and hand.

—produces a **"wrist drop."**

D. Injury to Long Thoracic Nerve

—is caused by a stab wound or during thoracic surgery.

—results in **"winging of the scapula"** due to paralysis of the serratus anterior muscle.

E. Injury to Musculocutaneous Nerve

—results in weakness of supination (biceps) and forearm flexion (brachialis and biceps).

F. Injury to Axillary Nerve

—is caused by fracture of the surgical neck of the humerus or inferior dislocation of the humerus.

—results in weakness of lateral rotation and abduction of the arm (the supraspinatus can abduct the arm but not to a horizontal level).

G. Injury to Radial Nerve

—is caused by fracture of the midshaft of the humerus.

—results in loss of the extensors of forearm, hand, metacarpals, and phalanges.

—results in loss of wrist extension, leading to **"wrist drop."**

—produces a weakness of abduction and adduction of the hand.

H. Injury to Ulnar Nerve

—is caused by fracture of the medial epicondyle.

—results in a **"claw hand,"** in which the ring and little fingers are hyperextended at the metacarpophalangeal joints and flexed at the interphalangeal joints.

—results in loss of abduction and adduction of fingers, flexion and metacarpophalangeal joints, due to paralysis of palmar and dorsal interossei and medial two lumbricals.

—results in loss of adduction of the thumb, due to paralysis of the adductor pollicis.

I. Injury to Median Nerve

—results in loss of pronation, flexion of lateral two interphalangeal joints, and impairment of medial two interphalangeal joints.

—produces a characteristic flattening of the thenar eminence, often referred to as an **"ape hand."**

Shoulder Region

I. Muscles

Muscle	Origin	Insertion	Nerve	Action
Deltoid	Lateral third of clavicle, acromion, and spine of scapula	Deltoid tuberosity of humerus	Axillary n.	Abducts, adducts, flexes, extends, and rotates arm
Supraspinatus	Supraspinous fossa of scapula	Superior facet of greater tubercle of humerus	Suprascapular n.	Abducts arm
Infraspinatus	Infraspinous fossa	Middle facet of greater tubercle of humerus	Suprascapular n.	Rotate arm laterally
Subscapularis	Subscapular fossa	Lesser tubercle of humerus	Upper and lower subscapular n.	Rotate arm medially
Teres major	Dorsal surface of inferior angle of scapula	Medial lip of intertubercular groove of humerus	Lower subscapular n.	Adducts and rotates arm medially
Teres minor	Upper portion of lateral border of scapula	Lower facet of greater tubercle of humerus	Axillary n.	Rotates arm laterally

Lateral rotators of arm: Infraspinatus. Teres minor (handwritten)

II. Quadrangular and Triangular Spaces

A. Quadrangular Space

—is bounded superiorly by the teres minor and subscapularis, inferiorly by the teres major, medially by the long head of the triceps, and laterally by the surgical neck of the humerus.

—transmits the axillary nerve and posterior circumflex humeral vessels.

B. Triangular Space

—is bounded superiorly by the teres minor, inferiorly by the teres major, and laterally by the long head of the triceps.

—contains the circumflex scapular vessels.

III. Arteries

A. Suprascapular Artery

—is a branch of the thyrocervical trunk.

—anastomoses with the deep branch of the transverse cervical artery (dorsal scapular) and scapular circumflex artery around the scapula, providing a collateral circulation.

—passes over the transverse scapular ligament (whereas, the suprascapular nerve passes under the ligament).

—supplies the supraspinatus, infraspinatus, shoulder, and acromioclavicular joints.

B. Dorsal Scapular or Descending Scapular Artery (a Deep Branch of the Transverse Cervical Artery)

—arises from the subclavian artery but may be a deep branch of the transverse cervical artery.

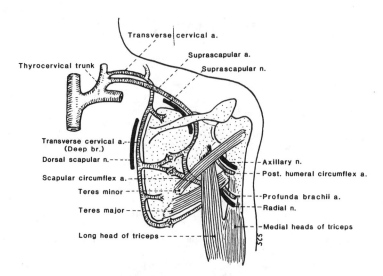

Figure 2.10. Blood supply to the dorsal scapular region.

—accompanies the dorsal scapular nerve and supplies the levator scapulae, rhomboids, and serratus anterior muscles.

C. Arterial Anastomoses around Scapula

—occur between:

1. **Suprascapular and circumflex scapular arteries.**
2. **Descending scapular and circumflex scapular arteries.**
3. **Descending scapular and posterior intercostal arteries.**
4. **Suprascapular, acromial, and posterior circumflex humeral arteries.**

IV. Nerves

A. Suprascapular Nerve

—arises from C5,6 and runs laterally across the posterior cervical triangle.
—passes under the transverse scapular ligament, whereas the suprascapular artery passes over the ligament.
—supplies the supraspinatus muscle and the shoulder joint, and then descends through the notch of the scapular neck to end at the infraspinatus muscle.

B. Dorsal Scapular Nerve

—arises chiefly from C5 and pierces the scalenus medius muscle.
—descends deep to the levator scapulae and the rhomboid minor and major to supply these muscles.

C. Spinal Accessory Nerve

—accompanies the superficial branch of the transverse cervical artery on the deep surface of the trapezius muscle.
—supplies the sternocleidomastoid and trapezius muscles.

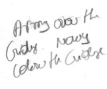

V. Shoulder Joint and Associated Structures

A. Shoulder (Glenohumeral) Joint

—is a multi-axial ball-and-socket joint between the glenoid cavity of the scapula and the head of the humerus.

—its articular surface consists of hyaline cartilage.

—its capsule lies deep to the tendon of the musculotendinous cuff.

—its cavity communicates with the subscapular bursa.

—is supplied by the axillary, suprascapular and lateral pectoral nerves.

—its capsule is attached to the margin of the glenoid cavity and to the anatomical neck of the humerus.

B. Acromioiclavicular Joint

—is a plane joint between the acromion and the lateral border of the clavicle.

—its articular surfaces are covered fibrous cartilages.

—its stability is provided by the coracoclavicular ligament, which consists of the conoid and trapezoid ligaments.

C. Rotator (or Musculotendinous) Cuff

—contributes the stability of the shoulder joint by keeping the head of the humerus pressed into the glenoid fossa.

—is formed by the tendons of the:

1. **Subscapularis.**
2. **Supraspinatus.**
3. **Infraspinatus.**
4. **Teres minor.**

D. Bursae around Shoulder

—form a lubricating mechanism between the rotator cuff and coracoacromial arch during movement of the shoulder joint.

1. Subacromial Bursa

—underlies the coracoacromial ligament.

—separates the acromion process and the supraspinatus muscle.

—frequently communicates with the subdeltoid bursa, which separates the deltoid muscle from the head of the humerus and the insertions of the rotator cuff.

—does not normally communicate with the synovial cavity of the glenohumeral joint.

—facilitates the movement of the deltoid muscle over the joint capsule and the supraspinatus tendon.

2. Subdeltoid Bursa

—lies between the deltoid and coracoacromial arch, and the tendon of the supraspinatus muscle.

—frequently communicates with the subacromial bursa.

E. Ligaments

1. Coracohumeral Ligament

—extends from the coracoid process to the greater tubercle of the humerus.

2. **Glenohumeral Ligaments**

   a. *Superior Glenohumeral Ligament*

      —extends from the supraglenoid tubercle to the upper part of the lesser tubercle of the humerus.

   b. *Middle Glenohumeral Ligament*

      —extends from the supraglenoid tubercle to the lower anatomical neck.

   c. *Inferior Glenohumeral Ligament*

      —extends from the supraglenoid tubercle to the lower part of the lesser tubercle.

3. **Transverse Humeral Ligament**

   —extends between the greater and lesser tubercles, and holds the tendon of the biceps in the intertubercular groove.

4. **Coracoacromial Ligament**

   —extends from the coracoid process to the acromion.

VI. Other Features

A. Referred Pain to Shoulder

—indicates most likely involvement of the phrenic nerve (or diaphragm).

—is due to the same origin of the phrenic nerve (C3,4, 5), which supplies the diaphragm, and supraclavicular (C3, 4) nerve, which supplies sensory fibers over the shoulder.

B. Suprascapular (or Transverse Scapular) Ligament

—bridges the scapular notch and converts it into a foramen that transmits the suprascapular nerve.

—is passed over by the suprascapular vessels.

—provides the site of origin for the omohyoid muscle.

C. Triangle of Auscultation

—is bounded by upper border of the latissimus dorsi, lateral border of the trapezius, medial border of the scapula.

—has its floor formed by the rhomboid major.

—is the site to hear breathing sounds most clearly.

D. Inferior Dislocation of Humerus

—is not uncommon, because the inferior aspect of the shoulder joint is not supported by muscles.

—may damage the axillary nerve and the posterior humeral circumflex vessels.

Arm and Forearm

I. Muscles of Arm

Muscle	Origin	Insertion	Nerve	Action
Coracobra-chialis	Coracoid process	Middle third of medial surface of humerus	Musculocuta-neous n.	Flexes and ad-ducts arm

Biceps brachii	Long head, supra-glenoid tubercle; short head, coracoid process	Radial tuberosity of radius	Musculocutaneous n.	Flexes arm and forearm, supinates forearm
Brachialis	Lower anterior surface of humerus	Coronoid process and ulnar tuberosity	Musculocutaneous and radial n.	Flexes forearm
Triceps	Long head, infraglenoid tubercle; lateral head, superior to radial groove of humerus; medial head, inferior to radial groove	Posterior surface of olecranon process of ulna	Radial n.	Extends forearm
Anconeus	Lateral eopcondyle of humerus	Olecranon and upper posterior surface of ulna	Radial n.	Extends forearm

II. Muscles of Anterior Forearm

Muscle	Origin	Insertion	Nerve	Action
Pronator teres	Medial epicondyle and coronoid process of ulna	Middle of lateral side of radius	Median n.	Pronates forearm
Flexor carpi radialis	Medial epicondyle of humerus	Bases of second and third metacarpals	Median n.	Flexes forearm, flexes and abducts hand
Palmaris longus	Medial epicondyle of humerus	Flexor retinaculum, palmar aponeurosis	Median n.	Flexes hand and forearm
Flexor carpi ulnaris	Medial epicondyle, medial olecranon, and posterior border of ulna	Pisiform, hook of hamate, and base of fifth metacarpal	Ulnar n.	Flexes and adducts hand, flexes forearm
Flexor digitorum superficialis	Medial epicondyle, coronoid process, oblique line of radius	Middle phalanges of finger	Median n.	Flexes middle phalanges, flexes hand and forearm
Flexor digitorum profundus	Anteromedial surface of ulna, interosseous membrane	Bases of distal phalanges of fingers	Ulnar and median n.	Flexes distal phalanges and hand
Flexor pollicis longus	Anterior surface of radius, interosseous membrane, and coronoid process	Base of distal phalanx of thumb	Median n.	Flexes thumb
Pronator quadratus	Anterior surface of distal ulna	Anterior surface of distal radius	Median n.	Pronates forearm

III. Muscles of Posterior Forearm

Muscle	Origin	Insertion	Nerve	Action
Brachioradialis	Lateral supracondylar ridge of humerus	Base of radial styloid process	Radial n.	Flexes forearm

III. Muscles of Posterior Forearm (Continued)

Muscle	Origin	Insertion	Nerve	Action
Extensor carpi radialis longus	Lateral supracondylar ridge of humerus	Dorsum of base of second metacarpal	Radial n.	Extends and abducts hand
Extensor carpi radialis brevis	Lateral epicondyle of humerus	Posterior base of third metacarpal	Radial n.	Extends and abducts hand
Extensor digitorum	Lateral epicondyle of humerus	Extensor expansion, base of middle and distal phalanges	Radial n.	Extends fingers and hand
Extensor digiti minimi	Common extensor tendon and interosseous membrane	Extensor expansion, proximal phalanx of little finger	Radial n.	Extends little finger
Extensor carpi ulnaris	Lateral epicondyle and posterior surface of ulna	Base of fifth metacarpal	Radial n.	Extends and adducts hand
Anconeus	Back of lateral eipcondyle	Olecranon and upper posterior surface of ulna	Radial n.	Extends forearm
Supinator	Lateral eipcondyle, radial collateral and annular ligaments	Lateral side of upper part of radius	Radial n.	Supinates forearm
Abductor pollicis longus	Interosseous membrane, middle third of posterior surfaces of radius and ulna	Lateral surface of base of first metacarpal	Radial n.	Abducts thumb and hand
Extensor pollicis longus	Interosseous membrane and middle third of posterior surface of ulna	Base of distal phalanx of thumb	Radial n.	Extends distal phalanx of thumb and abducts hand
Extensor pollicis brevis	Interosseous membrane and posterior surface of middle third radius	Base of proximal phalanx of thumb	Radial n.	Extends proximal phalanx of thumb and abducts hand
Extensor indicis	Posterior surface of ulna and interosseous membrane	Extensor expansion of index finger	Radial n.	Extends index finger

IV. Arteries

A. Brachial Artery

- —extends from the inferior border of the teres major muscle to its bifurcation in the cubital fossa.
- —lies on the triceps and brachialis, and medial to the coracobrachialis and biceps muscles.
- —is accompanied by the basilic vein in the middle of the arm.
- —lies in the center of the cubital fossa, medial to the biceps tendon, lateral to the median nerve, and deep to the bicipital aponeurosis.

−provides unnamed muscular and named branches and terminates by dividing into the radial and ulnar arteries in the cubital fossa.

1. Profunda Brachii Artery

−descends posteriorly in company with the radial nerve.
−its ascending branch anastomoses with the descending branch of the posterior circumflex humeral artery.
−divides into a middle collateral artery, which anastomoses with the interosseous recurrent artery, and the radial collateral artery, which follows the radial nerve through the lateral intermuscular septum and ends in front of the lateral epicondyle by anastomosing with the radial recurrent artery of the radial artery.

2. Superior Ulnar Collateral Artery

−pierces the medial intermuscular septum and descends with the ulnar nerve behind the septum and medial epicondyle, and anastomoses with the posterior ulnar recurrent branch of the ulnar artery.

3. Inferior Ulnar Collateral Artery

−arises a little above the elbow, descends in front of the medial epicondyle, and anastomoses with the anterior ulnar recurrent branch of the ulnar artery.

B. Radial Artery

−arises as the smaller lateral branch of the brachial artery in the cubital fossa.
−descends laterally under cover of the brachioradialis, with the superficial radial nerve on its lateral side, on the supinator and flexor pollicis longus.
−curves over the radial side of the carpal bones beneath the tendons of the abductor pollicis longus and the extensor pollicis longus and brevis and over the surface of the scaphoid and trapezium.
−runs through the anatomical snuff box, enters the palm by passing between the two heads of the first dorsal interosseous muscle and then between the heads of the adductor pollicis, and divides into the princeps pollicis artery and the deep palmar arch.
−gives off the radial recurrent, muscular, dorsal carpal, palmar carpal, and superficial palmar arteries.

1. Radial Recurrent Artery

−arises from the radial artery a little below its origin.
−anastomoses with the radial collateral branch of the profunda brachii artery.

2. Palmar Carpal Branch

−joins the palmar carpal branch of the ulnar artery and forms the palmar carpal arch.

3. Superficial Palmar Branch

−passes through the thenar muscle and anastomoses with the superficial branch of the ulnar artery to complete the superficial palmar arterial arch.

4. Dorsal Carpal Branch

–joins the dorsal carpal branch of the ulnar artery and the dorsal terminal branch of the anterior interosseous artery to form the dorsal carpal rete (or arch).

C. Ulnar Artery

–is the larger medial branch of the brachial artery in the cubital fossa.
–descends behind the ulnar head of the pronator teres and lies between the flexor digitorum superficialis and profundus muscles.
–enters the hand anterior to the flexor retinaculum, lateral to the pisiform, and medial to the hook of the hamate.
–divides into the superficial palmar arch and the deep palmar branch, which passes between the abductor and flexor digiti minimi brevis and runs medially to join the radial artery to complete the deep palmar arch.
–gives off the following named branches:

1. Anterior Ulnar Recurrent Artery

–anastomoses with the inferior ulnar collateral artery

2. Posterior Ulnar Recurrent Artery

–anastomoses with the superior ulnar collateral artery.

3. Common Interosseous Artery

–arises from the lateral side of the ulnar artery and divides into the anterior and posterior interosseous arteries.

  a. *Anterior Interosseous Artery*

  –descends with the anterior interosseous nerve in front of the interosseous membrane, between the flexor digitorum profundus and the flexor pollicis longus.
  –perforates the interosseous membrane to anastomose with the posterior interosseous artery and to join the dorsal carpal network.

  b. *Posterior Interosseous Artery*

  –gives off an interosseous recurrent artery, which anastomoses with a middle collateral branch of the profunda brachii artery.
  –descends behind the interosseous membrane in company with the posterior interosseous nerve.
  –anastomoses with the dorsal carpal branch of the anterior interosseous artery.

  c. *Palmar Carpal Branch*

  –joins the palmar carpal branch of the radial artery to form the palmar carpal arch.

  d. *Dorsal Carpal Branch*

  –passes around the ulnar side of the wrist and joins the dorsal carpal rete.

D. Anastomoses around the Elbow Joint

–occur between:

1. The radial collateral artery and the radial recurrent artery in front of the lateral epicondyle.

2. The middle collateral artery and the interosseous recurrent artery behind the lateral epicondyle.

3. The inferior ulnar collateral artery and the anterior ulnar recurrent artery in front of the medial epicondyle.

4. The superior ulnar collateral artery and the posterior ulnar recurrent artery behind the medial epicondyle.

V. Nerves

A. Musculocutaneous Nerve (C5–7)

–arises from the lateral cord of the brachial plexus.
–pierces the coracobrachialis muscle.
–descends between the biceps and brachialis muscles.
–innervates the coracobrachialis, biceps, and brachialis muscles.
–continues into the forearm as the lateral antebrachial cutaneous nerve.

B. Median Nerve (C5–T1)

–runs down the anteromedial aspect of the arm and has no branches in the brachium.
–enters the forearm between the two heads of the pronator teres muscle.
–passes through the cubital fossa, deep to the bicipital aponeurosis, medial to the brachial artery.
–may be injured by supracondylar fracture of the humerus.
–gives off its largest branch of the forearm, the anterior interosseous nerve.
–passes through the wrist deep to the flexor retinaculum and divides into a muscular branch to the thenar muscles and digital branches to the thumb and two and one-half fingers.

C. Axillary Nerve (C5,6)

–passes posteriorly through the quadrangular space accompanied by the posterior humeral circumflex artery.
–winds around the surgical neck of the humerus.
–innervates the deltoid by its anterior posterior branches and teres minor by its posterior branch.
–gives rise to the lateral brachial cutaneous nerve.

D. Radial Nerve (C5–T1)

–is the largest branch of the brachial plexus.
–runs down the posterior aspect of the arm.
–lies in the musculospiral groove on the back of the humerus with the profunda brachii artery.
–passes anterior to the medial epicondyle, between the brachialis and brachioradialis muscles, where it divides into superficial and deep branches.
–may be damaged by the midhumeral fracture, causing paralysis of the extensor muscles of the wrist and hand.
–gives off the posterior brachial and antebrachial cutaneous nerves.
–its superficial branch descends in the forearm under cover of the brachioradialis and then passes dorsally around the radius under the tendon of brachioradialis. The nerve runs distally to the dorsum of the hand to distribute the radial side of the hand and radial two and one-half digits.
–its deep branch enters the supinator muscle, winds laterally around the radius in the substance of the muscle, and continues as the posterior

interosseous nerve with the posterior interosseous artery. It supplies muscles of the back of the forearm.

E. Ulnar Nerve (C7–T1)

–runs down the medial aspect of the arm and has no branches in the brachium.

–descends behind the medial epicondyle in a groove, where it may be damaged by the fracture of the medial epicondyle, and produces funny-bone symptom.

–descends between the flexor digitorum superficialis and profundus muscles and supplies these two muscles.

–enters the hand superficial to the flexor retinaculum, lateral to the pisiform bone, and divides into superficial and deep branches. The deep branch passes medial to the hook of the hamate and runs medially across the interossei, supplying the hypothenar muscle as well as all the interossei, the third and fourth lumbricals, and the adductor pollicis. The superficial branch supplies the palmaris brevis and then divides into a proper digital nerve to the little finger and a common digital nerve to the little and ring fingers.

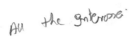
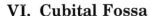

All the interosse

VI. Cubital Fossa

–is a V-shaped interval on the anterior aspect of the elbow.

–is bounded by the brachioradialis laterally and the pronator teres medially.

–its upper limit is an imaginary horizontal line connecting the epicondyles of the humerus.

–has its floor formed by the brachialis and the supinator.

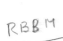

RBBM

–contains (from lateral to medial) the radial nerve, biceps tendon, brachial artery, and median nerve.

–has its lower end where the brachial artery divides into the radial and ulnar arteries.

–has its fascial roof strengthened by the bicipital aponeurosis.

VII. Aponeurosis and Ligaments

A. Bicipital Aponeurosis

–originates from the medial border of the biceps tendon.

–passes downward and medially to blend with the deep fascia of the forearm.

–lies on the brachial artery and the median nerve.

B. Interosseous Membrane of Forearm

–is a broad sheet of dense connective tissue extending between the radius and the ulna.

–forms the intermediate radioulnar joint and functions as a shock absorber.

–provides the attachment for the deep extrinsic flexor, extensor, and abductor muscles of the hand.

–is pierced by the anterior interosseous vessels.

–is slack when arm is used to break a fall.

C. Annular Ligament

–is fibrous band that forms nearly four-fifths of a circle around the head of the radius, the remainder being formed by the radial notch.

−attaches to the anterior and posterior lips of the radial notch of the ulna.

−forms a collar around the head of the radius and thus serves as a re-straining ligament, preventing withdrawal of the head of the radius from its socket.

−permits rotation of the radius relative to the ulna.

−fuses with the radial collateral ligament and blends with the articular capsule of the elbow joint.

−gives the attachment of the origin of the supinator muscle.

D. Radial Collateral Ligament

−a fibrous thickening that extends from the lateral epicondyle to the an-terior and posterior margins of the radial notch of the ulna and the an-nular ligament of the radius.

E. Ulnar Collateral Ligament

1. Anterior Band

−extends from the medial epicondyle to the medial edge of the coronoid process of the ulna.

2. Posterior Band

−extends from the medial epicondyle to the medial edge of the olecranon.

3. Oblique Band

−extends between the medial edges of the coronoid process and the olecranon.

VIII. Other Features

A. Carrying Angle

−is the angle formed by the axis of the arm and forearm when the forearm is extended, because the medial edge of the trochlea projects more infe-riorly than its lateral edge, and thus the long axis of the humerus lies at an angle of about 170° to the long axis of the ulna.

−carries the hand away from the sides of the body in extension and pron-ation.

−disappears when the forearm is flexed or pronated, because the trochlea runs in a spiral direction from anterior to poster aspect.

−is wider in women than in men.

B. Pronation and Supination   *Supination is stronger*

−are used to describe the twisting movements of the hand relative to the forearm: in supination, the palm is faced forward (lateral rotation), while in pronation the radius rotates over the ulna and thus the palm is faced backward (medial rotation about a longitudinal axis, in which the shafts of the radius and ulna cross each other).

−are movements in which the upper end of the radius nearly rotates within the annular ligament.

−have unequal strengths, supination being the stronger of the two.

C. Radial Pulse

−can be felt at the wrist between the tendons of the brachioradialis and flexor carpi radialis muscles.

—may also be palpated in the anatomical snuff-box between the tendons of the extensor pollicis longus and brevis muscles.

D. Ulnar Pulse

—is palpable just to the radial side of the insertion of the flexor carpi ulnaris into the pisiform bone.

Hand

I. Fascia, Aponeurosis, and Synovial Sheaths

A. Flexor Retinaculum

—serves as an attachment (origin) for muscles of the thenar eminence.
—forms a carpal (osteofacial) tunnel on the anterior aspect of the wrist.
—is attached medially to the pisiform and the hook of hamate, and laterally to the tubercles of the scaphoid and trapezium.

B. Extensor Retinaculum

—is a thickening of the antebrachial fascia on the back of the wrist.
—extends from the lateral margin of the radius to the styloid process of the ulna, the pisiform, and the triquetrum.
—is crossed by the superficial branch of the radial nerve.

C. Palmar Aponeurosis

—is a heavy fascia overlying the tendons in the palm.
—is continuous with the palmaris longus tendon, the thenar and hypothenar fasciae, the flexor retinaculum, and the palmar carpal ligament.

D. Facial Spaces of Palm

—are large facial spaces in the hand, divided by a midpalmar (oblique) septum into the thenar space and the midpalmar space.

1. Thenar Space

—is a palmar space lying between the middle metacarpal bone and the tendon of the flexor pollicis longus.

2. Midpalmar Space

—is a palmar space lying between the middle metacarpal bone and the radial side of the hypothenar eminence.

E. Synovial Flexor Sheaths

1. Common Synovial Flexor Sheath (Ulnar Bursa)

—envelops or contains both the tendons of the flexor digitorum superficialis and profundus muscles.

2. Synovial Sheath for Flexor Pollicis Longus (Radial Bursa)

—envelops the tendon of the flexor pollicis longus muscle.

F. Extensor Aponeurosis

—is the expansion of the extensor tendon over the metacarpophalangeal joint.
—is referred to by clinicians as the **extensor hood.**
—provides the insertion of the lumbrical and interosseous muscles.

II. Muscles

Muscle	Origin	Insertion	Nerve	Action
Abductor pollicis brevis	Flexor retinaculum, scaphoid, and trapezium	Lateral side of base of proximal phalanx of thumb	Median n.	Abducts thumb
Flexor pollicis brevis	Flexor retinaculum and trapezium	Base of proximal phalanx of thumb	Median n.	Flexes thumb
Opponens pollicis	Flexor retinaculum and trapezium	Lateral side of first metacarpal	Median n.	Opposes thumb to other digits
Adductor pollicis	Capitate and bases of second and third metacarpals (oblique head); palmar surface of third metacarpal (transverse head)	Medial side of base of proximal phalanx of the thumb	Ulnar n.	Adducts thumb
Palmaris brevis	Medial side of flexor retinaculum, palmar aponeurosis	Skin of medial side of palm	Ulnar n.	Wrinkles skin on medial side of palm
Abductor digiti minimi	Pisiform and tendon of flexor carpi ulnaris	Medial side of base of proximal phalanx of little finger	Ulnar n.	Abducts little finger
Flexor digiti minimi brevis	Flexor retinaculum and hook of hamate	Medial side of base of proximal phalanx of little finger	Ulnar n.	Flexes proximal phalanx of little finger
Opponens digiti minimi	Flexor retinaculum and hook of hamate	Medial side of fifth metacarpal	Ulnar n.	Opposes little finger
Lumbricals (4)	Lateral side of tendons of flexor digitorum profundus	Lateral side of extensor expansion	Median (two lateral), ulnar (two medial)	Flex MP[a] joints and extend IP joints
Dorsal interossei (4)	Adjacent sides of metacarpal bones	Lateral sides of bases of proximal phalanges; extensor expansion	Ulnar n.	Abduct fingers; flex MP joints; extend IP joints
Palmer interossei (3)	Medial side of second metacarpal; lateral sides of fourth and fifth metacarpals	Bases of proximal phalanges in same sides as their origins; extensor expansion	Ulnar n.	Adduct fingers; flex MP joints; extend IP joints

[a]MP, metacarpophalangeal; IP, interphalangeal.

III. Nerves

A. Median Nerve

—enters the palm of the hand deep to the flexor retinaculum.

—gives off an important muscular branch of the recurrent branch to the thenar muscles.

—terminates by dividing into three common palmar digital nerves (under cover of the palmar aponeurosis and the superficial palmar arterial arch), which then divides into the proper palmar digital branches.

—supplies the skin of the lateral side of palm and palmar side of the lateral three and one-half fingers as well as the dorsal side of the index, middle, and one-half ring fingers.

B. Ulnar Nerve

—enters the hand superficial to the flexor retinaculum.

—terminates by dividing into the superficial and deep branches at the root of the hypothenar eminence.

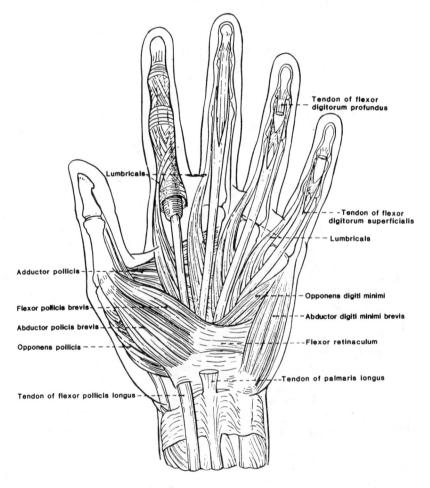

Figure 2.11. Superficial muscles of the hand.

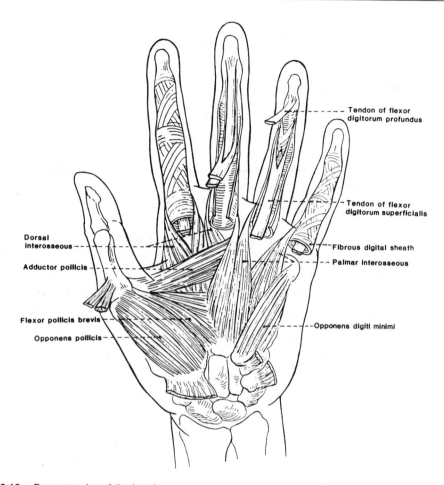

Figure 2.12. Deep muscles of the hand.

1. **Superficial Branch**

   –terminates in the palm by dividing into three palmar digital branches, which supply the skin of the little finger and the medial side of the ring finger.

2. **Deep Branch**

   –arises at about the level of the pisiform bone.

   –enters the palm under cover of the flexor digiti minimi brevis.

   –runs around the hook of hamate and turns laterally with the deep palmar arterial arch under cover of the flexor tendons.

   –supplies all three of the hypothenar muscles, the third and fourth lumbricals, all of the interossei, and the adductor pollicis.

IV. Arterial Arches

A. Superficial Palmar Arterial Arch

   –is formed by the main termination of the ulnar artery but is usually completed by the superficial palmar branch of the radial artery.

–lies immediately under the palmar aponeurosis.

–gives off three common palmar digital arteries, each of which bifurcates into proper palmar digital arteries.

B. Deep Palmar Arterial Arch

–is formed by the main termination of the radial artery, usually completed by the deep palmar branch of the ulnar artery.

–passes between the transverse and oblique heads of the adductor pollicis muscle.

–accompanies two venae comitantes and the deep branch of the ulnar nerve.

–gives off the following branches:

1. Princeps Pollicis Artery

–arises from the radial artery and descends along the ulnar border of the first metacarpal bone under the flexor pollicis longus tendon.

–divides into two proper digital arteries for each side of the thumb.

2. Radialis Indicis Artery

–arises from the deep palmar arch or the princeps pollicis artery.

–descends between the first dorsal interosseous muscle and the transverse head of the adductor pollicis muscle.

–runs distally along the radial side of the index finger.

–may communicate with the superficial palmar arch.

3. Palmar Metacarpal Arteries

–are three in number, descend on the interossei, and join the common palmar digital arteries.

IV. Other Features

A. Anatomical Snuff-box

–is a triangular interval between the tendon of the extensor pollicis longus medially and the tendons of the extensor pollicis brevis and abductor pollicis longus laterally.

–is limited proximally by the styloid process of the radius.

–its floor is formed by the scaphoid and trapezium and crossed by the radial artery.

B. Carpal Tunnel Syndrome

–is caused by the compression of the median nerve due to the reduced size of the osseofibrous carpal tunnel by:

1. Inflammation of the flexor retinaculum.

2. Anterior dislocations of the lunate bone.

3. Arthritic changes

4. Inflammation of tendon and its sheath by fibers of the flexor retinaculum.

–leads to pain and paresthesia (tingling, burning, and numbness) in the hand in the area of distribution of the median nerve.

–may even cause an atrophy of the thenar muscles in case of severe compression.

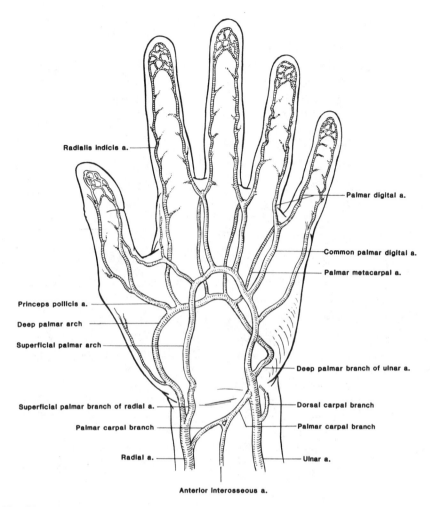

Radialis indicis a.

Palmar digital a.

Common palmar digital a.

Palmar metacarpal a.

Princeps pollicis a.

Deep palmar arch

Superficial palmar arch

Deep palmar branch of ulnar a.

Superficial palmar branch of radial a.

Dorsal carpal branch

Palmar carpal branch

Palmar carpal branch

Radial a.

Ulnar a.

Anterior Interosseous a.

Figure 2.13. Blood supply to the hand.

C. Following Structures Lie Inside the Anterior Carpal Tunnel:

1. Median Nerve.
2. Flexor Pollicis Longus.
3. Flexor digitorum profundus.
4. Flexor digitorum superficialis.

D. Structures Entering the Palm Superficial to Flexor Retinaculum:

1. Flexor carpi ulnaris tendon.
2. Ulnar nerve.
3. Ulnar artery.
4. Palmaris longus.
5. Superficial palmar branch of the radial artery.

V. Additional Characteristics of Some Muscles

A. Adductor Pollicis Muscle

–arises by two heads. (The oblique head arises from the capitate and trapezoid, and the base of the second metacarpal, whereas the transverse head arises from the front of the third metacarpal bone.)
–inserts on the proximal phalanx.
–is innervated by the deep branch of the ulnar nerve.
–is not considered as a thenar muscle.

B. Lumbricals

–originate from the tendons of the flexor digitorum profundus and pass on the thumb side (radial side) of each knuckle.
–insert on the base of the proximal phalanx along with tendons of extensor digitorum longus and interossei.
–are innervated by median nerve (lateral two) and ulnar nerve (medial two).
–can flex (along with interossei) the metacarpophalangeal joints and extend the interphalangeal joints.

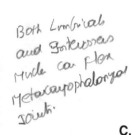
Both Lumbricals and Interosseous Muscle can flex Metacarpophalangeal Joints.

C. Interosseous (Dorsal and Palmar) Muscles

–originate by two heads from the adjacent sides of metacarpal bones (dorsal), and arise by a single head from the metacarpal shaft of the finger (palmar).
–insert into the extensor expansions.
–are innervated by the deep branch of the ulnar nerve.
–can flex the metacarpophalangeal joints, and extend the interphalangeal joints, when the metacarpophalangeal joints are extended by the extensor digitorum communis.
–also adduct (palmar, PAD) and abduct (dorsal, DAB) the fingers. (PAD—Palmar interosseous muscles *ad*duct fingers. DAB—Dorsal interosseus muscles *ab*duct fingers.)

Summary of Muscle Actions of Upper Limb (Muscles in Parentheses Are Less Important in Function)

Movement of Scapula

Elevation—trapezius (upper), levator scapulae
Depression—trapezius (lower), serratus anterior, pectoralis minor
Protrusion (forward or lateral movement: abduction)—serratus anterior
Retraction (backward or medial movement: adduction)—trapezius, rhomboids
Anterior or inferior rotation of glenoid fossa—rhomboid major
Posterior or superior rotation of glenoid fossa—serratus anterior (trapezius)

Movement at Shoulder Joint (Ball-and-Socket Joint)

Adduction—pectoralis major, latissimus dorsi (deltoid posterior)
Abduction—deltoid (supraspinatus)
Flexion—pectoralis major (clavicular part), deltoid anterior (coracobrachialis, biceps)
Extension—latissimus dorsi, deltoid posterior

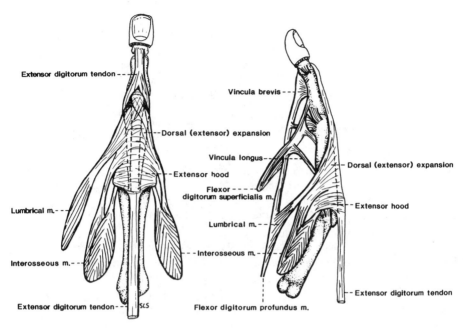

Extensor digitorum tendon

Dorsal (extensor) expansion

Vincula brevis

Vincula longus

Extensor hood

Flexor digitorum superficialis m.

Dorsal (extensor) expansion

Lumbrical m.

Extensor hood

Lumbrical m.

Interosseous m.

Interosseous m.

Extensor digitorum tendon

Extensor digitorum tendon

Flexor digitorum profundus m.

Figure 2.14. Dorsal (extensor) expansion of the middle finger.

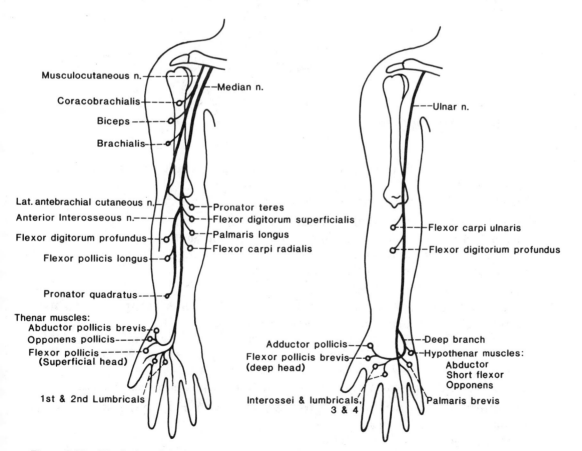

Musculocutaneous n.

Median n.

Coracobrachialis

Ulnar n.

Biceps

Brachialis

Lat. antebrachial cutaneous n.

Pronator teres

Anterior Interosseous n.

Flexor digitorum superficialis

Flexor digitorum profundus

Palmaris longus

Flexor carpi ulnaris

Flexor carpi radialis

Flexor digitorium profundus

Flexor pollicis longus

Pronator quadratus

Thenar muscles:
Abductor pollicis brevis
Opponens pollicis
Flexor pollicis
(Superficial head)

Adductor pollicis

Deep branch

Flexor pollicis brevis
(deep head)

Hypothenar muscles:
Abductor
Short flexor
Opponens

1st & 2nd Lumbricals

Interossei & lumbricals,
3 & 4

Palmaris brevis

Figure 2.15. Distribution of the musculocutaneous, median, and ulnar nerves.

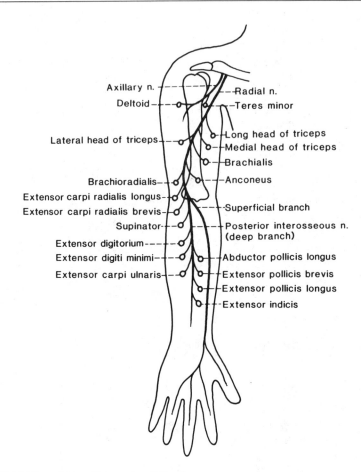

Figure 2.16. Distribution of the axillary and radial nerves.

Medial rotation—subscapularis (pectoralis major, deltoid anterior, latissimus dorsi, teres major)

Lateral rotation—infraspinatus, teres minor (deltoid posterior)

Movement at Elbow Joint (Hinge Joint)

Flexion—brachialis, biceps, brachioradialis (pronator teres)

Extension—triceps (medial head)

Pronation—pronator quadratus (pronator teres)

Supination—supinator (biceps)

Movement at Radiocarpal and Midcarpal Joints (Ellipsoid Joints)

Adduction—flexor carpi ulnaris, extensor carpi ulnaris

Abduction—flexor carpi radialis, extensor carpi radialis longus and brevis

Flexion—flexor carpi radialis, flexor carpi ulnaris, palmaris longus (adductor pollicis longus)

Extension—extensor carpi radialis longus and brevis, extensor carpi ulnaris

Movement at Metacarpophalangeal Joint (MPJ) (Ellipsoid Joint)

Adduction—palmar interossei (PAD)

Abduction—dorsal interossei (DAB)

Flexion—lumbricals and interossei
Extension—extensor digitorum

Movement at Interphalangeal Joint (IPJ) (Hinge Joint)

Flexion—flexor digitorum superficialis (proximal IPJ), flexor digitorum profundus (distal IPJ)

Extension—lumbricals and interossei (when MPJ is extended by extensor digitorum)

Extension—extensor digitorum (when MPJ is flexed by lumbricals and interossei)

Summary of Muscle Innervations of Upper Limb (*indicates exception or dual innervation)

Muscles of Anterior Compartment of Arm: Musculocutaneous Nerve

1. Biceps brachii
2. Coracobrachialis
3. Brachialis (musculocutaneous nerve and radial nerve)

Muscles of Posterior Compartment of Arm: Radial Nerve

1. Triceps
2. Anconeus

Muscles of Anterior Compartment of Forearm: Median Nerve

1. Superficial layer:
   a. Pronator teres
   b. Flexor carpi radialis
   c. Palmaris longus
   *d. Flexor carpi ulnaris (ulnar nerve)
2. Middle layer:
   a. Flexor digitorum superficialis
3. Deep layer:
   *a. Flexor digitorum profundus (median nerve and ulnar nerve)
   b. Flexor pollicis longus
   c. Pronator quadratus

Muscles of Posterior Compartment of Forearm: Radial Nerve

1. Superficial layer:
   a. Brachioradialis
   b. Extensor carpi radialis longus
   c. Extensor carpi radialis brevis
   d. Extensor carpi ulnaris
   e. Extensor digitorum communis
   f. Extensor digiti minimi
2. Deep layer:
   a. Abductor pollicis longus
   b. Extensor pollicis longus

    c. Extensor pollicis brevis
    d. Extensor indicis

Thenar Muscles: Median Nerve

1. Abductor pollicis brevis
2. Opponens pollicis
*3. Flexor pollicis brevis (median and ulnar nerves)

Adductor Pollicis: Ulnar Nerve

Hypothenar Muscles: Ulnar Nerve

1. Abductor digiti minimi
2. Opponens digiti minimi
3. Flexor digiti minimi

Lumbricals (Medial Two) and Interossei Muscles: Ulnar Nerve
Lumbricals (Lateral Two): Median Nerve

Axillary artery is divided by pectoralis minor muscle
Axillary vein begins at the lower border of Teres major
CSF is secreted and reabsorbed by the epithelial cells of the
Choroid plexus. These cells actively pump sodium into the CSF
water and chloride passively follow. the active sodium transport.
potassium is not actively transported into the CSF and intact
is reabsorbed to some extent by the choroid plexuses.

Review Test

UPPER LIMB

DIRECTIONS: For each of the questions or incomplete statements below, *one* or *more* of the answers or completions given is correct. Choose answer:

  A. if only **1, 2,** and **3** are correct
  B. if only **1** and **3** are correct
  C. if **2** and **4** are correct
  D. if only **4** is correct
  E. if all are correct

2.1. The lymphatic drainage of the breast
1. may constitute a pathway for spread of malignant tumors to axillary nodes.
2. includes rich drainage from cutaneous as well as glandular regions.
3. has pathways to the venous system.
4. includes collecting vessels that follow the perforating blood vessels through the pectoralis major muscle.

2.2. The pectoralis minor muscle
1. divides the axillary nerve into three parts.
2. is innervated by the medial pectoral nerve and acts to depress the shoulder.
3. originates from the coracoid process.
4. is attached to the ribs.

2.3. The intercostobrachial cutaneous nerve
1. is a lateral cutaneous branch of the second intercostal nerve which passes into the arm.
2. may communicate with the medial brachial cutaneous nerve.
3. pierces the intercostal and serratus anterior muscles.
4. is a branch of the medial cord of the brachial plexus.

2.4. The medial pectoral nerve
1. contains somatic motor fibers.
2. contains axons whose cell bodies are in the sympathetic ganglion.
3. supplies the pectoralis major muscle.
4. is not connected with the lateral pectoral nerve.

2.5. Nerves that originate from the posterior cord of the brachial plexus supply the following muscles:
1. subscapularis.
2. teres major.
3. latissimus dorsi.
4. teres minor.

2.6. Neuron cell bodies of nerve fibers in the medial brachial cutaneous nerve are located in
1. dorsal root ganglia.
2. anterior horn of the gray matter of the spinal cord.
3. sympathetic chain ganglia.
4. lateral horn of the gray matter of the spinal cord.

2.7. The musculocutaneous nerve
1. contains postganglionic sympathetic axons.
2. contains afferent axons.
3. does not contain preganglionic parasympathetic axons.
4. contains somatic efferent axons.

DIRECTIONS: Each of the questions or incomplete statements below is followed by suggested answers or completions. Select the *one best* in each case.

2.8. The brachial plexus

A. contains nerve fibers originating from ventral roots only and not from dorsal roots.
B. contains nerve fibers originating from ventral rami only and not from dorsal rami.
C. Each root of the brachial plexus is formed by fibers originating from more than one ventral ramus.
D. Each trunk of the brachial plexus is formed by fibers originating from more than one ventral ramus.
E. All trunks of the brachial plexus give off branches to innervate muscles.

2.9. Of the following arteries, which one would be *least* likely to be involved in the vascular anastomosis around the shoulder joint and scapula?

A. dorsal scapular.
B. thoracoacromial.
C. subscapular.
D. posterior circumflex humeral.
E. superior ulnar collateral.

2.10. Select the **incorrect** statement.

A. Part of the axillary artery lies posterior to the tendon of the pectoralis minor muscle.
B. The roots of the brachial plexus pass (lie) anterior to the middle scalene muscles.
C. Normally, for most of its course, in the axilla, the axillary vein will be found lying lateral and posterior to the axillary artery and the posterior cord of the brachial plexus.
D. The axillary sheath is a fascial extension of the prevertebral layer of cervical fascia and encloses the great vessels and nerves of the limb, which are closely grouped together.
E. Some of the roots of the brachial plexus give off nerves to the muscle that forms the medial wall of the axilla.

2.11. Select the **incorrect** statement.

A. The mammary gland is composed of from 15–20 lobes.
B. The mammary gland is invested by deep fascia and connected to the skin by strong connective tissue strands called suspensory ligaments.
C. Branches of the internal thoracic artery help to supply the mammary gland with arterial blood.
D. Each lobe of the mammary gland has a single lactiferous duct that opens onto the nipple.
E. The anterior branches of the lateral cutaneous branches of intercostal nerves (two to six) provide sensory fibers to the skin of the breast and autonomic fibers to the smooth muscles and blood vessels.

2.12. Select the **incorrect** statement.

A. Normally, the areolar area of the female breast has no adipose tissue immediately deep to it (in contact with its deep surface).
B. The clavipectoral fascia, costocoracoid membrane, and suspensory ligament of the axilla all represent different aspects of the same fascial layer.
C. The pectoralis major, pectoralis minor, and subclavius muscles either originate or insert on some part of the humerus.
D. The lateral lip of the intertubercular (bicipital) groove serves as a point of insertion for the pectoralis major muscle.

2.13. Which one would not be a branch of the thoracoacromial artery?

A. acromial.
B. pectoral.
C. clavicular.
D. deltoid.
E. superior thoracic.

2.14. In the defect known as winged scapula, which one of the following structures has probably been damaged?

A. roots of the eighth cervical and first thoracic spinal nerves.
B. thoracodorsal nerve.
C. subscapularis muscle.
D. serratus anterior muscle.
E. serratus posterior superior muscle.

2.15. The median nerve is formed by parts of the

A. lateral and posterior cords.
B. posterior divisions of the upper and middle trunks.
C. medial and lateral cords.
D. posterior divisions of the middle and lower trunks.
E. medial and posterior cords.

2.16. Select the correct statement. Which trunk of the brachial plexus has direct branches?

A. all three trunks.
B. only the upper trunk.
C. only the middle trunk.
D. only the lower trunk.
E. only the upper and middle trunks.

DIRECTIONS: For each of the questions or incomplete statements below, *one* or *more* of the answers or completions given is correct. Choose answer:

A. if only **1, 2,** and **3** are correct
B. if only **1** and **3** are correct
C. if only **2** and **4** are correct
D. if only **4** is correct
E. if all are correct

2.17. Find correct statement(s) concerning the intrinsic muscles of the hand.

1. The adductor pollicis is innervated by the median nerve.
2. The thenar muscles are innervated by the median nerve derived from the posterior cords of the brachial plexus.
3. The lumbrical muscles arise from the tendons of the flexor digitorum superficialis.
4. The dorsal interosseous muscles aid in flexion of the metacarpophalangeal joints and extension of the interphalangeal joints.

2.18. Which of the following muscles form(s) the floor of the cubital fossa?

1. brachioradialis.
2. brachialis.
3. pronator teres.
4. supinator.

A patient with a fracture of the clavicle at the junction of the inner and middle third of the bone exhibits overriding of the medial and lateral fragments. Answer questions 19–22.

2.19. The lateral portion of the fractured clavicle is displaced downward by the

1. deltoid muscle.
2. gravity of the arm.
3. pectoralis major muscle (clavicular portion).
4. trapezius muscle.

2.20. Which of the following muscles is responsible for the medial fragment being angulated upward?

1. pectoralis major.
2. deltoid muscle.
3. trapezius muscle.
4. sternocleidomastoid muscle.

2.21. If the arm is medially rotated, which of the following muscles are responsible for this action?

1. pectoralis major.
2. subscapularis.
3. teres major.
4. latissimus dorsi.

2.22. The fractured clavicle

1. may cause a fatal hemorrhage from the subclavian vein.
2. may be responsible for thrombosis of the subclavian vein, causing a pulmonary embolism.
3. may be responsible for thrombosis of the subclavian artery, causing an embolism to the brachial artery.
4. may damage the lower trunk of the brachial plexus.

2.23. The radial nerve is severely damaged as a result of fracture of the **lower third** of the humerus. Which of the following would result?

1. wrist extension is lost, leading to a "wristdrop."
2. weakness in pronating the forearm.
3. sensory loss over the dorsal aspect of the base of the thumb.
4. an inability to oppose the thumb.

2.24. Which of the following muscles is responsible for the flexion of the proximal interphalangeal joints?

1. palmar interossei.
2. flexor digitorum profundus.
3. extensor indicis.
4. flexor digitorum superficialis.

2.25. If the flexion of the distal interphalangeal joint of the index finger is paralyzed (impaired), one would also expect

1. similar paralysis of the third digit.
2. atrophy of the thenar eminence.
3. loss of sensation over the distal part of the second digit.
4. complete paralysis of the thumb.

2.26. Which of the following nerves supplies the muscle that is responsible for movement of the metacarpophalangeal joint of the ring finger?

1. median.
2. radial.
3. musculocutaneous.
4. ulnar.

2.27. Name the muscles that are capable of adduction of the arm.

1. pectoralis major.
2. supraspinatus.
3. latissimus dorsi.
4. infraspinatus.

2.28. Which of the following nerves supply the abductors of the arm?

1. suprascapular.
2. musculocutaneous.
3. axillary.
4. radial.

2.29. Retraction or adduction of the scapula is accomplished by the

1. latissimus dorsi.
2. trapezius.
3. serratus anterior.
4. rhomboids.

2.30. Select the correct statement(s).

1. All intrinsic muscles of the thumb but the opponens pollicis insert into the base of the proximal phalanx.
2. Both heads of the biceps brachii and two heads of the triceps move the shoulder joint.
3. The little finger does not have a named adductor.
4. The flexor digitorum profundus tendon attaches to the middle phalanx and the flexor pollicis longus to the terminal phalanx of the thumb.

DIRECTIONS: Each set of lettered headings below is followed by a list of numbered words or phrases. Choose answer:

    A. if the item is associated with **A** only.
    B. if the item is associated with **B** only.
    C. if the item is associated with both **A** and **B**.
    D. if the item is associated with neither **A** nor **B**.

    A. Pronation
    B. Supination
    C. Both
    D. Neither

2.31. The wrist joint is actively involved in this movement.

2.32. An important muscle involved in this movement would be paralyzed by severance of a nerve lying in the spiral groove in the humerus.

2.33. The proximal radioulnar and distal radioulnar joints participate in this movement.

2.34. The brachialis muscle strongly participates in this movement.

2.35. This movement would be virtually abolished by severance of the ulnar nerve as it crosses the posterior surface of the medial epicondyle of the humerus.

    A. Extensor digitorum communis
    B. Interossei
    C. Both
    D. Neither

2.36. Functions to extend the interphalangeal joints when the metacarpophalangeal joints are extended.

2.37. Functions to extend the interphalangeal joints when the metacarpophalangeal joints are flexed.

2.38. Motor innervation is derived from a branch of the posterior cord of the brachial plexus.

2.39. The median nerve innervates half of these muscles.

2.40. They arise from the flexor digitorum profundus tendons.

    A. Metacarpophalangeal joints
    B. Interphalangeal joints
    C. Both
    D. Neither

2.41. Flexion at these joints is produced by the flexor digitorum superficialis and profundus muscles.

2.42. The interossei and lumbricals act at these joints to produce flexion.

2.43. Muscles capable of extending these joints are the long extensor muscles of the fingers.

2.44. Extension at these joints may be produced either by the lumbricals and interossei muscles or the long extensor muscles of the fingers.

2.45. The movements of adduction and abduction of the fingers occur at these joints.

    A. Radius
    B. Ulnar
    C. Both
    D. Neither

2.46. rotates during supination and pronation.

2.47. does not articulate with carpal bones.

2.48. receives the attachment of the biceps brachii muscle.

2.49. has styloid process that normally projects more distally than the styloid process of the ulna.

2.50 provides attachment for the pronator quadratus muscles.

DIRECTIONS: Each of the questions or incomplete statements below is followed by suggested answers or completions. Select the *one* that is *best* in each case.

2.51. Abduction of the arm is carried out by muscles that are innervated by the
A. axillary and thoracodorsal nerves.
B. suprascapular and axillary nerves.
C. musculocutaneous and median nerves.
D. axillary nerve only.
E. radial nerve only.

2.52. Which of the following muscles do(es) not attach to the middle digit, that is, to the second finger?
A. flexor digitorum profundus.
B. extensor digitorum communis.
C. palmar interossei.
D. dorsal interossei.
E. lumbricals.

2.53. The important contents of the proximal portion of the cubital fossa lie in this order from medial to lateral
A. biceps, median nerve, brachial artery.
B. median nerve, biceps, brachial artery.
C. brachial artery, median nerve, biceps.
D. brachial artery, biceps, median nerve.
E. median nerve, brachial artery, biceps.

2.54. Select the correct statement:
A. All three heads of the triceps and the two heads of the biceps move the shoulder joint.
B. Both heads of the biceps and two heads of the triceps move the shoulder joint.
C. Both heads of the biceps and one head of the triceps move the shoulder joint.
D. Only one head of the biceps and one head of the triceps move the shoulder joint.
E. Only one head of the biceps and two heads of the triceps move the shoulder joint.

2.55. The extensor expansion or hood on the middle digit is related to
A. extensor digitorum communis, one lumbrical, one dorsal interosseous, and one palmar interosseous muscle.
B. extensor digitorum communis, two lumbricals, and two dorsal interossei muscles.
C. extensor digitorum communis, one lumbrical, and two dorsal interossei muscles.
D. extensor indicis, one lumbrical, and two dorsal interossei muscles.
E. None of the above that is a proper combination of muscles.

2.56. The axillary nerve
A. arises from the lateral cord of the brachial plexus.
B. lies adjacent to medial and posterior surface of the anatomical neck of the humerus.
C. supplies the deltoid and the teres major.
D. may be damaged by inferior dislocation of the head of the humerus.
E. accompanies the scapular circumflex artery.

2.57. The radial artery
A. passes through the carpal tunnel.
B. accompanies the posterior interosseous nerve in the forearm.
C. is principal source of blood to the superficial palmar arch.
D. The princeps pollicis artery is a branch of this artery.
E. passes distally between flexor digitorum superficialis and flexor digitorum profundus.

2.58. Which nerve group (below) is intimately related to some portion of the humerus and may be affected by fractures of the humerus? (To be injured in a fracture the nerve must lie close to, or be in contact with, the bone.)
A. axillary, musculocutaneous, and radial.
B. axillary, median, and ulnar.
C. axillary, radial, and ulnar.
D. axillary, median, and musculocutaneous.
E. median, radial, and ulnar.

2.59. Severance of the ulnar nerve at the wrist results in:
A. hyperextension at the metacarpophalangeal joints.
B. inability to abduct and adduct the fingers.
C. anesthesia over palmar surface of fifth finger.
D. all of the above.
E. Only B and C are correct.

2.60. The ulnar bursa, or common flexor sheath, contains

A. the tendons of the flexor digitorum superficialis only.
B. the tendons of the flexor digitorum profundus only.
C. the tendons of the flexor digitorum superficialis and profundus only.
D. the tendons of the flexor pollicis longus only.
E. the tendons of the flexor digitorum superficialis, flexor digitorum profundus, flexor pollicis longus, and flexor carpi radialis.

2.61. Which of the following muscles are not supplied by the median nerve?

A. flexor digitorum superficialis.
B. opponens pollicis.
C. two medial lumbricals.
D. pronator teres.
E. palmaris longus.

2.62. Muscles innervated by the ulnar nerve include:

A. all interossei.
B. abductor pollicis brevis.
C. all lumbricals.
D. pronator quadratus.
E. flexor digitorum superficialis.

2.63. Inflammation of the synovial sheath of the common flexor tendons causes damage to the nerve passing through the carpal tunnel, leading to the clinical syndrome called carpal tunnel syndrome. In this condition, all of the following are true except

A. The dorsal and palmar interosseous muscles are normal.
B. The flexor digitorum superficialis and profundus muscles are not normal.
C. There is flattening of the outer half of the thenar eminence.
D. There is diminished sensitivity in the medial one and one-half fingers.
E. The adductor pollicis muscle is not atrophied.

2.64. Select the correct statement.

A. Both ulnar and median nerves lie deep to the flexor retinaculum.
B. Both ulnar and median nerves lie superficial to the flexor retinaculum.
C. The ulnar nerve runs deep and the median nerve runs superficial to the flexor retinaculum.
D. The ulnar nerve runs superficial and the median nerve runs deep to the flexor retinaculum.
E. The ulnar nerve runs superficial and the ulnar artery runs deep to the flexor retinaculum.

2.65. Which one of the intrinsic muscles of the thumb attaches to the first metacarpal?

A. abductor pollicis brevis.
B. adductor pollicis.
C. opponens pollicis.
D. flexor pollicis brevis (superficial head).
E. flexor pollicis brevis (deep head).

DIRECTIONS: For each numbered item, select the *one* lettered heading that is most closely associated with it. Each lettered heading may be selected once, more than once, or not at all.

A. Axillary nerve
B. Radial nerve
C. Median Nerve
D. Musculocutaneous nerve
E. Ulnar nerve

2.66. It passes through the quadrangular space of the shoulder.

2.67. It innervates a muscle that draws the thumb back into the plane of the palm and originates on the third metacarpal.

2.68. It usually passes between the two heads of the pronator teres and innervates the flexor of the distal phalanx of the thumb.

2.69. It innervates muscles that function to abduct or adduct the fingers.

2.70. It is usually accompanied by the profunda brachii artery in part of its course.

A. Scapula
B. Clavicle
C. Humerus
D. Radius
E. Ulna

2.71. It has a rough area on the anterior surface of the coronoid process into which the brachialis muscle inserts.

2.72. It has its head at the distal end.

2.73. It has its head at the proximal end.

2.74. It provides an origin of the long head of the biceps brachii muscle.

2.75. It has a trochlea whose medial margin projects more than its lateral, so that its long axis is set obliquely to that of the shaft.

A. Teres minor
B. Latissimus dorsi
C. Biceps brachii
D. supraspinatus
E. Brachioradialis

2.76. It can supinate the forearm and originates from the scapula.

2.77 It helps to stabilize the glenohumeral joint and is innervated by the axillary nerve.

2.78. It receives its nerve supply from the posterior cord of the brachial plexus and forms a part of the posterior axillary fold.

2.79. It can flex the forearm and is innervated by the radial nerve.

2.80. It participates in the formation of the rotator cuff, attaches on the greater tuberosity of the humerus, and abducts the arm.

A. Palmar metacarpal artery
B. Anterior interosseous artery
C. Posterior interosseous artery
D. Radial artery
E. Ulnar artery

2.81. It gives off the princeps pollicis artery.

2.82. It lies superficial to the flexor retinaculum.

2.83. It is the most superficial structure that seen in the anatomical snuff-box.

2.84. It gives off an interosseous recurrent artery.

2.85. It descends between the flexor digitorum superficialis and profundus.

Answers and Explanations

UPPER LIMB

2.1. E. The lymphatic drainage in the lateral quadrants of the breast goes mostly to the axillary nodes, particularly the pectoral nodes. The lymphatic vessels in the medial quadrants follow the perforating vessels through the pectoralis major to enter the parasternal nodes. The remainder goes to the apical nodes as well as nodes of the opposite breast and of the anterior abdominal wall.

2.2. C. The pectoralis minor divides the axillary artery into three parts. It originates from the second to the fifth ribs and inserts on the coracoid process.

2.3. A. The intercostobrachial cutaneous nerve arises from the lateral cutaneous branch of the second intercostal nerve. It may communicate with the medial brachial cutaneous nerve, which is a branch of the medial cord of the brachial plexus.

2.4. A. The medial pectoral nerve forms a loop in front of the axillary artery with the lateral pectoral nerve. It contains somatic motor fibers that supply the pectoralis major muscle and postganglionic sympathetic fibers, with cell bodies in the sympathetic chain ganglia, which supply the blood vessels.

2.5. E. The subscapularis muscle is innervated by the upper and lower subscapular nerves; the teres major by the lower subscapular nerve; the latissimus dorsi by the thoracodorsal nerve; the teres major by the lower subscapular nerve; the teres minor by the axillary nerve. All of these nerves are originated from the posterior cord of the brachial plexus.

2.6. B. The medial brachial cutaneous nerve contains sensory fibers whose cell bodies are located in the dorsal root ganglia. It also contains postganglionic sympathetic fibers whose cell bodies are located in the sympathetic chain ganglia. The anterior horn contains neuron cell bodies of skeletal motor fibers, whereas the lateral horn contains those of preganglionic sympathetic fibers.

2.7. E. The musculocutaneous nerve contains (*a*) postganglionic sympathetic axons supplying blood vessels, hair follicles, and sweat glands; (*b*) afferent axons to innervate cutaneous tissues; and (*c*) somatic efferent fibers to innervate skeletal muscles.

2.8. B. The brachial plexus is formed by the ventral rami of the lower four cervical and first thoracic nerves. The spinal nerves are formed by the union of the dorsal and ventral roots. The root of the brachial plexus is the same as the ventral primary ramus of the spinal nerve. The only upper trunk of the brachial plexus sends branches to innervate muscles such as the suprascapular nerve and the nerve to the subclavius.

2.9. E. The superior ulnar collateral artery enters the anastomosis around the elbow joint.

2.10. C. The axillary vein ascends through the axilla, along the medial side of the axillary artery.

2.11. B. The mammary gland lies in the superficial fascia.

2.12. C. The pectoralis minor originates from the second to the fifth ribs and inserts on the coracoid process of the scapula. The subclavius muscle arises from the first rib and its costal cartilage and inserts on the clavicle.

73

2.13. E. The thoracoacromial artery has only four branches: pectoral, clavicular, acromial, and clavicular.

2.14. D. The winged scapula is caused by the paralysis of the serratus anterior muscle due to the damage of the long thoracic nerve that arises from the root of the brachial plexus (C5,6,7).

2.15. C. The medial and lateral heads of the median nerve arise from the medial and lateral cords, respectively.

2.16. B. The middle and lower trunks of the brachial plexus have no branches.

2.17. D. The adductor pollicis is innervated by the ulnar nerve. The median nerve is formed by the union of the lateral and medial heads from the lateral and medial cords, respectively. The lumbrical muscles arise from the tendons of the flexor digitorum profundus.

2.18. A. The floor of the cubital fossa is formed by the brachialis and supinator muscles. The brachioradialis and pronator teres muscles form the lateral and medial boundaries of the fossa, respectively.

2.19. A. The lateral fragment of the clavicle is displaced downward by the pull of the deltoid and pectoralis major muscle.

2.20. D. The sternocleidomastoid muscle is attached to the superior border of the medial third of the clavicle.

2.21. E. The pectoralis major, subscapularis, teres major, and latissimus dorsi muscles can rotate the arm medially.

2.22. E. The fractured clavicle may damage the subclavian vein, leading to a pulmonary embolism; cause the thrombosis of the subclavian artery, leading to emoblism of the brachial artery; and cause damage to the lower trunk of the brachial plexus.

2.23. B. The pronator teres, pronator quadratus, and oponens pollicis muscles are innervated by the median nerve.

2.24. D. The flexor digitorum profundus muscle flexes the distal interphalangeal joints, whereas the flexor digitorum superficialis flexes the proximal interphalangeal joints. The palmar interosseous muscles flex the metacarpophalangeal joint and adduct the fingers.

2.25. A. The flexion of the distal interphalangeal joints of the index and middle fingers is accomplished by the flexor digitorum profundus muscle, which is innervated by the median nerve. This nerve also innervates the skin over the distal part of the second digit and the thenar muscles, but the adductor pollicis and the deep head of the flexor pollicis brevis are innervated by the ulnar nerve.

2.26. C. The metacarpophalangeal joint of the ring finger is flexed by the interossei and lumbricals, which are innervated by the ulnar nerve, and extended by the extensor digitorum, which is innervated by the radial nerve.

2.27. B. The supraspinatus muscle abducts the arm, whereas the infraspinatus rotates the arm laterally.

2.28. B. The abductors of the arm are the deltoid and supraspinatus muscles, which are innervated by the axillary and suprascapular nerves, respectively.

2.29. C. The latissimus dorsi muscle is a strong adductor and extensor of the arm, whereas the serratus anterior muscle abducts and upwardly rotates the scapula.

2.30. B. The short head of the biceps brachii arises from the coracoid process of the scapula, and the long head of the triceps brachii arises from the infraglenoid tubercle of the scapula. The flexor digitorum profundus tendon attaches to the distal phalanx of the fingers and the flexor pollicis longus to the distal phalanx of the thumb.

2.31. D. Both pronation and supination occur at the proximal and distal radioulnar joints.

2.32. B. The radial nerve lying in the spiral groove of the humerus is severed, resulting in a paraylsis of the supinator muscle.

2.33. C. Both the proximal and distal radioulnar joints participate in pronation and supination.

2.34. D. The brachialis muscle flexes the forearm at the elbow joint.

2.35. D. The pronator teres and quadratus muscles are innervated by the median nerve. The supinator is innervated by the radial nerve and the biceps brachii (which can supinate) is innervated by the musculocutaneous nerve.

2.36. B. The interphalangeal joints are extended by the interossei and the lumbricals when the metacarpophalangeal joints are extended by the extensor digitorum communis.

2.37. A. The interphalangeal joints are extended by the extensor digitorum communis when the metacarpophalangeal joints are flexed by the lumbricals and the interossei.

2.38. A. The extensor digitorum communis is innervated by the radial nerve, which is derived from the posterior cord of the brachial plexus. However, the palmar and dorsal interossei are innervated by the ulnar nerve, which is derived from the medial cord of the brachial plexus.

2.39. D. The median nerve innervates the lateral one-half of the flexor digitorum profundus and lateral two lumbricals.

2.40. D. The lumbricals arise from the flexor digitorum profundus tendon.

2.41. B. The flexor digitorum superficialis flexes the proximal interphalangeal joints, whereas the flexor digitorum profundus flexes the distal interphalangeal joints.

2.42. A. The interossei and the lumbricals flex the metacarpophalangeal joints.

2.43. C. The extensor digitorum communis can extend to the metacarpophalangeal and interphalangeal joints.

2.44. B. The interossei and the lumbricals extend the interphalangeal joints when the metacarpophalangeal joints are extended by the extensor digitorum communis.

2.45. A. The palmar and dorsal interossei adduct and abduct the fingers at the metacarpophalangeal joints, respectively.

2.46. A. The radius rotates during supination and pronation.

Supinator — Bicep Bradi - Supinator

2.47. B. The radius but not the ulna articulates with carpal bones.

2.48. A. The biceps brachii muscle inserts on the tuberosity of the radius.

2.49. A. The radius has a styloid process that normally projects more distally than that of the ulna.

2.50. C. The pronator quadratus muscle arises from the anterior surface of the lower fourth of the ulna and inserts on the anterior surface of the lower fourth of the radius.

2.51. B. The abductors of the arm are the deltoid and supraspinatus muscles, which are innervated by the axillary and suprascapular nerves, respectively.   ABDSv

2.52. C. The palmar interossei are adductors of the fingers, and thus they have no attachment on the middle finger.

2.53. E. The contents of the cubital fossa from medial to lateral side are the median nerve, the brachial artery, the biceps tendon, and the radial nerve.

supraglenoid

2.54. C. Both heads of the biceps brachii and the long head of the triceps brachii are attached to the scapula.

2.55. C. The dorsal interossei abduct the fingers, whereas the palmar interossei adduct the fingers. Thus, the middle finger has an abductor on each side but no adductors.

2.56. D. The axillary nerve arises from the posterior cord of the brachial plexus, passes around the surgical neck of the humerus in company with the posterior humeral circumflex artery, and supplies the deltoid and teres minor muscles. Due to its close association with the surgical neck of the humerus, it may be damaged by inferior dislocation of the head of the humerus.

2.57. D. The radial artery runs distally beneath the brachioradialis, with the superficial radial nerve, passes through the anatomical snuff-box, enters the palm by passing between the two heads of the first dorsal interosseous muscle, and divides into the princeps pollicis artery and the deep palmar arch.

2.58. C. The axillary nerve passes posteriorly around the surgical neck of the humerus; the radial nerve lies in the radial groove of the middle of the shaft of the humerus; and the ulnar nerve passes behind the medial condyle.

2.59. E. The fingers are adducted by the palmar interossei and abducted by the dorsal interossei. These muscles are innervated by the ulnar nerve. This nerve also supplies skin over the palmar surface of the medial one and one-half fingers.

2.60. C. The ulnar bursa, or common flexor sheath, contains both the tendons of the flexor digitorum superficialis and profundus muscles, whereas the radial bursa envelops the tendon of the flexor pollicis longus.

2.61. C. The two medial lumbricals are innervated by the ulnar nerve, whereas the two lateral lumbricals are innervated by the median nerve.

2.62. A. All interossei (palmar and dorsal) and the two medial lumbricals are innervated by the ulnar nerve.

2.63. D. The carpal tunnel syndrome results from injury of the median nerve. The diminished sensitivity in the medial one and one-half fingers is caused by damage to the ulnar nerve.

2.64. D. The ulnar artery and the ulnar nerve pass superficial to the flexor retinaculum, whereas the median nerve passes deep to the retinaculum.

2.65. C. The opponens pollicis inserts on the first metacarpal, whereas all other short thumb muscles insert on the proximal phalanges.

2.66. A. The axillary nerve and the posterior humeral circumflex artery pass through the quadrangular space.

2.67. E. The abductor pollicis arises from the second and third metacarpals, inserts on the proximal phalanx, draws the thumb back into the plane of the palm (adduction of the thumb), and is innervated by the ulnar nerve.

2.68. C. The median nerve usually passes between the two heads of the pronator teres and innervates the flexor pollicis longus muscle.

2.69. E. The ulnar nerve supplies the dorsal interossei (abductors) and the palmar interossei (adductors).

2.70. B. The radial nerve turns around in the spiral groove on the back of the humerus with the profunda brachii artery.

2.71. E. The brachialis muscle inserts on a rough area on the anterior surface of the coronoid process and tuberosity of the ulna.

2.72. E. The ulna has its head at the distal end.

2.73. D. The radius has its head at the proximal end.

2.74. D. The long head of the biceps brachii originates from the supraglenoid tubercle of the scapula.

2.75. C. The humerus has a trochlea whose medial edge projects more inferiorly than its lateral edge, and thus the long axis of the humerus is set obliquely to the long axis of the ulna, forming an angulation, called a "carrying angle."

2.76. C. The long head of the biceps brachii muscle originates from the supraglenoid tubercle, whereas its short head arises from the coracoid process of the scapula. This muscle supinates the forearm.

2.77. A. The teres minor muscle forms part of the rotator cuff, which helps to stabilize the glenohumeral joint. This muscle is innervated by the axillary nerve.

2.78. B. The latissimus dorsi muscle forms part of the posterior axillary fold and is innervated by the thoracodorsal nerve, which arises from the posterior cord of the brachial plexus.

2.79. E. The brachioradialis flexes the forearm and is innervated by the radial nerve.

2.80. D. The supraspinatus arises from the supraspinous fossa and inserts on the superior facet of the greater tubercle of the humerus. This muscle is innervated by the suprascapular nerve and abducts the arm.

2.81. D. The radial artery divides into the princeps pollicis artery and the deep palmar arch.

2.82. E. The ulnar artery enters the hand superficial to the flexor retinaculum, lateral to the pisiform, where it divides into the superficial and deep branches.

2.83. D. The radial artery runs through the anatomical snuff-box and then enters the palm by passing between the two heads of the first dorsal interosseous muscle.

2.84. C. The posterior interosseous artery gives off an interosseous recurrent artery that anastomoses with a branch of the profunda brachii artery.

2.85. E. The ulnar artery descends between the flexor digitorum superficialis and profundus.

Development of Limbs

The limb Buds appear during the 4th week of development but the upper limb buds developing first. Lower limb structures rotate 90degrees Medially where as upper limb structure rotate 90 laterally. The Cranial Caudal and proximal and distal growth gradients. upper limb developing earlier than th lower and the girdle region developing before the digital region of each limb.

3
Lower Limb

Cutaneous Nerves, Superficial Veins, and Lymphatics

I. Cutaneous Nerves

A. Lateral Femoral Cutaneous Nerve

—arises from the lumbar plexus (L2-3), emerges from the lateral border of the psoas major, crosses the iliacus and passes under the lateral end of the inguinal ligament.

—divides into an anterior and a posterior branch and supplies the skin on the anterior and lateral aspects of the thigh as far as the knee.

B. Posterior Femoral Cutaneous Nerve

—arises from the sacral plexus (S1-S3), passes through the greater sciatic foramen below the piriformis, runs deep to the gluteus maximus, and emerges from the inferior border of this muscle.

—descends in the posterior midline of the thigh deep to the fascia lata and pierces the fascia lata near the popliteal fossa.

—supplies the skin of the buttock, the thigh and the calf.

C. Saphenous Nerve

—arises from the femoral nerve in the femoral triangle, descends with the femoral vessels through the femoral triangle and the adductor canal.

—descends in the leg in company with the greater saphenous vein and supplies the skin on the medial side of the leg and foot.

D. Lateral Sural Cutaneous Nerve

—arises from the common peroneal nerve in the popliteal fossa and supplies the skin on the posterolateral side of the leg.

—may have a communicating branch to join the medial sural cutaneous nerve.

E. Medial Sural Cutaneous Nerve

—arises from the tibial nerve in the popliteal fossa.

—may join the lateral sural nerve or its communicating branch to form the sural nerve.

—supplies the medial side of the heel and foot.

F. Sural Nerve

–is formed by the union of the medial sural and the lateral sural nerve (or the communicating branch of the lateral sural nerve).

–supplies the lateral side of the foot.

II. Superficial Veins

A. Great Saphenous Vein

–begins at the medial end of the dorsal venous arch of the foot.

–ascends in front of the medial maleolus and along the medial surface of the tibia and the femur.

–passes through the saphenous opening (fossa ovalis) in the deep fascia of the thigh to enter the femoral vein.

–passes through the fascia lata and pierces the femoral sheath to join the femoral vein.

–is accompanied by the saphenous nerve.

B. Small (or Short) Saphenous Vein

–begins at the lateral end of the dorsal venous arch.

–passes upward along the lateral side of the foot with the sural nerve, behind the lateral malleolus.

–passes to the popliteal fossa, where it perforates the deep fascia and terminates in the popliteal vein.

–is connected with the inferior gluteal vein by a communicating branch.

III. Lymphatics

A. Inguinal Group of Lymph Nodes

–drains the superficial thigh region directly.

–drains the lower limb indirectly via deep lymphatic channels from the popliteal nodes.

–drains the anterolateral abdominal wall below the umbilicus; the gluteal region; part of the uterus; the anus; and the external genitalia except the glans.

–consists of a superficial group (located subcutaneously near the saphenofemoral junction) and a deep group (medial to the femoral vein).

Bones

I. Coxal or Hip Bone

–consists of the ilium, ischium, and pubic bones.

–articulates with the sacrum to form the pelvic girdle.

A. Ilium

–forms the upper part of the acetabulum and the lateral part of the hip bone.

–presents the anterior superior iliac spine, the anterior inferior iliac spine, the posterior iliac spines, the greater sciatic notch, the iliac fossa, the gluteal lines, etc.

B. Pubis

–forms the anterior part of the acetabulum and the anteromedial part of the hip bone.

–presents the body, the superior and inferior rami, the obturator foramen, the pubic crest and tubercle, the pectineal line (or pecten pubis).

C. Ischium

–forms the posteroinferior part of the acetabulum and the lower posterior part of the hip bone.

–presents the body, the ischial spine, the ischial tuberosity, the lesser sciatic notch, the ramus, etc.

D. Acetabulum

–is a cup-shaped cavity on the external surface of the hip bone, in which the head of the femur fits.

–has a defect below at the acetabular notch.

–is formed by the ilium, the ischium, and the pubis.

II. Femur

A. Head

–forms about two-thirds of a sphere and is directed medially, upward and slightly forward to fit into the acetabulum.

–its articular surface has a depression, the fovea capitis femoris, to which the ligamentum capitis femoris is attached.

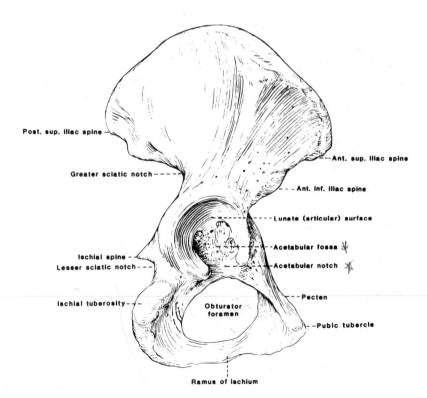

Figure 3.1. Lateral view of the hip bone.

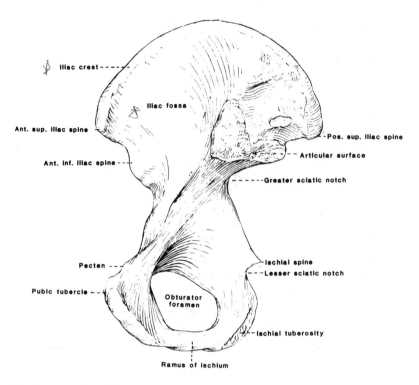

Figure 3.2. Medial view of the hip bone.

B. Neck
    –connects the head to the body (shaft) and forms an angle of about 125°.
    –is separated in front from the shaft by the intertrochanteric line, to which the iliofemoral ligament is attached.

C. Greater Trochanter
    –projects upward from the junction of the neck with the shaft.
    –provides an insertion for the gluteus medius and minimus.
    –the trochanteric fossa on its medial aspect receives the obturator externus tendon.

D. Lesser Trochanter
    –lies in the angle between the neck and the shaft.
    –projects at the inferior end of the intertrochanteric crest.
    –provides an insertion of the iliopsoas tendon.

E. Linea Aspera
    –is the rough line or ridge on the body (shaft).
    –exhibits lateral and medial lips that provide attachments for many muscles and three intermuscular septa.

F. Pectineal Line
    –runs from the lesser trochanter to the medial lip of the linea aspera.
    –provides an insertion of the pectineus muscle.

G. Adductor Tubercle
–is a tubercle at the uppermost part of the medial femoral condyle.
–provides an insertion of the adductor magnus.

III. Patella
–is the largest sesamoid bone.
–is found within a tendon (the quadriceps), like all sesamoid bones.
–articulates with the femur but not with the tibia.
–attaches to the tibial tuberosity by a continuation of the quadriceps tendon, called the patellar ligament.
–functions to increase the angle of pull of the quadriceps femoris, thereby magnifying its power.

IV. Tibia
–is the weight-bearing medial bone of the leg.
–its two condyles articulate with the condyles of the femur.
–has the tibial tuberosity into which the ligamentum patellae inserts.

A. Medial Malleolus
–has the malleolar groove for the tendons of the tibialis posterior and flexor digitorum longus.
–also has another groove (lateral to the malleolus groove) for the tendon of the flexor hallucis longus muscle.

V. Fibula
–has little or no function in weight bearing but serves for muscle attachments.

A. Lateral Malleolus
–its fossa gives attachment for the transverse tibiofibular and posterior talofibular ligaments.
–its anterior border provides attachment for the anterior tibiofibular and anterior talofibular ligaments.
–its posterior border gives attachment for the posterior talofibular ligament and the superior peroneal retinaculum.
–its tip gives attachment for the calcaneofibular ligament.

VI. Tarsus
–consists of seven tarsal bones including talus, calcaneus, cuboid, navicular, and three cuneiforms.

A. Talus
–consists of a body, a neck, and a head.
–transmits the weight of the body from the tibia to other weight-bearing bones of the foot.
–has a deep groove called the sulcus tali for the interosseous ligaments between the talus and the calcaneus.

B. Calcaneus
–is the largest and strongest bone of the foot, which lies below the talus.
–forms the heel and articulates with the talus superiorly and the cuboid anteriorly.

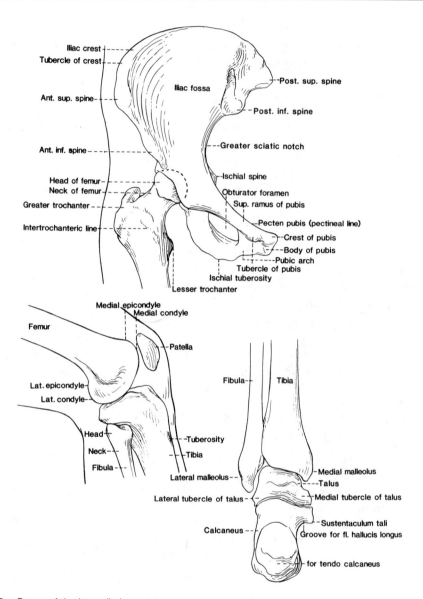

Figure 3.3. Bones of the lower limb.

–the **sustentaculum tali** is a bracket-like lateral projection from the medial surface of the calcaneus and supports the talus. On its inferior surface there is a groove for the flexor hallucis longus.

C. Navicular

–is a boat-shaped tarsal bone, lying between the head of the talus and the three cuneiform bones.

D. Cuboid

–is the most laterally placed tarsal bone.
–has a notch and groove for the tendon of the peroneus longus.

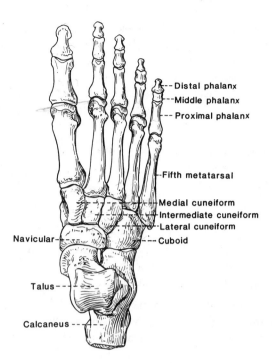

Figure 3.4. Bones of the foot.

E. Cuneiform Bones
–are wedge-shaped bones.
–articulate with the navicular bone posteriorly and with three metatarsals anteriorly.

VII. Metatarsus
–consists of five metatarsals.
–has prominent medial and lateral sesamoid bones on the first metatarsal.

VIII. Phalanges
–are 14 in number; each digit has three except the first, which has two.

Joints

I. Hip Joint
–is a multiaxial ball-and-socket type of synovial joint.
–its cavity is deepened by the acetabular rim and is completed below by the transverse ligament, which closes the acetabular notch.

A. Acetabular Labrum
–is a complete fibrocartilage rim.
–deepens the articular socket for the head of the femur and subsequently stabilizes the hip joint.

B. Fibrous Capsule of Hip Joint
–is attached proximally to the margin of the acetabulum and to the transverse acetabular ligament.

–is attached distally to the neck of the femur as follows: anteriorly to the intertrochanteric line and the root of the greater trochanter and posteriorly to the intertrochanteric crest.

–encloses the head and most of the neck of the femur.

–is reinforced anteriorly by the iliofemoral ligament, posteriorly by the ischiofemoral, and inferiorly by the pubofemoral ligaments.

C. Ligaments

1. Iliofemoral Ligament

–reinforces the fibrous capsule anteriorly and is in the form of an inverted Y.

–is the largest and most important ligament that covers the anterior aspect of the hip joint.

–is attached proximally to the anterior inferior iliac spine and the acetabular rim, and distally to the intertrochanteric line and the front of the greater trochanter of the femur.

–strongly resists hyperextension at the hip joint.

2. Ischiofemoral Ligament

–reinforces the fibrous capsule posteriorly.

–extends from the ischial portion of the acetabular rim to the neck of the femur, medial to the base of the greater trochanter.

3. Pubofemoral Ligament

–reinforces the fibrous capsule inferiorly.

–extends from the pubic portion of the acetabular rim and the superior pubic ramus to the lower part of the femoral neck.

4. Ligamentum Capitis Femoris

–arises from the floor of the acetabular fossa (more specifically, from the margins of the acetabular notch and from the transverse ligament) and attaches to the fovea of the femur.

5. Transverse Acetabular Ligament

–is a fibrous band that bridges the acetabular notch and converts it into a foramen.

D. Blood Supply

–is derived from branches of the medial and lateral femoral circumflex, and superior and inferior gluteal, and obturator arteries.

E. Nerve Supply

–is from branches of the femoral, obturator, and superior gluteal nerves and the nerve to the quadratus femoris.

II. Knee Joint

–is a hinge type of synovial joint permitting flexion, extension, and some rotation.

–is encompassed by a fibrous capsule that is rather thin, weak, and often incomplete.

Knee joint contain Menisci that do not Completely Compartmentalize the joint but most likely serve to assist in the distribution of synovial fluid

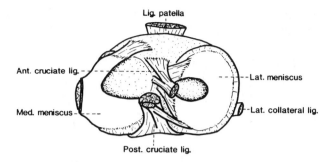

Figure 3.5. Ligaments of the knee joint.

—its capsule is attached to the margins of the femoral condyles and, to the patella and the ligamentum patella, and to the tibia at the margins of the tibial condyles.

—is stabilized on its lateral side by the biceps and gastrocnemius (lateral head) tendons, the iliotibial tract, and the fibular collateral ligaments.

—is stabilized on its medial side by the sartorius, gracilis, gastrocnemius (medial head), semitendinosus, and semimembranosus muscles, and the tibial collateral ligament.

A. Ligaments

1. Anterior Cruciate Ligament

—lies inside the knee joint capsule, but outside the synovial cavity of the joint.

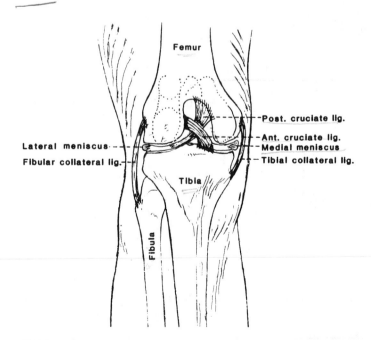

Figure 3.6. Ligaments of the knee joint, anterior view.

—attaches to the anterior intercondylar area of the tibia, hence the "anterior" part of its name.

—passes upward, backward, and laterally to be inserted into the posterior aspect of the medial surface of the lateral femoral condyle.

—prevents backward dislocation of the femur on the tibia.

—limits excessive anterior mobility of the tibia on the femur when the knee is extended.

—is lax when the knee is flexed.

2. Posterior Cruciate Ligament

—lies outside the synovial cavity, but within the fibrous joint capsule.

—attaches to the posterior impression of the intercondylar area.

—passes upward, forward, and medially to be inserted into the anterior part of the lateral surface of the medial femoral condyle.

—prevents forward displacement of the femur on the tibia when the knee is flexed.

—is lax when the knee is extended.

3. Medial Meniscus

—lies outside the synovial cavity, but within the joint capsule.

—is C-shaped (i.e., forms a semicircle).

—is attached to the interarticular area of the tibial or medial collateral ligament.

—is more frequently torn in injuries than the lateral meniscus.

—deepens the concavity of the tibial condyles.

—acts as a cushion or shock absorber.

—facilitates lubrication.

4. Lateral Meniscus

—lies outside the synovial cavity, but within the joint capsule.

—is circular in shape (i.e., it nearly forms a circle) and is incompletely attached to the upper aspect of the tibia.

—is separated laterally from the fibular (or lateral) collateral ligament by the tendon of the popliteus muscle.

—aids in forming a more stable base for the articulation of the femoral condyle.

5. Transverse Ligament

—binds the anterior horns (ends) of the lateral and medial semilunar cartilages (menisci).

6. Tibial Collateral Ligament

—is attached to the medial meniscus, as well as the medial aspects of the articular capsule and the tibial condyle.

—is a broad band, separated from the capsule anteriorly by a bursa.

—prevents medial displacement of the two long bones.

7. Fibular Collateral Ligament

—extends between the lateral femoral epicondyle and the head of the fibula.

—is a rounded cord that stands well away from the capsule of the joint.

B. Bursae

1. Suprapatellar Bursa

–lies deep to the quadriceps femoris.

–is the major bursa communicating with the knee joint cavity. (The semimembranosus bursa may also communicate with it).

2. Prepatellar Bursa

–lies over the superficial surface of the patella.

3. Infrapatellar Bursa

–consists of a subcutaneous infrapatellar bursa, which lies over the patellar ligament, and a deep infrapatellar bursa, which lies deep to the patellar ligament.

C. Blood Supply

–is provided by the genicular branches (superior medial and lateral, inferior medial and lateral, and middle) of the popliteal artery.

–is also provided by a descending branch of the lateral femoral circumflex artery, an articular branch of the descending genicular artery, and the anterior tibial recurrent artery.

D. Nerve Supply

–is from branches of the sciatic, femoral, and obturator nerves.

E. Movement of Knee Joint

–is largely limited to flexion and extension.

–includes rotation of the tibia on the femur and rotation of the femur on the tibia.

–is most free in rotation when the knee is flexed.

1. Full Extension

–is accompanied by medial rotation of the femur on the tibia.

–pulls all ligaments taut.

2. Rotation

–occurs when the knee is flexed.

F. Clinical Notes

1. The Unhappy Triad of the Knee Joint

–is characterized by:

  a. *Rupture of the tibial collateral ligament.*

  b. *Tearing of the anterior cruciate ligament.*

  c. *Injury to the medial meniscus.*

–can occur when a football player is tackled from the side.

–is indicated by a knee that is markedly swollen, particularly in the suprapatellar region.

–results in tenderness upon application of pressure along the extent of the tibial collateral ligament.

–can be treated in the following way: The medial meniscus is removed; the tibial collateral ligament is anchored by sutures through holes drilled in the tibia; and finally, the anterior cruciate ligament is anchored to the site of its original attachment by sutures run through holes drilled in the femur.

2. Knee Jerk (or Patellar Reflex)

—occurs when the ligamentum patellae is tapped, resulting in a sudden contraction of the quadriceps femoris.

3. Housemaid's Knee

—is an inflammation and swelling of the prepatellar bursa.

III. Ankle Joint

—is a synovial joint of the hinge (ginglymus) type between the tibia and fibula above and the trochlea of the talus below.

A. Articular Capsule

—is a thin fibrous capsule that lies anteriorly and posteriorly, allowing movement.
—is reinforced medially by the medial or deltoid ligament and laterally by the lateral ligament, which prevents anterior and posterior slipping of the tibia and fibula on the talus.

B. Medial (or Deltoid) Ligament

—forms the keystone for the lateral longitudinal arch.
—has four parts: the **tibionavicular, tibiocalcaneal, anterior tibiotalar,** and **posterior tibiotalar** ligaments.
—extends from the medial malleolus to the navicular, calcaneus, and talus.
—resists eversion of the foot.

C. Lateral Ligament

—consists of the **anterior talofibular, posterior talofibular,** and **calcaneofibular** ligaments.

IV. Intertarsal Joints

—consist of the talocalcanean (or subtalar), talocalcaneonavicular, calcaneocuboid, and transverse tarsal joints.

A. Talocalcanean (or Subtalar) Joint

—is part of the talocalcaneonavicular joint.
—allows inversion and eversion of the foot.
—is formed between the talus and calcaneus.

B. Talocalcaneonavicular Joint

—is a part of the transverse tarsal joint.
—resembles a ball-and-socket joint in which the head of the talus is in contact with a socket formed by the calcaneus and the navicular.
—is supported by the spring (or plantar calcaneonavicular) ligament.

C. Calcaneocuboid Joint

—is a part of the transverse tarsal joint.
—resembles a saddle joint, between the calcaneus and the cuboid.
—is supported by the short plantar (or plantar calcaneocuboid) and long plantar ligaments.
—is also supported by the tendon of the peroneus longus.

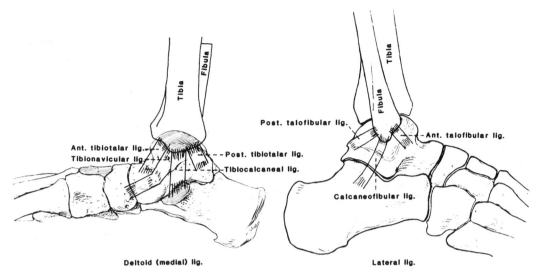

Figure 3.7. Ligaments of the ankle joint.

D. Transverse Tarsal Joint

—is a functional joint, consisting of the talonavicular part of the talocalcaneonavicular joint and the calcaneocuboid joint.

V. Tarsometatarsal Joints

—are plane joints and strengthen the transverse arch.

—are united by articular capsules, reinforced by the plantar, dorsal, and interosseous ligaments.

VI. Metatarsophalangeal Joints

—are ellipsoid (condyloid) joints.

—are joined by articular capsules, reinforced by the plantar and collateral ligaments.

VII. Interphalangeal Joints

—are hinge (ginglymus) joints.

—are enclosed by articular capsules, reinforced by the plantar and collateral ligaments.

Anterior Thigh

I. Femoral Triangle

—is bounded by:

    a. The inguinal ligament superiorly.

    b. The sartorius muscle laterally.

    c. The adductor longus muscle medially.

—contains the femoral nerve and vessels.

A. Femoral Ring

—is bounded by:

    a. The inguinal ligament anteriorly.

b. The femoral vein laterally.

c. The lacunar ligament medially.

d. The pectineal ligament posteriorly.

B. Femoral Canal

–lies medial to the femoral vein in the femoral sheath.

–is occupied by fat, areolar connective tissue, and lymph nodes.

–is a potential weak area and site of femoral herniation.

C. Femoral Sheath

–is a funnel-shaped extension of the transversalis and iliopsoas fasciae into the thigh, deep to the inguinal ligament.

–contains (from lateral to medial) the femoral artery, femoral vein, and femoral canal.

*The femoral nerve lies outside the femoral sheath, lateral to the femoral artery.

D. Femoral Hernia

–its neck lies deep to the inguinal ligament.

–lies lateral to the public tubercle and inferior to the inguinal ligament.

–its sac is formed by the parietal peritoneum.

–is more common in women than in men.

–passes through the femoral ring and canal.

E. Adductor Canal

–begins at the apex of the femoral triangle and ends at the tendinous hiatus.

–lies between the adductor magnus and longus and the vastus medialis.

–is covered by the satorius muscle and fascia.

–contains the femoral vessels, saphenous nerve, and nerve to the vastus medialis.

II. Anterior Muscles of Thigh

Muscle	Origin	Insertion	Nerve	Action
Iliacus	Iliac fossa; ala of sacrum	Lesser trochanter	Femoral n.	Flexes and rotates thigh medially
Sartorius	Anterior superior iliac spine	Upper medial side of tibia	Femoral n.	Flexes and rotates thigh laterally; flexes and rotates leg medially
Rectus femoris	Anterior inferior iliac spine; posterior-superior rim of acetabulum	Base of patella; tibial tuberosity	Femoral n.	Flexes thigh; extends leg
Vastus medialis	Intertrochanteric line; linea aspera; medial intermuscular septum	Medial side of patella; tibial tuberosity	Femoral n.	Extends leg
Vastus lateralis	Intertrochanteric line, greater trochanter, linea	Lateral side of patella; tibial tuberosity	Femoral n.	Extends leg

	aspera; gluteal tuberosity; lateral intermuscular septum			
Vastus intermedius	Upper shaft of femur; lower lateral intermuscular septum	Upper border of patella; tibial tuberosity	Femoral n.	Extends leg

III. Medial Muscles of Thigh

Muscle	Origin	Insertion	Nerve	Action
Adductor longus	Body of pubis below its crest	Middle third of linea aspera	Obturator n.	Adducts, flexes, and rotates thigh laterally
Adductor brevis	Body and inferior ramus of pubis	Pectineal line; upper part of linea aspera	Obturator n.	Adducts, flexes, and rotates thigh laterally
Adductor magnus	Ischiopubic ramus; ischial tuberosity	Linea aspera medial supracondylar line; adductor tubercle	Obturator and sciatic n.	Adducts, flexes, and extends thigh
Pectineus	Pectineal line of pubis	Pectineal line of femur	Obturator and femoral n.	Adducts and flexes thigh
Gracilis	Body and inferior ramus of pubis	Medial surface of upper quarter of tibia	Obturator n.	Adducts and flexes thigh; flexes and rotates leg medially
Obturator externus	Margin of obturator foramen and obturator membrane	Intertrochanteric fossa of femur	Obturator n.	Rotates thigh laterally

IV. Blood Vessels

A. Obturator Artery

–arises from the internal iliac artery in the pelvis.

–passes through the obturator foramen where it divides into anterior and posterior branches.

–its anterior branch descends in front of the adductor brevis and gives off muscular branches.

–its posterior branch descends behind the adductor brevis, supplies the adductor muscles, and gives off the acetabular branch, which passes through the acetabular notch and provides a small artery to the head of the femur.

B. Femoral Artery

–begins as the continuation of the external iliac artery below the inguinal ligament.

–descends through the femoral triangle and enters the adductor canal.

1. Superficial Epigastric Artery

–runs subcutaneously upward toward the umbilicus.

2. Superficial Circumflex Iliac Artery

—runs laterally toward the anterior superior iliac spine, more or less parallel with the inguinal ligament.

3. External Pudendal Artery

—emerges through the saphenous ring, goes medially over the spermatic cord (or the round ligament of the uterus), and sends inguinal branches to the skin above the pubis and anterior scrotal (or labial) branches to the skin of the scrotum (or labium majus).

4. Profunda Femoris (or Deep Femoral) Artery

—arises from the femoral artery within the femoral triangle.
—descends in front of the pectineus, adductor brevis, and magnus muscles but behind the adductor longus.
—gives off the medial and lateral femoral circumflex and muscular branches.
—provides, in the adductor canal, four perforating arteries that perforate and supply the adductor magnus and hamstring muscles.
—its first perforating branch anastomoses with the inferior gluteal, and the transverse branches of the medial and lateral femoral circumflex arteries. This is known as the cruciate anastomosis of the buttock.

5. Medial Circumflex Femoral Artery

—arises from the femoral or profunda femoris artery in the femoral triangle.
—runs between the pectineus and iliopsoas muscles, continues between the obturator externus and adductor brevis, and enters the gluteal region between the adductor magnus and quadratus femoris.
—gives off muscular branches and an acetabular branch and then divides into an ascending branch, which anastomoses with the gluteal arteries, and a transverse branch, which joins the cruciate anastomosis.

6. Lateral Circumflex Femoral Artery

—arises from the femoral or from the profunda.
—passes laterally deep to the satorius and rectus femoris muscles.
—divides into ascending, transverse, and descending branches.

a. Ascending Branch

—ascends deep to the tensor fasciae latae and then between the gluteus medius and minimum muscles to anastomose with the superior gluteal artery.

b. Transverse Branch

—penetrates the vastus lateralis, winds around the femur, and joins the cruciate anastomosis.

c. Descending Branch

—descends with the nerve to the vastus lateralis muscle beneath the rectus femoris.
—anastomoses with the superior lateral genicular branch of the popliteal artery.

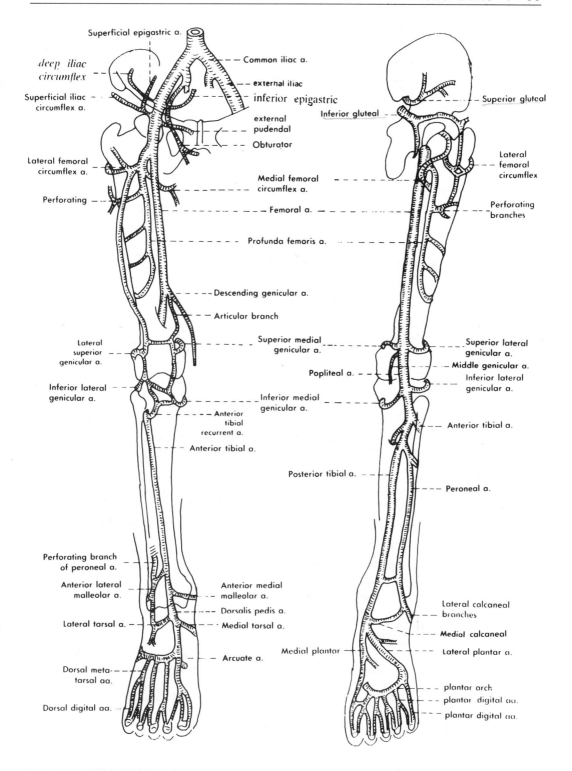

Figure 3.8. Blood supply to the lower limb.

7. **Descending Genicular Artery**
   –arises from the femoral artery just before it passes through the adductor canal.
   –divides into the articular branch, which enters the anastomosis around the knee, and the saphenous branch, which supplies the superficial tissue and skin on the medial side of the knee.

V. Nerves

A. Obturator Nerve
–arises from the plexus (L3-4) and enters the thigh through the obturator foramen.
–divides into an anterior branch and a posterior branch.

1. **Anterior Branch**
   –descends between the adductor longus and brevis and supplies the adductor longus and brevis, gracilis, and pectineus muscles.

2. **Posterior Branch**
   –descends between the adductor brevis and magnus muscles and supplies the obturator externus and adductor magnus muscles.

B. Femoral Nerve
–arises from the lumbar plexus (L2-4) in the substance of the psoas major, emerges between the iliacus and the psoas major, and enters the thigh by passing deep to the inguinal ligament, lateral to the femoral sheath.
–gives off **muscular branches**, **articular branches** to the hip and knee joints, and **cutaneous branches**, including the anterior femoral cutaneous nerve and the saphenous nerve, which descends through the femoral triangle and accompanies the femoral artery in the adductor canal.

Gluteal Region and Posterior Thigh
I. Bony Landmarks and Ligaments of Gluteal Region

1. Sacrotuberous Ligament
–extends from the ischial tuberosity to the posterior iliac spines, the lower sacrum, and coccyx.
–converts, with the sacrospinous ligament, the lesser sciatic notch into the lesser sciatic foramen.

B. Sacrospinous Ligament
–extends from the ischial spine to the lower sacrum and the coccyx.
–converts the greater sciatic notch into the greater sciatic foramen.

C. Greater Sciatic Foramen transmits:
1. The piriformis muscle.
2. The superior and inferior gluteal vessels and nerves.
3. The internal pudendal vessels and pudendal nerve.
4. The sciatic nerve.
5. The posterior femoral cutaneous nerve.
6. The nerves to the obturator internus and quadratus femoris muscles.

D. Lesser Sciatic Foramen transmits:

1. The tendon of the obturator internus.
2. The nerve to the obturator internus.
3. The internal pudendal vessels and pudendal nerve.

E. Structures that Pass Through Both the Greater and Lesser Sciatic Foramina are:

1. The pudendal nerve.
2. The internal pudendal vessels.
3. The nerve to the obturator internus.

F. Iliotibial Tract

−is a particularly strong lateral portion of the fascia lata.
−is derived from the insertion of the gluteus maximus and tensor fasciae latae.
−helps to form the fibrous capsule of the knee joint.

G. Fascia Lata

−is a strong membranous fascia, covering muscles of the thigh.
−forms the lateral and medial intermuscular septa by its inward extension to the femur.
−is attached to the pubic symphysis, crest and ramus, the ischial tuberosity, the inguinal and sacrotuberous ligaments, and the sacrum and coccyx.

II. Muscles of Gluteal Region

Muscle	Origin	Insertion	Nerve	Action
Gluteus maximus	Ilium; sacrum; coccyx; sacrotuberous ligament	Gluteal tuberosity; iliotibial tract	Inferior gluteal n.	Extends and rotates thigh laterally
Gluteus medius	Ilium between iliac crest, anterior and posterior gluteal lines	Greater trochanter	Superior gluteal n.	Abducts and rotates thigh medially
Gluteus minimus	Ilium between anterior and inferior gluteal lines	Greater trochanter	Superior gluteal n.	Abducts and rotates thigh medially
Tensor fasciae latae	Iliac crest; anterior superior iliac spine	Iliotibial tract	Superior gluteal n.	Flexes, abducts, and rotates thigh medially
Piriformis	Pelvic surface of sacrum; sacrotuberous ligament	Upper end of greater trochanter	Sacral n. (S1-2)	Rotates thigh laterally
Obturator internus	Ischiopubic rami; obturator membrane	Greater trochanter	N. to obturator internus	Abducts and rotates thigh laterally
Superior gemellus	Ischial spine	Obturator int. tendon	N. to obturator internus	Rotates thigh laterally
Inferior gemellus	Ischial tuberosity	Obturator int. tendon	N. to quadratus femoris	Rotates thigh laterally
Quadratus femoris	Ischial tuberosity	Intertrochanteric crest	N. to quadratus femoris	Rotates thigh laterally

All the Gluteal Muscles Rotate the thigh laterally Except G. Medius
and G. Minimum. Tensor fascia lata
Abducts of the thigh GGOT

III. Posterior Muscles of Thigh[a]

Muscle	Origin	Insertion	Nerve	Action
Semitendinosus	Ischial tuberosity	Medial surface of upper part of tibia	Tibial portion of sciatic n.	Extends thigh; flexes and rotates leg medially
Semimembranosus	Ischial tuberosity	Medial condyle of tibia	Tibial portion of sciatic n.	Extends thigh; flexes and rotates leg medially
Biceps femoris	Long head from ischial tuberosity; short head from linea aspera and upper supracondylar line	Head of fibula	Tibial (long head) and common peroneal (short head) divisions of sciatic n.	Extends thigh; flexes and rotates leg laterally

[a]These three muscles are collectively called **hamstrings.**

IV. Blood Vessels

A. Superior Gluteal Artery

—arises from the internal iliac artery and passes between the lumbosacral trunk and the first sacral nerve.

—enters the buttock through the greater sciatic foramen above the piriformis.

—runs deep to the gluteus maximus and divides into a superficial branch, which divides into numerous branches to supply the gluteus maximus, and a deep branch, which runs between the gluteus medium and minimus muscles and supplies these muscles and the tensor fasciae latae.

B. Inferior Gluteal Artery

—arises from the internal iliac artery and usually passes between the first and second sacral nerves.

—enters the buttock through the greater sciatic foramen below the piriformis.

—enters the deep surface of the gluteus maximus and descends on medial side of the sciatic nerve, in company with the posterior femoral cutaneous nerve.

V. Nerves

A. Superior Gluteal Nerve

—arises from the sacral plexus (L4-S1).

—enters the buttock through the greater sciatic foramen above the piriformis.

—passes between the gluteus medius and minimus and divides into numerous branches to innervate the gluteus medius and minimus, the tensor fasciae latae, and the hip joint.

B. Inferior Gluteal Nerve

—arises from the sacral plexus (L5-S2).

—enters the buttock through the greater sciatic foramen below the piriformis.

–divides into numerous branches to supply the overlying gluteus maximus.

C. Posterior Femoral Cutaneous Nerve

–arises from the sacral plexus (S1-3), enters the buttock through the greater sciatic foramen below the piriformis.

–runs deep to the gluteus maximus and emerges from the inferior border of this muscle.

–descends on the posterior thigh and supplies the skin of the thigh and over the calf.

D. Sciatic Nerve

–arises from the sacral plexus (L4-S3) and is the largest nerve in the body, consisting of the tibial and common peroneal components.

–enters the buttock through the greater sciatic foramen below the piriformis.

–descends over the obturator internus gemelli and quadratus femoris muscles between the ischial tuberosity and the greater throchanter.

–innervates the hamstring muscles by its tibial division except for the short head of the biceps femoris, which is innervated by its common peroneal division.

–provides articular branches to the hip and knee joints.

VI. Popliteal Fossa

–is bounded superiorly by the semitendinosus and semimembranosus muscles (medially) and the biceps muscle (laterally).

–is bounded inferiorly by the plantaris and the lateral head of the gastrocnemius (laterally) and the medial head of the gastrocnemius (medially).

–contains the popliteal vessels, the common peroneal and tibial nerves, the small saphenous vein, etc.

–its floor is composed of the femur, the oblique popliteal ligament, and the popliteus muscle.

A. Popliteal Artery

–is a continuation of the femoral artery at the adductor hiatus and runs through the popliteal fossa.

–terminates at the lower border of the popliteus muscle by dividing into the anterior and posterior tibial arteries.

–gives off five genicular arteries:

1. Superior Lateral Geniculate Artery

–passes deep to the biceps femoris tendon.

2. Superior Medial Geniculate Artery

–passes deep to the semimembranosus and semitendinosus muscles and enters the substance of the vastus medialis.

3. Inferior Lateral Geniculate Artery

–passes laterally above the head of the fibula and then deep to the fibular collateral ligament.

4. Inferior Medial Geniculate Artery

–passes medially along the upper border of the popliteus muscle, deep to the popliteus fascia.

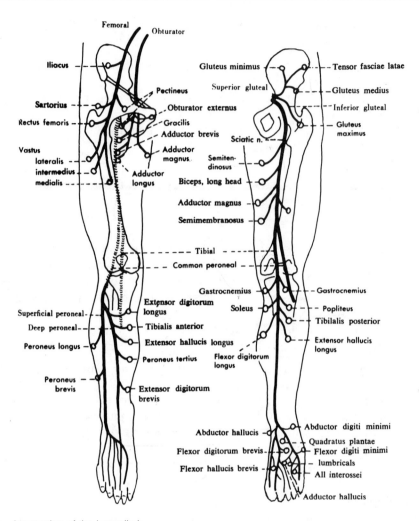

Figure 3.9. Innervation of the lower limb.

5. Middle or Azygos Genicular Artery

—pierces the oblique popliteal ligament and enters the knee joint, where it supplies the cruciate ligaments and the synovial membrane of the joint cavity.

B. Popliteal Vein

—ascends through the popliteal fossa behind the popliteal artery.

—receives the small saphenous vein and veins corresponding to the branches of the popliteal artery.

C. Ligaments

1. Arcuate Popliteal Ligament

—arises from the head of the fibula and passes upward and medially over the tendon of the popliteus muscle on the back of the knee joint.

2. Oblique Popliteal Ligament

—is an oblique expansion of the tendon of the semimembranosus and passes upward obliquely across the posterior surface of the knee joint from the medial condyle of the tibia.

Leg and Foot

I. Anterior and Lateral Muscles of Leg

Muscle	Origin	Insertion	Nerve	Action
Anterior:				
Tibialis anterior	Lateral tibial condyle; interosseous membrane	First cuneiform; first metatarsal	Deep peroneal n.	Dorsiflexes and inverts foot
Extensor hallucis longus	Middle half of anterior surface of fibula; interosseous membrane	Base of distal phalanx of big toe	Deep peroneal n.	Extends big toe; dorsiflexes and inverts foot
Extensor digitorium longus	Lateral tibial condyle; upper two-thirds of fibula; interosseous membrane	Bases of middle and distal phalanges	Deep peroneal n.	Extends toes; dorsiflexes and everts foot
Peroneus tertius	Distal one-third of fibula; interosseous membrane	Base of fifth metatarsal	Deep peroneal n.	Dorsiflexes and everts foot
Lateral:				
Peroneus longus	Lateral tibial condyle; head and upper lateral side of fibula	Base of first metatarsal; medial cuneiform	Superficial peroneal n.	Everts and plantar flexes foot
Peroneus brevis	Lower lateral side of fibula; intermuscular septa	Base of fifth metatarsal	Superficial peroneal n.	Everts and plantar flexes foot

II. Posterior Muscles of Leg

Muscle	Origin	Insertion	Nerve	Action
Superficial group:				
Gastrocnemius	Lateral (lateral head) condyle and medial (medial head) condyles of femur	Posterior aspect of calcaneus via tendo calcaneus	Tibial n.	Flexes knee; plantar flexes foot
Soleus	Upper fibula head; soleal line on tibia	Posterior aspect of calcaneus via tendo calcaneus	Tibial n.	Plantar flexes foot
Plantaris	Lower lateral supracondylar line	Posterior surface of calcaneus	Tibial n.	Plantar flexes foot
Deep group:				
Popliteus	Lateral condyle of femur; popliteal ligament	Upper posterior side of tibia	Tibial n.	Flexes and rotates leg medially

Flexor hallucis longus	Lower two thirds of fibula; interosseous membrane; intermuscular septa	Base of distal phalanx of big toe	Tibial n.	Flexes distal phalanx of big toe
Flexor digitorum longus	Middle posterior aspect of tibia	Distal phalanges of lateral four toes	Tibial n.	Flexes distal phalanges of lateral four toes
Tibialis posterior	Interosseous membrane; upper parts of tibia and fibula	Tuberosity of navicular; sustentacula tali; 3 cuneiforms; cuboid; bases of 2-4 metatarsals	Tibial n.	Plantar flexes and inverts foot

III. Blood Vessels

A. Posterior Tibial Artery

—arises from the popliteal artery at the lower border of the popliteus, between the tibia and the fibula.

—is accompanied by two vena commitantes and the tibial nerve.

—gives off the **peroneal artery** which descends between the tibialis posterior and the flexor hallucis longus and supplies the lateral muscles of the leg. It passes behind the lateral malleolus and ends in branches to the ankle and heel.

—also gives off the posterior lateral and medial malleolar, perforating, muscular branches.

—terminates by dividing into the medial and lateral plantar arteries of the sole.

B. Medial Plantar Artery

—is the smaller terminal branch of the posterior tibial artery.

—runs between the abductor hallucis and the flexor digitorum brevis.

—gives off a superficial branch, which supplies the big toe, and a deep branch, which sends three superficial digital branches.

C. Lateral Plantar Artery

—is the larger terminal branch of the posterior tibial artery.

—runs forward laterally in company with the lateral plantar nerve between the quadratus plantae and the flexor digitorum brevis and then the flexor digitorum brevis and the adductor digiti minimi.

—forms the plantar arch by joining the deep plantar branch of the dorsalis pedis artery. The plantar arch gives off four plantar metatarsal arteries.

D. Anterior Tibial Artery

—arises from the popliteal artery and enters the anterior compartment by passing through the gap at the upper end of the interosseous membrane.

—descends on the interosseous membrane, between the tibialis anterior and extensor digitorum longus muscles.

—runs distally across the ankle midway between the lateral and medial malleoli and continues onto the dorsum of the foot as the dorsalis pedis artery.

—gives off the anterior tibial recurrent artery, which ascends to the knee joint.

—also gives off the anterior medial and lateral malleolar arteries at the ankle.

E. Dorsalis Pedis Artery

—begins anterior to the ankle joint midway between the two malleoli as the continuation of the anterior tibial artery.

—gives off the medial and lateral tarsal arteries and divides into a deep plantar artery to the deep plantar arch and an arcuate artery, which gives off the second, third, and fourth dorsal metatarsal arteries.

IV. Nerves

A. Common Peroneal Nerve

—is separated from the tibial portion at the apex of the popliteal fossa and descends through the fossa.

—superficially crosses the lateral head of the gastrocnemius, then turns laterally around the neck of the fibula deep to the peroneus longus where it divides into the deep peroneal (or anterior tibial) and superficial peroneal nerves.

—gives off the **lateral sural cutaneous nerve** to supply the skin on the lateral part of the back of the leg, and the **recurrent articular branch** to the knee joint.

B. Superficial Peroneal Nerve

—arises from the common peroneal nerve, between the peroneus longus and the neck of the fibula.

—descends in the lateral compartment and supplies the peroneus longus and brevis muscles.

—emerges between the peroneus longus and brevis by piercing the deep fascia at the lower third of the leg to become subcutaneous and supplies the skin of the lower leg and foot.

C. Deep Peroneal (or Anterior Tibial) Nerve

—arises from the common peroneal nerve, between the peroneus longus and the neck of the fibula.

—gives off a recurrent branch to the knee joint.

—passes around the neck of the fibula and through the extensor digitorum longus.

—descends on the interosseous membrane between the extensor digitorum longus and the tibialis anterior and then between the extensor digitorum longus and the extensor hallucis longus.

—supplies the anterior muscles of the leg and divides into medial and lateral branches.

D. Tibial Nerve

—descends through the popliteal fossa and then lies on the popliteus muscle.

—gives off three articular branches that accompany the medial superior genicular, middle genicular, and medial inferior genicular arteries to the knee joint.

–supplies the muscular branches to the posterior muscles of the leg.

–gives rise to the **medial sural cutaneous** nerve, the medial calcaneal branch to the skin of heel and sole, and articular branches to the ankle joint.

–terminates beneath the flexor retinaculum by dividing into the medial and lateral plantar nerves.

E. Medial Plantar Nerve

–arises beneath the flexor retinaculum, deep to the posterior portion of the abductor hallucis, as the larger terminal branch from the tibial nerve.

–passes distally between the abductor hallucis and flexor digitorum brevis, and supplies these muscles.

–gives off common digital branches that divide into proper digital branches which supply the flexor hallucis brevis and the first lumbrical and the skin of the medial three and one-half toes.

F. Lateral Plantar Nerve

–is the smaller terminal branch of the tibial nerve.

–runs distally and laterally between the quadratus plantae and the flexor digitorum brevis, supplying the quadratus plantae and the adductor digiti minimi.

–divides into a **superficial branch**, which supplies the flexor digiti minimi brevis, and a **deep branch**, which supplies the plantar and dorsal interossei, the lateral three lumbricals, and the adductor hallucis.

V. Muscles of Foot

Muscle	Origin	Insertion	Nerve	Action
Dorsum of foot:				
Extensor digitorum brevis	Dorsal surface of calcaneus	Base of proximal phalanx of big toe; tendons of extensor digitorum longus	Deep peroneal n.	Extends toes
Sole of Foot:				
Abductor hallucis	Medial turbercle of calcaneus	Base of proximal phalanx of big toe	Medial plantar n.	Abducts big toe
Flexor digitorum brevis	Medial tubercle of calcaneus	Middle phalanges of lateral four toes	Medial plantar n.	Flexes middle phalanges of lateral four toes
Abductor digiti minimi	Medial and lateral tubercles of calca neus	Proximal phalanx of little toe	Lateral plantar n.	Abducts little toe
Quadratus plantae	Medial and lateral side of calcaneus	Tendons of flexor digitorum longus	Lateral plantar n.	Aids to flex toes
Lumbricals (4)	Tendons of flexor digitorum longus	Proximal phalanges; extensor expansion	First by medial plantar n.; lateral three by lateral plantar n.	Flex metatarsophalangeal joints and extend interphalangeal joints

Flexor hallucis brevis	Cuboid; third cuneiform	Proximal phalanx of big toe	Medial plantar n.	Flexes big toe
Adductor hallucis	Oblique head from bases of 2-4 metatarsals; transverse heat from capsule of lateral four metatarsophalangeal joints	Proximal phalanx of big toe	Lateral plantar n.	Adducts big toe
Flexor digiti minimi brevis	Base of fifth metatarsal	Proximal phalanx of little toe	Lateral plantar n.	Flexes little toe
Plantar interossei (3)	Medial sides of metatarsals 3-5	Medial sides of base of proximal phalanges of 3-5	Lateral plantar n.	Adduct toes; flex proximal, and extend distal phalanges
Dorsal interossei (4)	Adjacent shafts of metatarsals	Proximal phalanges of toes 2 (medial and lateral sides), 3-4 (lateral sides)	Lateral plantar n.	Abduct toes; flex proximal, and extend distal phalanges

VI. Retinacula, Ligaments, and Arches

A. Flexor Retinaculum

–is a deep fascial band that passes between the medial malleolus and the medial surface of the calcaneus.

–holds three tendons in place beneath it: tibialis posterior, flexor digitorum longus, and flexor hallucis longus.

–transmits the tibial nerve and posterior tibial artery beneath it.

B. Plantar Aponeurosis

–is a thick fascia investing the plantar muscles.

–radiates from the calcaneal tuberosity (or tuber calcanei) toward the toes and gives attachment to the short flexor muscles of the toes.

C. Transverse (Metatarsal) Arch

–is formed by the navicular, all three cuneiforms, cuboid, and all five metatarsal bones of the foot.

–is maintained anteriorly by the transverse head of the adductor hallucis muscle.

D. Lateral Longitudinal Arch

–is formed by the calcaneus, cuboid, and lateral two metatarsal bones.

–its "keystone" is the cuboid bone.

–is supported by the peroneus longus tendon and the long and short palmar ligaments.

E. Medial Longitudinal Arch

–is formed by the talus, calcaneus, navicular, cuneiforms, and medial three metatarsals.

–is supported by the spring ligament.

F. Long Plantar Ligament

–extends from the calcaneus to the tuberosity of the cuboid and the base of the metatarsals.

–forms a canal for the tendon of the peroneous longus.

–supports the lateral side of the longitudinal arch of the foot.

G. Short Plantar (Plantar Calcaneocuboid) Ligament

–extends from the front of the inferior surface of the calcaneus to the plantar surface of the cuboid bone.

–lies deep to the long plantar ligament.

–supports the lateral side of the longitudinal arch.

H. "Spring" (Plantar Calcaneonavicular) Ligament

–passes from the sustentaculum tali of the calcaneous to the navicular.

–supports the head of the talus.

–supports the medial side of the longitudinal arch.

VII. Clinical Considerations

A. Damage to Common Peroneal Nerve

–results in **"foot-drop"** and loss of sensation from the dorsum of the foot.

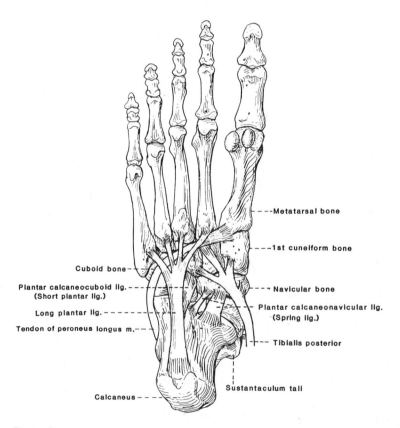

Figure 3.10. Plantar ligaments.

B. Damage to Deep Peroneal Nerve

–results in "foot drop" and, thus, a characteristic high-stepping gait.

C. Damage to Tibial Nerve above the ankle

–results in:

    a. Secondary loss on the sole of the foot, affecting posture and locomotion of the lower limb.

    b. A characteristic "clawing" of the toes.

D. Anterior Tibial Syndrome

–is caused by an acute impairment of the intramuscular circulation in the muscles of the anterior compartment of the leg.

–is also caused by an injury of the deep peroneal nerve.

–involves both the anterior tibialis muscle and the extensor hallucis longus muscles.

–results in a severely limited dorsiflexion of the foot and toes.

–is accompanied by extreme tenderness and pain on the anterolateral aspect of the leg.

E. Ankle Jerk

–is a reflex twitch of the triceps surae (i.e., the medial and lateral heads of the gastrocnemius and the soleus muscles).

–is induced by tapping the tendo calcaneus.

–its reflex center is in the fifth lumbar and first sacral segment of the spinal cord.

F. Patient with Flat Foot

–waddles with his feet turned out in a kind of duck-walk.

–is characterized by disappearance of the medial portion of the longitudinal arch, which appears completely flattened.

–wears shoes that are worn much more on the inner border of the soles and heels than on the outer border.

–feels pain due to stretching of the spring and plantar ligaments.

G. Talipes Equinovarus (Clubfoot)

–is characterized by the:

    a. Plantar flexion.

    b. Inversion.

    c. Adduction of the foot.

–is a congenitally deformed foot that is twisted from its natural position.

Summary of Muscle Actions of Lower Limb (Muscles in Parenthesis Are Less Important In Function)

Movements at Hip Joint (ball-and socket joint)

Flexion—iliopsoas, tensor fasciae latae, rectus femoris (adductor, sartorius, pectineus)

Extension—hamstrings, gluteus maximus (adductor magnus)

Adduction—adductors (pectineus, gracilis)

Abduction—gluteus medius and minimus
Medial rotation—tensor fasciae latae, gluteus medius and minimus
Lateral rotation—obturator internus and externus, gemelli, piriformis, quadratus femoris, gluteus maximus

Movements at Knee Joint (Hinge Joint)

Flexion—hamstrings (gracilis, sartorius, gastrocnemius, popliteus)
Extension—Quadriceps femoris
Medial rotation—semitendinosus (popliteus)
Lateral rotation—biceps femoris

Movements at Ankle Joint (Hinge Joint)

Dorsiflexion—anterior tibialis, extensor digitorum longus (extensor hallucis longus, peroneus tertius)
Plantar flexion—1. Triceps surae (plantaris)
                    2. Posterior tibialis, peroneus longus (flexor digitorum longus, flexor, hallucis longus) (when knee is fully flexed)

Movements at Intertarsal Joint (Talocalcanean, Transverse Tarsal Joint)

Inversion—tibialis posterior, tibialis anterior (triceps surae)
Eversion—Peroneus longus and brevis, extensor digitorum longus (peroneus tertius)

Movements at Metatarsophalangeal Joint (Ellipsoid Joint)

Flexion—lumbricals, interossei, flexor hallucis brevis, flexor digiti minimi brevis
Extension—extensor digitorum longus and brevis, extensor hallucis longus

Movements at Interphalangeal Joint (Hinge Joint)

Flexion—flexor digitorum longus and brevis, flexor hallucis longus
Extension—extensor digitorum longus and brevis, extensor hallucis longus

Summary of Muscle Innervations of Lower Limb (* indicated exception)

Muscles of Thigh

Muscles of Anterior Compartment: Femoral Nerve

    1. Sartorius
    2. Quadriceps femoris

       a. Rectus femoris
       b. Vastus medialis
       c. Vastus intermedius
       d. Vastus lateralis

Muscles of Medial Compartment: Obturator Nerve

    1. Adductor longus
    2. Adductor brevis
  *3. Adductor magnus (obturator and tibial nerves)
    4. Gracilis
    5. Obturator externus
  *6. Pectineus (femoral and obturator nerves): lies on border of anterior and posterior compartment

Muscles of Posterior Compartment: Tibial Nerve of Sciatic Nerve

1. Semitendinosus
2. Semimembranosus
3. Biceps femoris, long head
*4. Biceps femoris, short head (common peroneal nerve)
*5. Adductor magnus (lies in both medial and posterior compartments)

Muscles of Lateral Compartment:

1. Gluteus maximus (inferior gluteal nerve)
2. Gluteus medius (superior gluteal nerve)
3. Gluteus minimus (superior gluteal nerve)
4. Tensor fasciae latae (superior gluteal nerve)
5. Piriformis (nerve to piriformis)
6. Obturator internus (nerve to obturator internus)
7. Superior gemellus (nerve to obturator internus)
8. Inferior gemellus (nerve to quadratus femoris)
9. Quadratus femoris (nerve to quadratus femoris)

Muscles of Leg

Muscles of the Anterior Compartment: Deep Peroneal Nerve

1. Tibialis anterior
2. Extensor digitorum longus
3. Extensor hallucis longus
4. Peroneus tertius

Muscles of Lateral Compartment: Superficial Peroneal Nerve

1. Peroneus longus
2. Peroneus brevis

Muscles of Posterior Compartment: Tibial Nerve

1. Superficial layer
   a. Gastrocnemius
   b. Soleus
   c. Plantaris
2. Deep layer
   a. Popliteus
   b. Tibialis posterior
   c. Flexor digitorum longus
   d. Flexor hallucis longus

Review Test

LOWER LIMB

DIRECTIONS: For each of the questions or incomplete statements below, *one* or *more* of the answers or completions given is correct. Choose answer:

    A. if only **1, 2**, and **3** are correct.
    B. if only **1** and **3** are correct.
    C. if only **2** and **4** are correct.
    D. if only **4** is correct
    E. if **all** are correct.

3.1. The adductor canal (in the lower extremity) is bounded by the

1. sartorius.
2. vastus medialis.
3. adductor longus and magnus.
4. gracilis.

3.2. The adductor canal contains

1. femoral vessels.
2. saphenous nerve.
3. nerve to the vastus medialis.
4. saphenous vein.

3.3. Concerning the superior gluteal nerve, it

1. innervates the gluteus medius and minimus muscles.
2. leaves the pelvis through the greater sciatic foramen, above the piriformis.
3. runs primarily in the plane between the gluteus medius and minimus muscles.
4. innervates the gluteus maximus muscle.

3.4. Concerning the great saphenous vein, it

1. ascends posterior to the medial malleolus.
2. empties into the femoral vein.
3. courses anterior to the medial condyles of the tibia and femur.
4. passes superficial to the fascia lata of the thigh.

3.5. Inability to extend the leg at the knee joint would indicate paralysis of the

1. semitendinosus and semimembranosus muscles.
2. sartorius muscle.
3. gracilis muscle.
4. quadriceps femoris muscle.

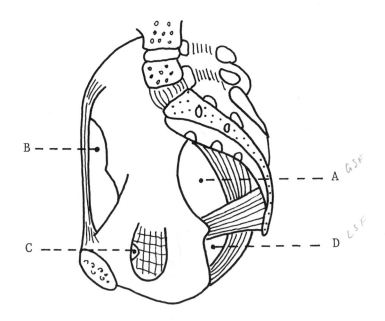

3.6. Identify the structure(s) that pass(es) through the space indicated by A.

1. piriformis muscle.
2. superior gluteal nerve.
3. sciatic nerve.
4. pudendal nerve.

3.7. Identify the structure(s) that pass(es) through the space indicated by B.

1. inferior epigastric artery.
2. iliopsoas muscle.
3. external pudendal artery.
4. femoral vein.

3.8. Identify the structure(s) that pass(es) through the space indicated by C.

1. iliolumbar artery.
2. lumbosacral trunk.
3. ilioinguinal nerve.
4. obturator nerve.

3.9. Identify the structure(s) that pass(es) through the space indicated by D.

1. pudendal nerve.
2. posterior cutaneous nerve of thigh.
3. obturator internus tendon.
4. inferior gluteal artery.

3.10. Identify the structure(s) that pass(es) through the spaces indicated by both A and D.

1. nerve to quadratus femoris muscle.
2. pudendal nerve.
3. sciatic nerve.
4. nerve to the obturator internus.

DIRECTIONS: For each numbered item, select *one* lettered heading that is most closely associated with it. Each lettered heading may be selected once, more than once, or not at all.

A. Calcaneofibular ligament
B. Long plantar ligament
C. Plantar calcaneonavicular (spring) ligament
D. Short plantar ligament
E. Deltoid ligament

3.11. The thickened medial part of the ankle joint capsule.

3.12. Forms a canal for the tendon of the peroneus longus muscle.

3.13. The cord-like ligament that reinforces the lateral side of the ankle joint.

3.14. Extends from the front of the inferior surface of the calcaneous to the plantar surface of the cuboid and supports the longitudinal arch.

3.15. Supports the head of the talus in maintaining the medial longitudinal arch.

A. Biceps femoris
B. Gluteus medius muscle
C. Iliopsoas muscle
D. Rectus femoris muscle
E. Tensor fasciae latae

3.16. Functions to rotate the leg laterally.

3.17. It is the chief flexor of the thigh.

3.18. Functions to flex the thigh and extend the leg.

3.19. Can flex and medially rotate the thigh in running and climbing.

3.20. Paralysis of this abductor and medial rotator of the thigh results in a tilt of the pelvis toward the opposite side of the body when the body weight is totally supported by the leg on the side of the paralyzed muscle.

DIRECTIONS: Each of the questions or incomplete statements below is followed by suggested answers or completions. Selection *one* that is *best* in each case.

3.21. The medial plantar nerve is a direct branch of the

A. common peroneal.
B. tibial nerve.
C. superficial peroneal nerve.
D. deep peroneal nerve.
E. anterior tibial nerve.

3.22. The dorsalis pedis artery is a continuation of the

A. posterior tibial artery.
B. popliteal artery.
C. femoral artery.
D. peroneal artery.
E. none of the above.

3.23. The ligament of the hip joint that transmits medial epiphysial vessels to the head of the femur is the

A. transverse acetabular ligament.
B. pubofemoral ligament.
C. ischiofemoral ligament.
D. iliofemoral ligament.
E. ligamentum teres femoris.

3.24. Which of the following ligaments prevents forward displacement of the femur on the tibia when the knee is flexed is the

A. anterior cruciate ligament.
B. fibular collateral ligament.
C. patellar ligament.
D. posterior cruciate ligament.
E. tibial collateral ligament.

3.25. The femoral nerve

A. innervates the psoas major muscle.
B. provides a branch that supplies the skin on the lateral side of the foot.
C. innervates the skin over the greater trochanter.
D. is lateral to the femoral artery.
E. innervates the tensor fasciae latae.

3.26. Which of the following muscles does **not** contribute directly to the stability of the knee joint?

A. soleus.
B. semimembranosus.
C. sartorius.
D. biceps femoris.
E. gastrocnemius.

3.27. The artery most likely to send a branch to the ligamentum teres femoris is the

A. superficial circumflex iliac.
B. inferior gluteal.
C. superficial epigastric.
D. superficial external pudendal.
E. obturator.

3.28. Select the correct statement.

A. The tendon of the flexor digitorum longus passes superficial to the tendon of the tibialis posterior as they pass around the medial malleolus.
B. The tendon of the flexor hallucis longus passes superficial to the tendon of the flexor digitorum longus as they cross the sole of the foot.
C. The flexor digitorum longus arises mainly from the middle half of the posterior shaft of the fibula.
D. The flexor hallucis longus arises mainly from the middle half of the posterior shaft or body of the tibia.
E. The tibialis posterior is a strong evertor of the foot.

3.29. One of the following structures does *not* pass under (deep to) the inferior or superior extensor retinaculum of the ankle. Identify it.

A. tibialis anterior.
B. extensor digitorum longus.
C. extensor hallucis longus.
D. peroneus tertius.
E. superficial peroneal nerve.

3.30. Select the correct statement.

A. The peroneus longus muscle inserts on the proximal end of the first metatarsus and the medial cuneiform bone.
B. Tendons of the flexor digitorum brevis muscle insert into the base of the proximal phalanx of each toe except the first (big) toe.
C. The quadratus plantae muscle inserts into the medial border of the flexor digitorum brevis muscle.
D. The flexor hallucis longus inserts into the base of the proximal phalanx of the first (big) toe.
E. The tibialis anterior muscle inserts on the calcaneus.

3.31. The longitudinal arches of the foot

A. include the poximal phalanges distally.
B. are primarily dependent on muscles for their support.
C. The lateral longitudinal arch includes the navicular bone.
D. Weight is transmitted from the tibia to the longitudinal arches by means of the talus.
E. is supported in part by a ligament that extends from the calcaneus to the sustentaculum tali.

3.32. The knee joint

A. Its medial meniscus is closer to a full circle than is the lateral one.
B. is supported medially by a collateral ligament that is completely free of the capsule.
C. is strengthened internally by the paired cruciate ligaments, the anterior one of which resists posterior movement of the tibia on the femur.
D. Its medial collateral ligament is firmly attached to the medial meniscus.
E. Its synovial cavity is usually continuous with the prepetallar bursa.

3.33. Select one incorrect statement. The femoral triangle

A. is covered superficially by fascia lata.
B. contains the femoral artery, vein, and nerve.
C. is bounded medially by the adductor longus muscle.
D. The femoral nerve is covered by the femoral sheath in this region.
E. is bounded superiorly by the inguinal ligament.

3.34. Of the following arteries involved in the vascular anastomosis around the hip joint, which one usually gives off the branch that follows the ligament of the head of the femur?

A. medial circumflex femoral.
B. inferior gluteal.
C. lateral circuflex femoral.
D. obturator.
E. superior gluteal.

3.35. A patient who on one side exhibits a slight weakness in the lateral arch of the foot and cannot dorsiflex the foot probably has damage to the

A. superficial peroneal nerve.
B. lateral plantar nerve.
C. deep peroneal nerve.
D. sural nerve.
E. posterior tibial nerve.

3.36. When the common peroneal nerve is severed in the popliteal fossa, but the tibial nerve is spared, the foot will be

A. plantar flexed and inverted.
B. dorsiflexed and everted.
C. dorsiflexed and inverted.
D. plantar flexed and everted.
E. dorsiflexed only.

3.37. To avoid damage to the sciatic nerve when giving an intramuscular injection in the gluteal region, the needle should be inserted

A. in the area over the sacrospinous ligament.
B. at a point midway between the ischial tuberosity and the lesser trochanter.
C. at midpoint of the gemelli muscles.
D. in the upper right quadrant of the gluteal region.
E. in the lower right quadrant of the gluteal region.

3.38. Select the correct statement. The peroneal artery

A. ends in branches to the ankle and heel.
B. continues into the foot as the dorsalis pedis artery.
C. gives rise to the medial plantar artery in the foot.
D. is a branch of the anterior tibial artery.
E. continues into the foot as the lateral plantar artery.

3.39. The groove in the lower surface of the cuboid bone is occupied by the tendon of

A. peroneus tertius.
B. peroneus brevis.
C. peroneus longus.
D. tibialis anterior.
E. tibialis posterior.

3.40. the groove on the undersurface of the sustentaculum tali is occupied by the tendon of

A. flexor digitorum brevis.
B. flexor digitorum longus.
C. flexor hallucis brevis.
D. flexor hallucis longus.
E. tibialis posterior.

DIRECTIONS: Each set of lettered headings below is followed by a list of numbered words or phrases. Choose answer.

    A. if the item is associated with A only.
    B. if the item is associated with B only.
    C. if the item is associated with both A and B.
    D. if the item is associated with neither A nor B.

A. Inversion of the foot
B. Eversion of the foot
C. Both
D. Neither

3.41. This movement takes place at the ankle joints.

3.42. Severance of the superficial peroneal nerve at its origin in the leg would greatly weaken this movement.

3.43. The tibialis posterior and anterior muscle bring about this movement.

3.44. This movement occurs primarily at the talocalcaneal and transverse tarsal joints.

3.45. Damage to a nerve passing around the lateral side of the neck of the fibula would weaken or abolish this movement.

A. Medial femoral circumflex artery
B. Lateral femoral circumflex artery

3.46. May arise from the femoral or profunda femoral artery.

3.47. Runs between the iliopsoas and the pectineus muscles.

3.48. Runs deep to the sartorius and rectus femoris muscles.

3.49. Enters the cruciate anastomosis.

3.50. Gives rise to an acetabular branch that anastomoses with the posterior branch of the obturator artery.

A. Rectus femoris muscle
B. Adductor magnus muscle of the thigh

3.51. Functions to extend the leg.

3.52. Crosses hip and knee joints and consequently acts on both the knee and hip joints.

3.53. Is innervated by the obturator nerve.

3.54. Is innervated by the tibial portion of the sciatic nerve.

3.55. Receives its blood supply from branches of the femoral artery.

A. Femoral nerve
B. Obturator nerve
C. Both
D. Neither

3.56. Innervates the pectineus muscle.

3.57. Innervates a muscle that inserts on the lesser trochanter.

3.58. Severance of this nerve would severely weaken the adduction of the thigh.

3.59. A branch of this nerve conducts sensation from the medial side of the thigh.

3.60. Lies within the femoral sheath during its course.

Answers and Explanations

LOWER LIMB

3.1 A. The adductor canal is bounded by the sartorius, vastus medialis, and adductor longus and magnus muscles.

3.2 A. The adductor canal contains the femoral vessels, the saphenous nerve, and the nerve to the vastus medialis.

3.3. A. The superior gluteal nerve leaves the pelvis through the greater sciatic foramen above the piriformis, runs between the gluteus medius and minimus muscles, and innervates these muscles and the tensor fasciae latae.

3.4. C. The greater saphenous vein courses anterior to the medial malleolus and medial to the medial condyles of the tibia and femur, ascends superficial to the fascia lata, and terminates in the femoral vein.

3.5. D. The quadriceps femoris muscle consists of the rectus femoris and the vastus medialis, intermedialis, and lateralis. They extend the leg at the knee joint. The semitendinosus and semimembranosus extend the thigh and flex the leg. The sartorius and gracilis can flex the leg.

3.6. E. The piriformis muscle, the superior gluteal, sciatic, and pudendal nerves pass through the greater sciatic foramen.

3.7. C. The iliopsoas muscle and the femoral vein enter the thigh by passing deep to the inguinal ligament.

3.8. D. The obturator nerve passes through the obturator foramen where it divides into anterior and posterior branches.

3.9. B. The pudendal nerve and the obturator internus tendon pass through the lesser sciatic foramen.

3.10. C. The pudendal nerve and the nerve to the obturator internus pass through both the greater and lesser sciatic foramina.

3.11. E. The deltoid ligament is the thickened medial part of the ankle joint capsule and consists of the anterior tibiotalar, tibionavicular, tibiocalcaneal, and posterior tibiotalar ligaments.

3.12. B. The long plantar ligament forms a canal for the tendon of the peroneus longus muscle.

3.13. A. The calcaneofibular ligament is the cord-like ligament that reinforces the lateral side of the ankle joint.

3.14. D. The short plantar ligament extends from the front of the inferior surface of the calcaneous to the plantar surface of the cuboid and supports the longitudinal arch.

3.15. C. The spring ligament supports the head of the talus in maintaining the medial longitudinal arch.

3.16. A. The biceps femoris muscle rotates the leg laterally, when the knee is flexed.

3.17. C. The iliopsoas is the chief flexor of the thigh.

3.18. D. The rectus femoris muscle crosses both the hip and knee joints, and thus it can flex the thigh and extend the leg.

3.19. E. The tensor fasciae latae can flex and medially rotate the thigh in running and climbing.

116

3.20. B. The gluteus medius muscle supports the pelvis, keeping it from tilting to the opposite side and swinging it forward when the opposite leg is raised from the ground, as in walking.

3.21. B. The medial plantar nerve is a branch of the tibial nerve.

3.22. E. The dorsalis pedis artery is a continuation of the anterior tibial artery.

3.23. E. The ligamentum teres femoris transmits medial epiphysial vessels to the head of the femur. These vessels originate from the posterior branch of the obturator artery.

3.24. D. The posterior cruciate ligament is an important ligament in preventing forward displacement of the femur on the tibia when the knee is flexed.

3.25. D. The femoral nerve lies outside the femoral sheath lateral to the femoral artery. The second and third lumbar nerves innervate the psoas major muscle. The sural nerve innervates the skin on the lateral side of the foot. The iliohypogastric nerve and superior cluneal nerves supply the skin over the greater trochanter. The superior gluteal nerve innervates the tensor fasciae latae.

3.26. A. The soleus muscle arises from the fibula and tibia below the knee joint; thus, this muscle does not contribute to the stability of the knee joint.

3.27. E. The posterior branch of the obturator artery sends a branch to the ligamentum teres femoris.

3.28. A. The tendon of the flexor digitorum longus passes superficial to the tendon of the tibialis posterior as they pass around the medial malleolus. The tendon of the flexor hallucis longus passes deep to the tendon of the flexor digitorum longus as they cross in the sole of the foot. The flexor digitorum longus arises mainly from the tibia, whereas the flexor hallucis longus arises from the fibula. The tibialis posterior inverts the foot.

3.29. E. The superficial peroneal nerve emerges between the peroneus longus and brevis and descends superficial to the extensor retinaculum of the ankle, supplying the skin of the lower leg and foot.

3.30. A. The peroneus longus muscle inserts on the proximal end of the first metatarsus and the medial cuneiform bone. The flexor digitorum brevis inserts into the base of the middle phalanges of the lateral four toes. The quadratus plantae inserts into the tendons of the flexor digitorum longus. The flexor hallucis longus inserts into the base of the distal phalanx of the first (big) toe. The tibialis anterior inserts on the first cuneiform and the first metatarsal.

3.31. D. Weight is transmitted from the tibia to the longitudinal arch by means of the talus. The longitudinal arches include the metatarsals distally. The medial longitudinal arch includes the navicular bone and is supported by the spring ligament, which extends from the sustentaculum tali of the calcaneous to the navicular. The lateral longitudinal arch is supported by the long and short plantar ligaments.

3.32. D. The medial collateral ligament of the knee joint is firmly attached to the medial meniscus, the articular capsule, and the tibia. The medial meniscus forms a semicircle (C-shaped). The anterior cruciate ligament resists posterior movement of the femur on the tibia. The synovial cavity of the knee joint is not usually continuous with the prepatellar bursa.

3.33. D. The femoral nerve lies outside the femoral sheath, lateral to the femoral artery. The femoral sheath contains (from lateral to medial) the femoral artery, femoral vein, and femoral canal.

3.34. D. The obturator artery gives off a branch that follows the ligament of the head of the femur.

3.35. C. The deep peroneal nerve supplies the anterior muscles of the leg, including the tibialis anterior, extensor hallucis longus, extensor digitorum longus, and peroneus tertius, which dorsiflex the foot.

3.36. A. The common peroneal nerve supplies the anterior and lateral muscles of the leg, whereas the tibial nerve supplies the posterior muscles of the leg. The muscles for dorsiflexion and eversion of the foot are paralyzed due to the severance of the common peroneal nerve, and thus the foot is plantar flexed and inverted.

3.37. D. For an intramuscular injection, the needle should be inserted in the upper right quadrant of the gluteal region to avoid damage to the sciatic nerve.

3.38. A. The peroneal artery is a branch of the posterior tibial artery, supplies the lateral muscles of the leg, passes behind the lateral malleolus, and ends in branches to the ankle and heel.

3.39. C. The groove in the lower surface of the cuboid bone is occupied by the tendon of the peroneus longus muscle.

3.40. D. The groove on the undersurface of the sustentaculum tali is occupied by the tendon of the flexor hallucis longus muscle.

3.41. D. The dorsiflexion and plantar flexion take place at the ankle joint.

3.42. B. The superficial peroneal nerve innervates the peroneus longus and brevis muscles, which evert the foot.

3.43. A. Both the tibialis anterior and posterior muscles invert the foot.

3.44. C. Both the inversion and eversion occur primarily at the talocalcaneal and transverse tarsal joints.

3.45. C. The common peroneal nerve passes around the lateral side of the neck of the fibula and deep to the peroneus longus where it divides into the deep and superficial peroneal nerves. The deep peroneal nerve supplies the anterior muscles of the leg, which invert the foot, whereas the superficial peroneal nerve innervates the lateral muscles of the leg, which evert the foot.

3.46. C. The medial and lateral femoral circumflex arteries may arise from the femoral or profunda femoris artery.

3.47. A. The medial femoral circumflex artery runs between the iliopsoas and pectineus muscles and continues between the obturator externus and adductor brevis.

3.48. B. The lateral femoral circumflex artery runs laterally deep to the sartorius and rectus femoris muscles, and divides into ascending, transverse, and descending branches.

3.49. C. The transverse branches of the medial and lateral circumflex femoral arteries, and ascending branch of the first perforating artery, and the inferior gluteal artery form the cruciate anastomosis.

3.50. A. The medial circumflex artery gives rise to an acetabular branch that anastomoses with the posterior branch of the obturator artery.

3.51. A. The rectus femoris muscle flexes the thigh and extends the leg because it crosses both the hip and knee joints.

3.52. A. See above, 3.51.

3.53. B. The adductor magnus muscle is innervated by the obturator and sciatic (tibial portion) nerves.

3.54. B. See above, 3.53.

3.55 C. The rectus femoris and adductor magnus muscles receive blood from branches of the femoral artery.

3.56. C. The pectineus muscle is innervated by the femoral and obturator nerves.

3.57. A. The femoral nerve innervates the iliacus muscle which inserts on the lesser trochanter of the femur.

3.58. B. The obturator nerve innervates the adductor muscles of the thigh.

3.59. C. Both the femoral and obturator nerves innervate the skin on the medial side of the thigh.

3.60. D. The femoral nerve lies outside the femoral sheath.

4
Thorax

Thoracic Wall

I. Skeleton of Thorax

A. Sternum

1. Manubrium
–has a jugular notch that can readily be palpated at the root of the neck.
–has a clavicular notch for articulation with a clavicle.
–also articulates with the first rib and the body of the sternum at the manubriosternal joint or at the sternal angle.

a. Sternal Angle (Angle of Louis)
–is the junction of the manubrium and the body of the sternum.
–is located at the level where:
    (1). The second rib articulates with the sternum.
    (2). The aortic arch begins and ends.
    (3). The trachea bifurcates into the right and left bronchi.
    (4). The inferior border of the superior mediastinum is demarcated.
    (5). A transverse plane would pass through the vertebral column between T4 and T5.

2. Body
–articulates with the second to seventh costal cartilages.
–also articulates with the xiphoid process at the xiphosternal joint.

3. Xiphoid Process
–is a flat cartilaginous process surrounding the bony center.

B. Ribs
–are 12 pairs that form the main part of the thoracic cage.
–extend from vertebrae to or toward the sternum.
–are divided into the heads, necks, tubercles, and shafts (bodies).
–their heads articulate with the corresponding vertebral bodies and intervertebral discs and subjacent vertebral bodies.
–their tubercles articulate with transverse processes of the corresponding vertebrae.

1. True Ribs
—are the first seven (1–7) ribs, which are attached to the sternum by their costal cartilages.

2. False Ribs
—are the lower five (8–12) ribs, which are connected to the costal cartilages immediately above to form the anterior costal margin.

3. Floating Ribs
—are the last two (11–12) ribs, which are connected only with the vertebrae.

4. Cervical Rib
—is a mesenchymal or a cartilaginous elongation of the transverse process of the seventh cervical vertebra.
—may end freely or articulate with the first throacic rib.
—may compress the lower trunk of the brachial plexus and the subclavian artery, leading to "neurovascular compression" or "thoracic outlet syndrome."

5. Lumbar (Gorilla) Rib
—is a rib that present on the vertebra below the twelfth thoracic rib.

II. Articulation of Thorax

A. Sternoclavicular Joint
—contains two separate synovial cavities.
—provides the only bony attachment between the appendicular and axial skeletons.
—is a saddle joint but has the movements of a ball-and-socket joint.
—has a fibrocartilaginous articular surface.

B. Sternocostal (Sternochondral) Joints
—are synchondroses in which the sternum articulates with the first seven costal cartilages.

C. Costochondral Joints
—are synchondroses in which the ribs articulate with their costal cartilages.

D. Interchondral Joints
—are gliding joints that are formed by the articulation of costal cartilages of ribs 6–10 with the cartilage immediately below.

E. Costovertebral Joints

1. Joints of Heads of Ribs
—are gliding joints in which the heads of ribs articulate with the bodies of two adjacent vertebrae and the intervertebral disc in between.

2. Costotransverse Joints
—are articulations between the tubercles of the ribs and the transverse processes of the corresponding vertebrae.

III. Muscles

Muscle	Origin	Insertion	Nerve	Action
External intercostals	Lower border of ribs	Upper border of rib below	Intercostal n.	Elevate ribs in inspiration
Internal intercostals	Lower border of ribs	Upper border of rib below	Intercostal n.	Elevate ribs
Innermost intercostals	Lower border of ribs	Upper border of rib below	Intercostal n.	Elevate ribs
Transversus thoracis	Posterior surface of lower sternum and xiphoid	Inner surface of second to sixth costal cartilages	Intercostal n.	Depress ribs
Subcostalis	Inner surface of lower ribs near their angles	Upper borders of second or third rib below	Intercostal n.	Elevate ribs

IV. Blood Vessels

A. Internal Thoracic Artery

—arises usually from the first part of the subclavian artery.

—descends directly behind the first six costal cartilages, just lateral to the sternum.

—gives off two anterior intercostal arteries in each of the upper six intercostal spaces.

—terminates at the sixth intercostal space by dividing into the superior epigastric and musculophrenic arteries.

1. Pericardiacophrenic Artery

—accompanies the phrenic nerve to the diaphragm.

—supplies the pleura, pericardium, and diaphragm (upper surface).

2. Anterior Intercostal Arteries

—supply the upper six intercostal spaces and anastomose with the posterior intercostal arteries.

—provide muscular branches to the intercostal, serratus anterior, and pectoral muscles.

3. Anterior Perforating Branches

—perforate the internal intercostal muscles in the upper six intercostal spaces.

—courses with the anterior cutaneous branches of the intercostal nerves and supply the pectoralis major muscle and the skin and subcutaneous tissue over it.

—provide medial mammary branches by their second, third, and fourth perforating branches.

4. Musculophrenic Artery

—follows the costal arch on the inner surface of the costal cartilages.

—gives off two anterior intercostal arteries in the seventh, eighth, and ninth spaces, perforates the diaphragm, and ends in the tenth intercostal space, where it anastomoses with the deep circumflex iliac artery.

—supplies the pericardium, diaphragm, and muscles of the abdominal wall.

5. Superior Epigastric Artery PAᵖ

—descends on the deep surface of the rectus abdominis muscle within the rectus sheath, supplies this muscle and anastomoses with the inferior epigastric artery.

—supplies the diaphragm, peritoneum, and anterior abdominal wall.

B. Thoracoepigastric Vein

—is a venous connection between the lateral thoracic vein and the superficial epigastric vein.

V. Lymphatic Drainage

A. Sternal or Parasternal (Internal Thoracic) Nodes

—are placed along the internal thoracic artery.

—receive lymph from the medial portion of the breast, the intercostal spaces, the diaphragm, and the supraumbilical region of the abdominal wall.

—drain into the junction of the internal jugular and subclavian veins.

B. Intercostal Nodes

—lie near the heads of the ribs.

—receive from the intercostal spaces and the pleura.

—drain into the cisterna chyli or the thoracic duct.

C. Phrenic Nodes

—lie on the thoracic surface of the diaphragm.

—receive from the pericardium, diaphragm, and liver.

—drain into the sternal and posterior mediastinal nodes.

VI. Nerves

A. Intercostal Nerves

—are the anterior primary rami of the first 11 thoracic spinal nerves.

—are called typical intercostal nerves for third to sixth nerves.

—run between the internal and innermost layers of muscles, with the intercostal veins and arteries above (**van**, veins-arteries-nerves).

—are lodged in the costal grooves on the inferior surface of the ribs.

—give off lateral and anterior cutaneous branches and muscular branches.

B. Subcostal Nerve

—is the anterior ramus of the twelfth thoracic nerve.

C. Thoracoabdominal Nerves

—are the anterior primary rami of the seventh to eleventh thoracic nerves.

Organs of Respiration

I. Mediastinum

—is an **interpleural space** (area between the pleural cavities) in the thorax bounded laterally by the pleural cavities, anteriorly by the sternum, and posteriorly by the vertebral column.

—consists of superior mediastinum and inferior mediastinum, which is further divided into the anterior, middle, and posterior mediastina.

—the superior mediastinum is bounded superiorly by the oblique plane of first rib and inferiorly by the imaginary line running from the sternal angle to the intervertebral disc between the fourth and fifth thoracic vertebrae.

—the **superior mediastinum** contains the superior vena cava, brachiocephalic veins, arch of the aorta, thoracic duct, trachea, esophagus, vagus nerve, left recurrent laryngeal nerve, phrenic nerve, etc.

—the **posterior mediastinum** contains the esophagus, thoracic aorta, azygos and hemiazygos veins, thoracic duct, vagus nerves, splanchnic nerves, etc.

—the **middle mediastinum** contains the heart, pericardium, phrenic nerves, vagus nerves, roots of great vessels, arch of the azygos vein, and main bronchi.

—the **anterior mediastinum** contains the remnants of the thymus gland, lymph nodes, fat, and connective tissue.

II. Trachea and Bronchi

A. Trachea

—begins at the inferior border of the cricoid cartilage (CV 6).

—has 16–20 incomplete hyaline cartilaginous rings that prevent the trachea from collapsing.

—is about 9–15 cm in length, about one-half the length of the esophagus.

—bifurcates into the right and left main bronchi at the level of the sternal angle (TV 5 or 6).

B. Right Main (Primary) Bronchus

—is shorter, wider, and more vertical than the left one.

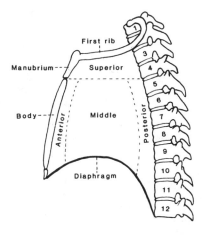

Figure 4.1. Mediastinum.

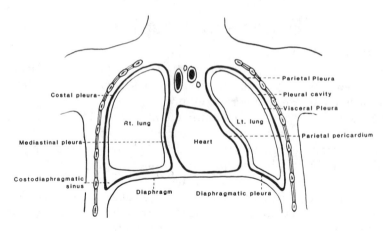

Figure 4.2. Frontal section of the thorax.

–receives more foreign bodies through the trachea.
–runs over the pulmonary vein and under the arch of the azygos vein.
–divides into the superior, middle, and inferior lobar (secondary) bronchi.

C. **Left Main (Primary) Bronchus** — Smaller diamete

Smaller in diameter
twice as long as th

Rt. Bronchus

–crosses anterior to the esophagus.
–divides into two lobar (secondary) bronchi, the upper and lower.

D. **Right Superior Lobar (Secondary) Bronchus**

–is known as the **eparterial** bronchus. (All others are the hyparterial bronchi.)
–is higher than any other bronchus.
–is even higher than the pulmonary artery.

III. Pleurae and Pleural Cavities

A. Pleura

–is a thin serous membrane that lines the inner surface of the thoracic wall and the mediastinum.

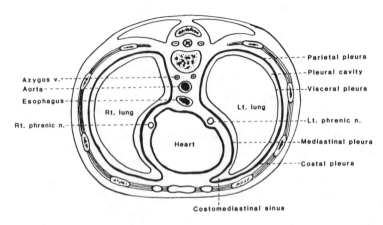

Figure 4.3. Horizontal section through the thorax.

–is innervated by the intercostal nerves for the costal and peripheral portions of the diaphragmatic pleura, whereas the remainder of the diaphragmatic pleura and mediastinal pleura are supplied by the phrenic nerve.

1. Parietal Pleura

–lines the wall of the thorax and has costal, diaphragmatic, mediastinal, and cervical (cupola) parts.

–is supplied by branches of the internal thoracic, superior phrenic, posterior intercostal, and superior intercostal arteries. However, the visceral pleura is supplied by the bronchial arteries.

–is very sensitive to pain.

2. Visceral Pleura

–intimately invests the lungs and dips into all of the fissures.

–is supplied by bronchial arteries, but its venous blood is drained by pulmonary veins.

–is insensitive to pain but contains vasomotor fibers and sensory endings of vagal origin, which may be involved in respiratory reflexes.

3. Cupola of Pleura (Cervical Pleura)

–is the dome of the parietal pleura, projecting into the neck.

–is strengthened by the suprapleural membrane (Sibson's fascia), which is a thickening of the endothoracic fascia.

–is at the level of the first rib behind and has the sympathetic trunk just behind it.

4. Pulmonary Ligament

–is a double layer of mediastinal pleura, extending from the hilus of the lung to the base (diaphragmatic surface).

–is a reflection (fusion) of the visceral and parietal pleurae, ending below in a free edge.

–supports the lung in the pleural sac.

B. Pleural Cavity

–is a potential space between the parietal and visceral pleurae.

–contains a film of fluid that lubricates the surface of the pleurae and facilitates the movement of the lungs.

1. Costodiaphragmatic Recess

–is the pleural recess formed by the reflection of the costal and diaphragmatic pleurae.

–can accumulate fluid in the erect position.

2. Costomediastinal Recess

–is part of the pleural cavity, where the costal and mediastinal pleurae meet.

3. Endothoracic Fascia

–is a small amount of loose connective tissue that separates the parietal pleurae from the thoracic wall.

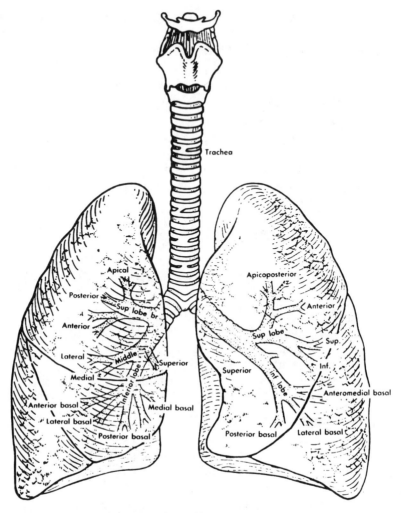

Figure 4.4.   Anterior view of the trachea, bronchi, and lungs.

IV. Lungs

  —are the essential organs of respiration.

  —their nonrespiratory tissues are nourished by the bronchial arteries and drained by the pulmonary veins.

  —receive parasympathetic fibers that supply the smooth muscle and glands of the bronchial tree and are probably excitatory to these structures.

  —receive sympathetic fibers that supply blood vessels, smooth muscle, and glands of the bronchial tree and are probably inhibitory.

  —have some sensory endings of vagal origin, which are stimulated by the stretching of the lung during inspiration and are concerned in the reflex control of respiration.

  —their bases rest upon the convex surface of the diaphragm, descend during inspiration, and ascend during expiration.

secondary bronchi are lined each ciliated, pseudostratified epithelium containing Goblet cells and have Cartilage plates. mucus gland and smooth musc. Bronchioles have Ciliated columnar epithelium. Terminal bronchioles lined by Ciliated cuboidal epithelium invested by smooth musc.

A. Right Lung

–its apex projects into the root of the neck and is smaller than that of the left.

–usually receives a single bronchial artery.

–is heavier and shorter than the left, due to the higher right dome of the diaphragm, and wider because the heart bulges more to the left.

–is divided into upper, middle, and lower lobes by the oblique and horizontal fissures.

–has three lobar (secondary) bronchi and 10 segmental (tertiary) bronchi.

B. Left Lung

–usually receives two bronchial arteries.

–has two lobes, upper and lower

–has an oblique fissure that follows the line of the sixth rib.

–has a **lingula**, which is a tongue-shaped portion of its upper lobe that corresponds to the middle lobe of the right lung and is formed by the more pronounced cardiac incisura in the left lung.

C. Bronchopulmonary Segment

–is the anatomical, surgical, and functional unit (subdivision) of the lungs.

–consists of a tertiary bronchus, the portion of the lung it ventilates, an artery, and a vein.

–refers to the portion of the lung supplied by the direct branches of the lobar bronchi.

–is separated from adjacent segments by connective tissue septa.

–is supplied by each segmental bronchus and segmental artery.

–has clinical importance for surgical removal of a diseased segment of the lung.

V. Lymphatic Vessels of Lung

–drain the bronchial tree, the pulmonary vessels, and the connective tissue septa.

–run along the bronchiole and bronchi toward the hilus, where they end in the pulmonary and bronchopulmonary nodes, which in turn drain into the tracheobronchial nodes.

–are not present in the walls of the pulmonary alveoli.

VI. Blood Vessels

A. Pulmonary Trunk

–extends upward from the conus arteriosus of the right ventricle.

–is invested with fibrous pericardium.

–has much less blood pressure than in the aorta.

B. Left Pulmonary Artery

–carries unoxygenated blood to the left lung.

–is shorter and narrower than the right one.

–is connected to the aorta by the ligamentum arteriosum, the fibrous remains of the ductus arteriosus.

C. Right Pulmonary Artery

–runs horizontally toward the hilus of the right lung under the arch of the

Both pulmonary arteries and Bronchial arteries accompany Bronchi

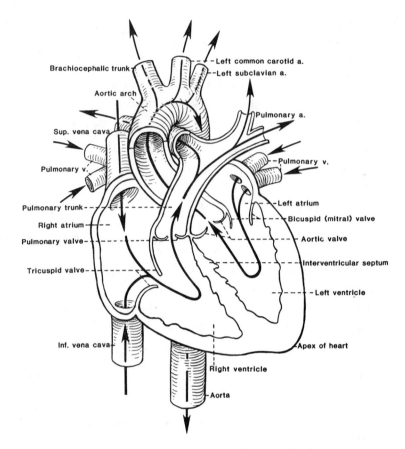

Figure 4.5. The pulmonary circulation and circulation through the heart chambers.

aorta behind the ascending aorta and superior vena cava and anterior to
of the right bronchus.

D. Pulmonary Veins

–do not accompany the bronchi (they are intersegmental in drainage).
–are five in number as they leave the lung, consisting of one from each
lobe of the lungs, although the right upper and middle veins usually join
so that only four enter the left atrium.
–carry oxygenated blood and enter the left atrium.
–do not have valves.
–their occlusion leads to ischemia of heart muscle and subsequent infarction.
–collect arterial blood from the respiratory part of the lung and venous
blood from the visceral pleura and from the bronchi.

E. Bronchial Arteries

–usually arise from the thoracic aorta.
–are usually one in number for the right lung, and usually two for the left
lung.
–supply oxygenated blood to the nonrespiratory conducting tissues of the
lungs.

5 vein

~they drain
Both Pulmonary
and Bronchial arteria

1 one for Rt Lung
2 Left Lung

F. Bronchial Veins — *Drain blood from Bronchial arteries only*

—receive blood from the larger subdivisions of the bronchi and empty into the azygos on the right and into the accessory hemiazygos vein on the left. (Other venous blood is drained by the pulmonary veins.)
—may receive twigs from the tracheobronchial lymph nodes.

VII. Respiration

—is the vital exchange of oxygen and carbon dioxide that occurs in the lungs.

A. During Inspiration

1. the diaphragm contracts, pulling the dome inferiorly into the abdomen, thereby increasing the thoracic cavity and decreasing intrathoracic pressure.
2. the pleural cavities and the lungs enlarge, the intraalveolar pressure is reduced, and the air possibly rushes into the lungs, due to atmospheric pressure.
3. the bronchial tree elongates, the root of the lungs moves downward, and the trachea and main bronchi descend.
4. the abdominal pressure is increased with decreased abdominal cavity.
5. the ribs are elevated.

B. During Expiration

1. the diaphragm, the intercostals, and other muscles relax; the thoracic volume is decreased; and the intrathoracic pressure is increased.
2. the stretched elastic tissue of the lungs recoils and much of the air is forced out.
3. the abdominal pressure is decreased and the ribs are depressed.

C. Muscles of Inspiration

—include the diaphragm, external intercostal, sternocleidomastoid, levator scapulae, serratus anterior, scalenus, pectoralis major and minor, erector spinae, and serratus posterior superior muscles.

D. Muscles of Expiration

—include the muscles of the abdominal wall, internal intercostals, and serratus posterior inferior muscles.

VIII. Nerve Supply

A. Pulmonary Plexus

—receives afferent and efferent (parasympathetic) fibers from the vagus nerve, joined by branches from the sympathetic trunk and cardiac plexus.
—is divided into the **anterior pulmonary plexus**, which lies in front of the root of the lung, and the **posterior pulmonary plexus**, which lies behind the root of the lung.
—its branches accompany the blood vessels and bronchi into the lung.

B. Phrenic Nerve

—arises from the third through fifth cervical nerves.
—lies in front of the scalenus anterior muscle.
—enters the thorax by passing deep to the subclavian vein and superficial to the subclavian arteries.

–runs anterior to the root of the lung, whereas the vagus nerve runs posterior to the root of the lung.

–is accompanied by the pericardiacophrenic vessels of the internal thoracic vessels.

–descends between the mediastinal pleura and pericardium.

–supplies the pericardium, the mediastinal and diaphragmatic pleurae, and the diaphragm.

IX. Clinical Considerations

A. Pneumothorax

–is the presence of air or gas and blood in the thoracic cavity.

B. Emphysema

–reduces the surface area available for gas exchange and thereby reduces oxygen absorption.

C. Pneumonia

–is an inflammation of the lungs.

Pericardium and Heart

I. Pericardium

–is a fibroserous sac that encloses the heart and the roots of the great vessels and occupies the middle mediastinum.

–is composed of the fibrous pericardium and serous pericardium.

–receives blood from the pericardiacophrenic arteries of the internal thoracic artery and from pericardial branches of the bronchial and esophageal arteries.

–is supplied with vasomotor and sensory fibers from the phrenic and vagus nerves, and the sympathetic trunks.

A. Fibrous Pericardium

–is a strong, dense, fibrous layer that blends with the adventitia of the great vessels and the central tendon of the diaphragm.

B. Serous Pericardium

–consists of the parietal layer, which lines the inner surface of the fibrous pericardium, and the visceral layer, which forms the outer layer (or epicardium) of the heart wall.

C. Pericardial Cavity

–is a potential space between the visceral layer of the serous pericardium (epicardium) and parietal layer of the serous pericardium lining the inner surfaces of the fibrous pericardium.

D. Pericardial Sinuses

1. Transverse Sinus of Pericardium

–is a subdivision of the pericardial sac, lying behind the aorta and pulmonary trunk but in front of the left atrium and superior vena cava.

–is formed by the serous pericardium covering the above structures.

2. Oblique Sinus

    —is a subdivision of the pericardial sac behind the heart.

    —is bounded by the reflection of the serous pericardium around the right and left pulmonary veins and inferior vena cava.

II. Heart

A. General Characteristics

    —its **apex** lies in the left fifth intercostal space slightly medial to the nipple line and is clinically useful for determining the posterior of the left border of the heart and for the auscultation of the mitral valve.

    —its wall consists of three layers: inner **endocardium**, middle **myocardium**, and outer **epicardium**.

1. Acute Margin of Heart

    —is the right margin, largely inferior, being the fairly sharp edge between the diaphragmatic and sternocostal surfaces.

2. Obtuse Margin of Heart

    —is the curved left side, which is the pulmonary surface.

    —passes from sternocostal to diaphragmatic surface without any sharp boundaries.

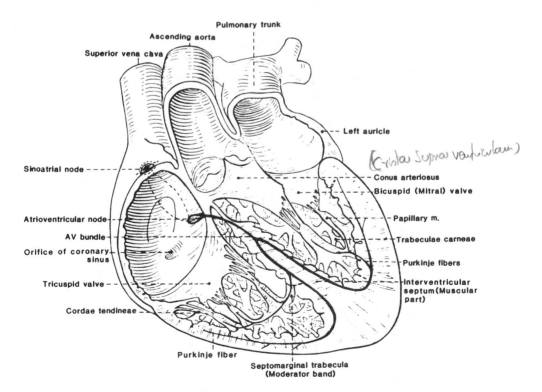

Figure 4.6. Internal anatomy of the heart and conducting system.

B. Internal Anatomy

1. Right Atrium

–its walls are relatively smooth except for the presence of the musculi pectinati.
–gives off the right auricular appendage.
–its pressure is normally slightly lesser than the left atrial pressure.

Musuli pectinati

a. *Right Auricle*

–is the conical muscular pouch of the superior extremity of the right atrium.
–covers the first part of the right coronary artery.

b. *Sinus Venarum (Cavarum)*

–is a smooth-walled portion of the right atrium, posterior and to the right of the crista terminalis by which it is separated from the rest of the atrium.
–represents the embryonic sinus venosus.
–receives the superior vena cava, inferior vena cava, coronary sinus, and anterior cardiac veins.

c. *Pectinate Muscles*

–are prominent bands of atrial myocardium located in the interior of both auricles and right atrium. The inner surface of the left atrium is smooth.

d. *Crista Terminalis*

–is a vertical muscular ridge running anteriorly along the right atrial wall from the opening of the superior vena cava to the inferior vena cava.
–represents the line of junction between the primitive sinus venosus and the right atrium proper.
–gives origin to the pectinate muscles, which run across the right atrial wall.
–is indicated externally by the sulcus terminalis.

e. *Venae Cordis Minimae*

–begins in the substance of the heart (endocardium and innermost layer of the myocardium).
–ends chiefly in the atria at **foramina venarum minimarum**.

f. *Fossa Ovalis*

–represents the position of the foramen ovale, through which blood runs from the right to the left atrium before birth.

2. Left Atrium

–lies more posterior than the right atrium.
–exhibits a smaller auricle, pectinate muscle, and venae cordis minimae.
–receives oxygenated blood through four pulmonary veins.

3. Right Ventricle

–normally makes up the major portion of the anterior surface of the heart.

—shows the following structures:

a. *Trabeculae Carneae*
   —are anastomosing muscular ridges of myocardium in the ventricles.

b. *Papillary Muscles*
   —are cone-shaped muscles enveloped by endocardium.
   —extend from the ventricular wall and their apices are attached to the chordae tendineae.
   —spring from the anterior and posterior walls and the septum.
   —prevent the cusps of the valve from being everted into the atrium by the pressure developed by the pumping action of the heart.

c. *Chordae Tendineae*
   —extend from the papillary muscles to the cusps.
   —prevent eversion of the valve during the ventricular contraction.

d. *Conus Arteriosus or Infundibulum* (Crista Supra ventricularis)
   —is the upper end of the right ventricle.
   —usually has smooth walls.
   —leads into the pulmonary orifice.

e. *Septomarginal Trabecula (Moderator Band)*
   —is an isolated trabecula of the bridge type.
   —extends from the interventricular septum to the base of the anterior papillary muscle of the right ventricle.
   —carries the right limb of the atrioventricular bundle from the septum to the sternocostal wall of the ventricle.

f. *Interventricular Septum*
   —gives an attachment of the septal cusp of the tricuspid valve.
   —is mostly muscular, though it has a small membranous upper part.
   —is the usual site of ventricular septal defects.

4. **Left Ventricle**
   —is divided into the left ventricle proper and the **aortic vestibule**, which is the upper and anterior part of the left ventricle and leads into the aorta.
   —shows the trabeculae carneae, two papillary muscles (anterior and posterior) with their cordae tendineae.
   —performs more work than the right; its wall usually measures twice as thick.
   —has a meshwork of muscular ridges called the trabeculae carneae.
   —contains the well-oxygenated blood.
   —is longer, narrower, and more conical in shape than the right ventricle.

C. Valves

1. **Pulmonary Valve**
   —lies behind the medial end of the third left costal cartilage and adjoining part of the sternum.

2. **Aortic Valve**
   —lies behind the left half of the sternum opposite the third intercostal space.

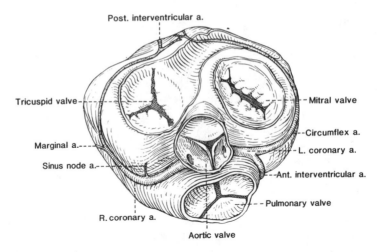

Figure 4.7. Superior view of the heart.

3. Tricuspid (Atrioventricular) Valve

Rt 4th intercostal space

—lies behind the right half of the sternum opposite the fourth intercostal space.
—has three cusps: an anterior, a posterior, and a septal.
—is covered by endocardium.
—is attached by the chordae tendineae to three papillary muscles that keep the valves against the pressure developed by the pumping action of the heart.

4. Mitral (Left Atrioventricular) Valve

Lt 4th Costal Cartilage

—lies behind the left half of the sternum opposite the fourth costal cartilage.
—is a bicuspid valve located at the left atrioventricular orifice.
—is similar to a bishop's mitre by Vesalius (16th century), and thus it is called the "mitral valve."
—makes a sound that is most audible at the apex of the heart over the left fifth intercostal space.

D. Heart Sound

—does not coincide with the anatomical position of the valve.
—for a particular valve is best heard in the area where its chamber is nearest to the chest wall and as far away as possible from the other valves.

1. Major Cause of Heart Sounds

a. *First ("Lubb") Heart Sound*

—is caused by the ventricular contraction and the closure of the tricuspid and bicuspid valves.

b. *Second ("Dupp") Heart Sound*

—is caused by the closure of the aortic and pulmonary valves.

2. Best Audible Place for Valve Sounds

a. *Mitral Valve Sound*

—is most audible over the left fifth intercostal space (apical region).

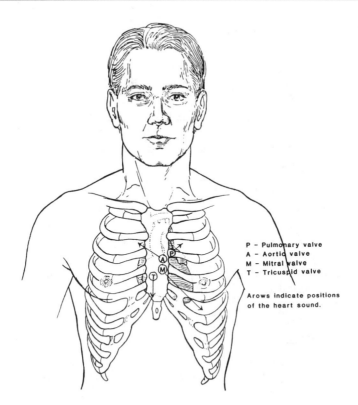

P – Pulmonary valve
A – Aortic valve
M – Mitral valve
T – Tricuspid valve

Arows indicate positions
of the heart sound.

Figure 4.8. Positions of valves of the heart and their sounds.

b. *Tricuspid Valve Sound*
–is most audible over the lower right part of the body of the sternum.

c. *Pulmonary Valve Sound*
–is most audible over the left second intercostal space.

d. *Aortic Valve Sound*
–is most audible over the right second intercostal space.

E. Conducting System

1. **Sinoatrial Node** → Supplied by Rt vagal and Rt Sympathetic Branch
   –is modified heart muscle.
   –initiates the heart beat and is called the "pacemaker."
   –lies in the myocardium at the cephalic end of the crista terminalis, near the opening of the superior vena cava.
   –is supplied by the sinus node artery, which is usually a branch of the right coronary artery.
   –gives rise to the atrioventricular bundle.

2. **Atrioventricular Node** — Left vagus and Left Sympathetic trunk.

Specialized Myocardium.

   –lies beneath the endocardium in the septal wall, above the opening of coronary sinus in the right atrium.
   –is supplied by the posterior interventricular artery branch of the right coronary artery.

—is supplied by autonomic nerve fibers, though the cardiac muscle fibers all lack motor endings.

3. Atrioventricular Bundle

—begins at the atrioventricular node.

—follows along the membranous septum.

—splits into right and left branches that descend into the interventricular septum and spread out into the ventricular walls.

—breaks up into terminal conducting fibers or Purkinje fibers.

F. Coronary Arteries

1. Right Coronary Artery

—arises from the anterior (right) aortic sinus and runs between the root of the pulmonary trunk and the right auricle.

—gives off branches to the right atrium and ventricle and also a marginal artery to the right ventricular wall.

—gives off a branch termed the **sinus node artery** that passes between the right atrium and the opening of the superior vena cava and supplies the sinuatrial node.

—is supplied by sensory and autonomic nerve fibers of the coronary plexuses.

2. Left Coronary Artery

—arises from the left aortic sinus, just above the aortic semilunar valve.

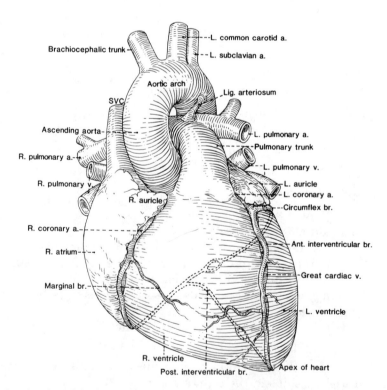

Figure 4.9. Anterior view of the heart with coronary arteries. *SVC,* superior vena cava.

–is larger (in diameter) than the right coronary artery.

–gives rise to the **circumflex** branch and **anterior interventricular** branch.

3. **Blood Flow in the Coronary Arteries**

–is maximal during diastole and minimal in systole, due to the compression of the arterial branches in the myocardium during systole.

G. Cardiac Veins and Coronary Sinus

1. **Coronary Sinus**

–lies in the posterior portion of the coronary sulcus.

–is the largest vein draining the heart.

–opens into the right atrium between the opening of the inferior vena cava and the atrioventricular opening.

–its one-cusp valve is located at the right margin of its aperature.

–receives the great, middle, and small cardiac veins; the oblique vein of the left atrium; and the posterior vein of the left ventricle.

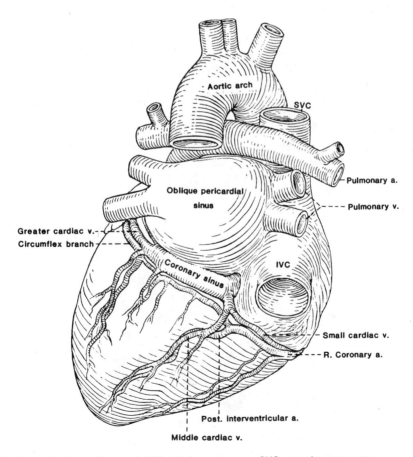

Figure 4.10. Posterior view of the heart. *IVC*, inferior vena cava; *SVC*, superior vena cava.

2. **Great Cardiac Vein**

   –begins at the apex of the heart, ascends in the anterior interventricular groove, and drains upward alongside the anterior interventricular branch of the left coronary artery.

   –turns to the left to lie in the coronary sulcus, and thus continues as the coronary sinus, encircling the pulmonary surface of the heart.

3. **Middle Cardiac Vein**

   –begins at the apex of the heart and ascends in the posterior interventricular groove, accompanying the posterior interventricular branch of the right coronary artery.

   –drains into the right end of the coronary sinus.

4. **Small Cardiac Vein**

   –runs along the right margin of the heart in company with the marginal artery.

   –runs posteriorly in the coronary sulcus to end in the right end of the coronary sinus.

5. **Oblique Vein of Left Atrium**

   –descends to empty into the left end of the coronary sinus.

6. **Anterior Cardiac Vein**

   –drains the anterior right ventricle.

   –crosses the coronary groove.

   –ends directly in the right atrium.

7. **Smallest Cardiac Veins (Venae Cordis Minimae)**

   –begin in wall of the heart and empty directly into its chambers.

H. **Lymphatic Vessels**

   –receive lymph from the myocardium and epicardium and follow the right coronary artery to empty into the anterior mediastinal nodes and follow the left coronary artery to empty into a node of the tracheobronchial group.

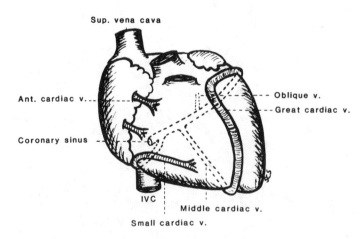

Figure 4.11. Anterior view of the heart. *IVC*, inferior vena cava.

I. Cardiac Plexus

- —receives the superior, middle, and inferior cervical and thoracic cardiac nerves from the sympathetic trunks and vagus nerves.
- —is divisible into the **superior cardiac plexus**, which lies beneath the arch of the aorta, in front of the pulmonary artery, and the **deep cardiac plexus**, which lies posterior to the arch of the aorta, in front of the bifurcation of the trachea.
- —gives branches to the atria, pulmonary plexuses, and coronary plexuses that distribute to the areas supplied by the arteries.
- —richly supplies the conducting system of the heart. (The cardiac muscle fibers are devoid of motor endings and are activated only by the conducting system.)
- —supplies the heart with sympathetic fibers, which increase the heart rate, and parasympathetic fibers, which decrease the heart rate.

J. Angina Pectoris

- —is characterized by attacks of chest pain originating in the heart.
- —is a pain felt beneath the sternum that often radiates to the left shoulder and down the arm.
- —is caused by an insufficient supply of oxygen to the heart muscle due to coronary arterial disease.
- —its pain impulses travel in visceral sensory fibers through the middle and inferior cervical and thoracic cardiac branches of the sympathetic nervous system before entering the thoracic segment of the spinal cord.

III. Special Features of Fetal Circulation

A. Foramen Ovale

- —is an opening in the septum secundum.
- —usually closes functionally at birth, but anatomical closure occurs later.
- —shunts blood from the right atrium into the left atrium before birth, without passing through the lung (pulmonary circulation).

B. Ductus Arteriosus

- —is derived from the sixth aortic arch.
- —connects the bifurcation of the pulmonary trunk with the aorta.
- —becomes functionally closed shortly after birth, but anatomical closure requires several weeks.
- —becomes the ligamentum arteriosum, which connects the left pulmonary artery (at its origin from the pulmonary trunk) to the concavity of the arch of the aorta.
- —shunts blood from the pulmonary trunk to the aorta before birth, bypassing the pulmonary circulation.

C. Ductus Venosus

- —shunts blood from the umbilical vein to the inferior vena cava before birth, without passing through the liver.
- —becomes the ligamentum venosum (fibrous cord), which joins the left branch of the portal vein to the inferior vena cava.

D. Placenta

- —serves the purpose of nutrition and excretion, receiving deoxygenated

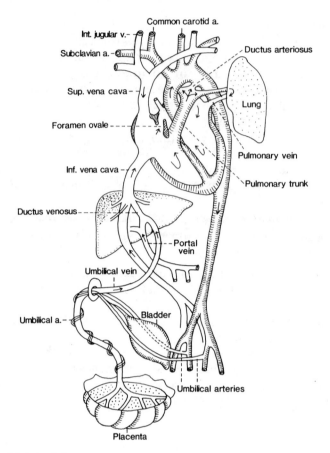

Figure 4.12. The fetal circulation.

blood from the fetus (through the umbilical artery) and returning it charged with oxygen and nutritive value material.

E. Tetralogy of Fallot

–is the most common form of cyanotic heart disease and consists of:

1. pulmonary stenosis.
2. ventricular septal defect.
3. overriding aorta (dextraposition of the aorta).
4. hypertrophy of the right ventricle.

Structures in Posterior Mediastinum

I. Posterior Mediastinum

–is bounded superiorly by the oblique plane of the first rib and inferiorly by an imaginary line running from the sternal angle to the disc between the fourth and fifth thoracic vertebrae.

–contains the azygos and hemiazygos veins, sympathetic trunk, vagus and splanchnic nerves, thoracic aorta, thoracic duct, esophagus, and posterior intercostal vessels.

II. Esophagus

—is a muscular tube, which is continuous with the pharynx in the neck and enters the thorax behind the trachea.

—has three constrictions: one at the level of the sixth cervical vertebra where it begins, one at the crossing of the left bronchus, and the third one at the tenth thoracic vertebra where it pierces the diaphragm.

—receives blood from three branches of the aorta (the inferior thyroid, bronchial, and esophageal arteries) as well as from the left gastric and inferior phrenic arteries.

III. Blood Vessels and Lymphatic Vessels

A. Thoracic Aorta

—begins at the level of the fourth thoracic vertebra.

—descends on the left side of the vertebral column and then approaches the median plane to end in front of the vertebral column by passing through the aortic hiatus of the diaphragm.

—gives off pericardial, bronchial, esophageal, mediastinal, posterior intercostal, subcostal, and superior phrenic branches.

B. Coarctation of Aorta

—takes place distal to the point of the entrance of the ductus arteriosus into the aorta, in which case an adequate collateral circulation develops before birth. If this condition occurs proximal to the origin of the left subclavian artery of ductus arteriosus, an adequate collateral circulation does not develop.

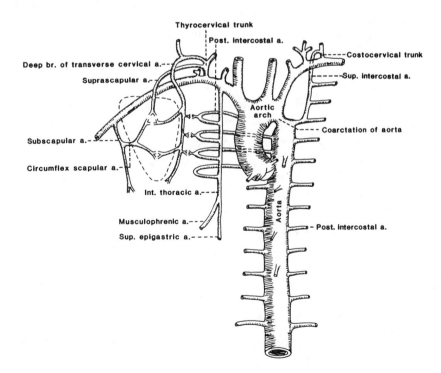

Figure 4.13. Coarctation of the aorta.

—results in tortuous and enlarged blood vessels, especially the internal thoracic, intercostal, epigastric and scapular arteries.

—results in an elevated blood pressure in the radial artery, with a decreased pressure in the femoral artery.

—results in the femoral pulse occurring after the radial pulse. (Normally, the femoral pulse occurs slightly before the radial pulse and is under about the same pressure.)

—is accompanied by the important collateral arterial circulation over the thorax which is as follows:

1. the anterior intercostal branches of the internal thoracic artery anastomose with posterior intercostal arteries.
2. the superior epigastric branch of the internal thoracic artery anastomoses with the inferior epigastric artery.
3. the posterior superior intercostal branch of the costocervical trunk anastomoses with the third posterior intercostal artery.
4. the posterior intercostal arteries anastomose with the descending scapular (or dorsal scapular) artery, which anastomoses with suprascapular and circumflex scapular arteries around the scapula.

C. Azygos Venous System

1. Azygos Vein

—receives the right posterior superior intercostal vein.

—is formed by the union of the right ascending lumbar and right subcostal veins.

—enters the thorax through the aortic opening of the diaphragm.

—arches over the root of the right lung.

—empties into the superior vena cava, of which it is the first tributary.

2. Hemiazygos Vein

—is formed by the junction of the left subcostal and ascending lumbar veins.

—ascends on the left side of the vertebral bodies behind the thoracic aorta, receiving the lower four posterior intercostal veins.

3. Accessory Hemiazygos Vein

—begins at the fourth intercostal space and receives the fourth to seventh or eighth intercostal veins.

—descends in front of the posterior intercostal arteries and terminates in the azygos vein.

4. Posterior Intercostal Vein

a. its first intercostal vein on each side drains into the corresponding brachiocephalic vein.

b. its second, third, and often fourth intercostal veins join to form the **superior intercostal vein**, which drains into the azygos vein on the right and into the brachiocephalic vein on the left.

c. the rest of the vein drains into the azygos vein on the right and the hemiazygos or accessory hemiazygos vein on the left.

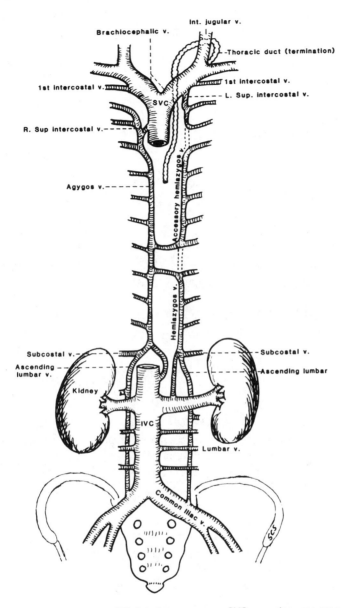

Figure 4.14. The azygos venous system. *IVC*, inferior vena cava. *SVC*, superior vena cava.

D. Thoracic Duct

—begins in the abdomen at the cisterna chyli, which is the dilated junction of the intestinal, lumbar, and descending intercostal trunks.

—drains the lower limbs, pelvis, abdomen, left thorax, left upper limb, and left side of head and neck.

—passes through the aortic opening of the diaphragm.

—ascends through the posterior mediastinum between the aorta and azygos vein.

—arches over the cupula of the left pleura to lie posterior to the left sub-clavian vein.

—empties usually into the junction of the left internal jugular and subcla-vian veins.

IV. Nerves

A. Sympathetic Trunk

—descends in front of the neck of the ribs and the posterior intercostal vessels.

—shows the cervicothoracic or stellate ganglion, which is formed by the fusion of the inferior cervical ganglion with the first thoracic ganglion.

—enters the abdomen through the crus of the diaphragm or behind the medial lumbocostal arch.

—gives rise to cardiac, pulmonary, mediastinal, and splanchnic branches.

—is connected to the thoracic spinal nerves by rami communicantes, gray and white.

1. Rami Communicantes

a. *Gray Rami Communicantes*

—contain postganglionic sympathetic fibers that supply the blood ves-sels, sweat glands, and hair follicles.

—contain fibers whose cell bodies are located in the sympathetic trunk.

—are connected to every spinal nerve.

b. *White Rami Communicantes*

—contain preganglionic sympathetic fibers whose cell bodies are lo-cated in the lateral horn of the spinal cord, and visceral afferent fibers whose cell bodies are located in the spinal (dorsal root) gan-glia.

—are limited to the spinal cord segments between T1 and L2.

2. Splanchnic Nerves

—contain largely preganglionic sympathetic fibers whose cell bodies are located in the lateral horn of the spinal cord, and visceral afferent fibers whose cell bodies are located in the dorsal root ganglia.

a. *Greater Splanchnic Nerve*

—arises usually from the fifth through ninth thoracic ganglia, per-forates the crus of the diaphragm or occasionally passes through the aortic hiatus, and ends in the celiac ganglion.

b. *Lesser Splanchnic Nerve*

—is usually derived from the tenth and eleventh thoracic ganglia, pierces the crus of the diaphragm, and ends in the aorticorenal ganglion.

c. *Least Splanchnic Nerve*

—is usually derived from the twelfth thoracic ganglion, pierces the crus of the diaphragm, and ends in the renal plexus.

b. Vagus Nerve

–its right one crosses anterior to the right subclavian artery, runs posterior to the superior vena cava, and descends at the right surface of the trachea and then posterior to the right main bronchus.

–its left one enters the thorax between the left common carotid and subclavian arteries and behind the left brachiocephalic vein, and descends on the arch of the aorta.

–gives off the thoracic cardiac branches, breaks up into the pulmonary plexuses, and then continues into the esophageal plexus.

–forms the vagal trunks (or gastric nerves) at the lower part of the esophagus and enters the abdomen through the esophageal hiatus.

–can be cut at the lower portion of the esophagus (vagotomy) to reduce gastric secretion in the treatment of peptic ulcer.

–also gives off:

1. Recurrent Laryngeal Nerve

–hooks around the subclavian artery on the right and around the arch of the aorta (lateral to the ligamentum arteriosum) on the left.

–ascends in the groove between the trachea and the esophagus.

–may be damaged on the left by an **aneurysm** of the aortic arch, leading to coughing, hoarseness, and paralysis of the ipsilateral vocal cord.

Review Test

THORAX

DIRECTIONS: For each of the questions or incomplete statements below, **one** or **more** of the answers or completions are correct. Choose answer:

A. if only **1**, **2**, and **3** are correct.
B. if only **1** and **3** are correct.
C. if only **2** and **4** are correct.
D. if only **4** is correct.
E. if all are correct.

4.1. The sternal angle is at a level where

1. the second rib articulates with the sternum.
2. the trachea bifurcates into the right and left bronchi.
3. the aortic arch both begins and ends.
4. the inferior border of the superior mediastinum is demarcated.

4.2. Assuming the arterial supply to the heart is normal, if the circumflex branch of the left coronary artery is blocked by a blood clot, which portion of the heart musculature would most likely be ischemic?

1. anterior portion of left ventricle.
2. anterior interventricular region.
3. posterior interventricular region.
4. posterior portion of left ventricle.

4.3. The ductus arteriosus

1. is anatomically closed about 3 months after birth.
2. carries poorly oxygenated blood during prenatal life.
3. is derived from the sixth aortic arch.
4. connects the left pulmonary vein with the aorta.

4.4. The thoracic duct

1. originates from the cisterna chyli in the abdomen.
2. passes upward through the aortic opening in the diaphragm.
3. drains into the junction of the left internal jugular vein and the left subclavian vein.
4. receives drainage from the right cervical lymph nodes.

4.5. The right lung

1. has 10 bronchopulmonary segments.
2. usually receives a single bronchial artery.
3. has three lobar (secondary) bronchi.
4. has a lingula, which is a tongue-shaped portion of its upper lobe.

4.6. The following nerves supply muscles that participate in forced inspiration:

1. intercostal nerves.
2. nerve to the scalenus anterior muscle.
3. medial pectoral nerve.
4. spinal accessory nerve.

4.7. Muscles that function to elevate the ribs in inspiration are

1. the sternocleidomastoid.
2. the scalenus anterior.
3. the external intercostals.
4. the internal intercostals.

146

4.8. Expiration can be accomplished by
1. elastic contraction of the lung.
2. contraction of muscles that elevate the rib cage.
3. contraction of the abdominal muscles.
4. contraction of the diaphragm.

4.9. More than the normal amount of blood could be found in the right ventricle if
1. the pulmonary artery was constricted (stenosed).
2. the left atrioventricular opening was abnormally small.
3. the pulmonary valves would not close properly.
4. the right atrioventricular opening was abnormally large.

4.10. Of the following structures, which are found in the superior mediastinum?
1. the brachiocephalic veins.
2. the trachea.
3. part of the left common carotid artery.
4. the arch of the aorta.

4.11. The posterior intercostal veins are tributaries to
1. the intervertebral veins.
2. the azygos veins.
3. the left subclavian vein.
4. the brachiocephalic veins.

4.12. Of the following, which are true statements?
1. The part of the heart that presents the greatest surface area of the sternocostal surface of the thorax is the left ventricle.
2. The right main bronchus forms a less acute angle with the trachea than does the left.
3. Normally, the anterior interventricular artery of the heart is a branch of the right coronary artery.
4. The septomarginal trabecula (moderator band) leads to the base of the anterior papillary muscle of the right ventricle.

4.13. The third rib articulates posteriorly with the
1. transverse process of the third thoracic vertebra.
2. body of the second thoracic vertebra.
3. body of the third thoracic vertebra.
4. transverse process of the second thoracic vertebra.

4.14. The right primary (or main) bronchus
1. is larger in diameter than the left one.
2. receives more foreign bodies through the trachea.
3. gives rise to the eparterial bronchus.
4. is longer than the left one.

4.15. The azygos vein
1. receives the left superior intercostal vein.
2. receives the right superior intercostal vein.
3. empties directly into the right brachiocephalic vein.
4. empties directly into the superior vena cava.

4.16. The phrenic nerve
1. enters the thorax by passing in front of the subclavian vein.
2. passes anterior to the root of the lung in its course through the thorax.
3. contains only the somatic motor nerve fibers.
4. supplies the pericardium and diaphragm.

4.17. The left recurrent laryngeal nerve
1. hooks below the aortic arch distal to the ligamentum arteriosum.
2. ascends into the neck, passing in front of the subclavian artery.
3. may be damaged by aortic aneurysms, leading to hoarseness.
4. forms the major part of the esophageal plexus.

4.18. The left vagus nerve
1. enters the thorax, passing in front of the left subclavian artery.
2. contributes to the anterior esophageal plexus.
3. forms the anterior vagal trunk or anterior gastric nerve at the lower part of the esophagus.
4. can be cut on the lower part of the esophagus to reduce gastric secretion.

4.19. The myocardial infarction within the interventricular septum may result in
1. a tricuspid valve insufficiency.
2. a pulmonary valve insufficiency.
3. a defect in conduction of cardiac impulses.
4. a mitral valve insufficiency.

4.20. Changes that take place in the circulation at (and after) birth normally include
1. an increased blood flow through the lungs.
2. a closure of the ductus arteriosus.
3. an increased left atrial pressure.
4. a closure of the foramen ovale.

DIRECTIONS: Each set of lettered headings below is followed by a list of numbered words or phrases. Choose answer:

    A. if the item is associated with **A** only.
    B. if the item is associated with **B** only.
    C. if the item is associated with both **A** and **B**.
    D. if the item is associated with neither **A** nor **B**.

    A. Oblique sinus
    B. Transverse sinus
    C. Both
    D. Neither

4.21. Is a subdivision of the pericardial cavity.

4.22. Lies largely between the visceral pericardium on the dorsal surface of the left atrium and parietal pericardium.

4.23. The aorta and pulmonary artery lie immediately anterior to this sinus near their origin from the heart.

4.24. The phrenic nerve passes through this sinus.

4.25. The esophagus is separated from this sinus by parietal pericardium.

    A. Right ventricle
    B. Left ventricle
    C. Both
    D. Neither

4.26. Normally makes up the major portion of the anterior surface of the heart.

4.27. This chamber has trabeculae carneae in its wall.

4.28. The mitral valve separates this chamber from its corresponding atrium.

4.29. The coronary sinus opens into this chamber.

4.30. Highly oxygenated blood is found in this chamber.

    A. Gray ramus
    B. White ramus
    C. Both
    D. Neither

4.31. Contains sympathetic postganglionic nerve fibers.

4.32. Is found *only* in the thoracic and upper lumbar region.

4.33. Afferent fibers from the viscera pass through this structure to the central nervous system.

4.34. Contains preganglionic parasympathetic neurons.

4.35. Postganglionic fibers forming this structure innervate the sweat glands.

    A. Ventricular systole
    B. Ventricular diastole
    C. Both
    D. Neither

4.36. The period of maximum blood flow to the myocardium.

4.37. Contraction of the atria occurs during this part of the cycle.

4.38. The pressure in the aorta is less than that in the left ventricle during this part of the cycle.

4.39. Transmission of the impulse from the sinoatrial node to the atrioventricular node occurs during this part of the cycle.

4.40. Contraction of the papillary muscles occurs during this part of the cycle.

A. Pulmonary valve
B. Aortic valve
C. Both
D. Neither

4.41. Normally consists of two cusps.

4.42. Is best heard through a stethoscope in the second intercostal space at the left border of the sternum.

4.43. Is the first to close at the end of the systole.

4.44. Is situated closer to the anterior surface of the heart.

4.45. Lies anterior to transverse sinus of pericardium.

DIRECTIONS: For each numbered item, select the *one* lettered heading that is most closely associated with it. Each lettered heading may be selected once, more than once, or not at all.

A. Vagus nerve
B. Phrenic nerve
C. Sympathetic trunk
D. Left recurrent laryngeal nerve
E. Greater splanchnic nerve

4.46. Breaks up into a plexus on the esophagus superior to the diaphragm.

4.47. Loops around the arch of the aorta near the ligamentum arteriosum.

4.48. Arises in the posterior mediastinum and enters the celiac ganglion.

4.49 Lies between the fibrous pericardium and parietal mediastinal pleura during part of its course.

4.50. Connected to the intercostal nerves by white and gray rami.

DIRECTIONS: Select the *one* numbered heading that is most closely associated with a question. Each numbered heading may be selected once, more than once, or not at all. Diagram of the heart valves, their cusps, and the coronary arteries, showing their usual position in situ.

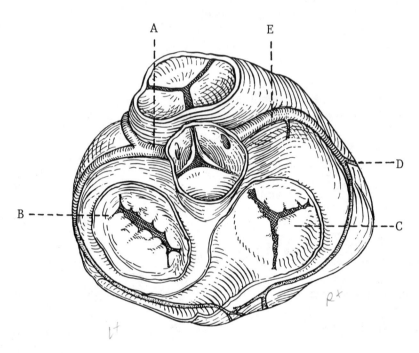

4.51.   Runs toward the apex of the heart and supply arterial blood to the anterior part of the right ventricle.

4.52.   Supply arterial blood to the sinoatrial node.

4.53.   Arises from the left aortic sinus.

4.54.   Provides the anterior interventricular artery.

4.55.   Is best heard through a stethoscope in the left fifth intercostal space at the midclavicular line (or nipple line).

A. Right atrium
B. Left atrium
C. Right ventricle
D. Left ventricle
E. Auricle

4.56.   The valve through which blood leaves this chamber can be auscultated (listened to) over the second left intercostal space just lateral to the sternum.

4.57.   Receives blood from the anterior cardiac veins.

4.58.   The apex of the heart is associated with this chamber.

4.59.   Would initially become enlarged as a result of coarctation (narrowing) of the aorta.

4.60.   The sinoatrial node is in the wall of this chamber.

A. Crista terminalis
B. Septomarginal trabecula
C. Chordae tendineae
D. Pectinate muscle
E. Anulus fibrosus

4.61. Contracts to maintain constant tension on the cusps. *C*

4.62. Gives an attachment of the cusps of the atrioventricular valves. *E*

4.63. *B* Extends from the interventricular septum to the base of the anterior papillary muscle of the right ventricle.

A **4.64.** Is a vertical muscular ridge, representing the line of junction between the primitive sinus venosus and the atrium proper.

B **4.65.** Contains Purkinje fibers from the right limb of the atrioventricular bundle.

DIRECTIONS: Each of the questions or incomplete statements below is followed by suggested answers or completions. Choose the *one* that is *best* in each case.

4.66. The posterior intercostal arteries
A. arise from esophageal branches of the aorta.
B. supply blood to the visceral pleura of the lung.
C. are embedded in the parietal pleura.
D. are accompanied by veins.
E. do not anastomose with branches of the internal thoracic artery.

4.67. The ligamentum arteriosum
A. is located on the visceral surface of the liver.
B. connects the left umbilical vein to the left portal vein.
C. connects the left pulmonary artery to the aortic arch.
D. becomes the median umbilical ligament in the adult.
E. becomes the round ligament of the liver in the adult.

4.68. If the borders of the normal heart are projected onto the surface of the chest, the apex is found
A. at the level of the xiphoid process of the sternum.
B. at the level of the sternal angle.
C. in the left fifth intercostal space.
D. in the right fifth intercostal space.
E. in the left fourth intercostal space.

4.69. Normal, quiet expiration is achieved by contraction of the following:
A. extensible tissue in the thoracic wall and lungs.
B. the posterior superior serratus muscles.
C. the pectoralis major muscle.
D. abdominal muscles.
E. the rhomboid muscles.

4.70. Fibers in the greater splanchnic nerves are primarily
A. somatic afferent and preganglionic visceral efferent.
B. visceral afferent and postganglionic visceral efferent.
C. visceral afferent and preganglionic visceral efferent.
D. somatic efferent and postganglionic visceral efferent.
E. visceral afferent and somatic efferent.

4.71. Identify the correct statement:
A. Some anterior intercostal arteries are branches of the costocervical trunk.
B. All posterior intercostal arteries are direct branches of the aorta.
C. The upper two posterior intercostal arteries are branches of the internal thoracic artery.
D. The anterior intercostal arteries are either direct or indirect branches of the internal thoracic artery.
E. The highest posterior intercostal arteries are branches of the thyrocervical trunk of the subclavian artery.

4.72. White rami communicantes contain
A. preganglionic efferent fibers only.
B. postganglionic efferent fibers only.
C. preganglionic efferent and postganglionic efferent fibers only.
D. preganglionic efferent and visceral afferent fibers only.
E. preganglionic efferent, postganglionic efferent, and visceral afferent fibers only.

4.73. The mitral (left atrioventricular) valve can be heard best

A. in the left fifth intercostal space approximately 3 1/2 inches from the midline.
B. over the medial end of the second left intercostal space.
C. over the medial end of the second right intercostal space.
D. over the right half of the lower end of the body of the sternum.
E. none of the above.

4.74. Select the correct statement.

A. The great cardiac vein is the companion vein to the posterior descending interventricular artery.
B. The middle cardiac vein is the companion vein to the anterior descending interventricular artery.
C. Anterior cardiac veins end directly in the chamber of the right atrium.
D. The small cardiac vein is a companion vein to the circumflex branch of the left coronary artery.
E. None of the above.

4.75. The sternocostal surface of the heart is made up in a large part by the

A. left atrium.
B. right atrium.
C. left ventricle.
D. right ventricle.
E. base of the heart.

4.76. The opening between the right atrium and the right ventricle is guarded by the

A. pulmonary semilunar valves.
B. mitral valve.
C. valve of the coronary sinus.
D. tricuspid valve.
E. aortic semilunar valves.

4.77. The conductive tissue of the heart known as the cardiac pacemaker is the

A. atrioventricular bundle (of His).
B. atrioventricular node.
C. sinoatrial node.
D. Perkinje fibers.
E. moderator band.

4.78. The heart is situated in the

A. superior mediastinum.
B. anterior mediastinum.
C. middle mediastinum.
D. posterior mediastinum.
E. none of these.

4.79. The middle lobe bronchus on the right side leads to the following bronchopulmonary segments:

A. medial and lateral.
B. anterior and posterior.
C. anterior basal and medial basal.
D. anterior basal and posterior basal.
E. none of the above.

4.80. The eparterial bronchus is the

A. left superior bronchus.
B. left inferior bronchus.
C. right superior bronchus.
D. right middle bronchus.
E. right inferior bronchus.

Answers and Explanations

THORAX

4.1. E. The sternal angle is the junction of the manubrium and the body of the sternum and is located at the level where: (*a*) the second rib articulates with the sternum; (*b*) the trachea bifurcates into the right and left bronchi; (*c*) the aortic arch both begins and ends; (*d*) the inferior border of the superior mediastinum is demarcated.

4.2. D. The circumflex branch of the left coronary artery supplies the posterior portion of the left ventricle. The right coronary artery gives rise to the marginal branch, which supplies the anterior portion of the left ventricle, and the posterior interventricular artery, which supplies the septum and the adjacent ventricles.

4.3. A. The ductus arteriosus is derived from the sixth aortic arch. The anterior interventricular artery arises from the left coronary artery. It connects the bifurcation of the pulmonary trunk with the aorta but it becomes the ligamentum arteriosum after birth, which connects the arch to the left pulmonary artery. The ductus arteriosus becomes functionally closed shortly after birth but anatomical closure requires several weeks or months. It carries poorly oxygenated blood during prenatal life.

4.4. A. The thoracic duct has a lower dilated end, called the cisterna chyli, passes through the aortic opening of the diaphragm, ascends between the aorta and the azygos vein, and empties into the junction of the left internal jugular and subclavian vein. The thoracic duct drains most of the lymph in the body except for that of the left head and neck, the left upper limb, and the left thorax.

4.5. A. The right lung is divided into upper, middle, and lower lobes by the oblique and horizontal fissures. Thus, the right lung has three lobar (secondary) bronchi and 10 lobar bronchopulmonary segments. The left lung has a lingula, which is a tongue-shaped portion of its upper lobe.

4.6. E. The muscles of expiration include the diaphragm, the external intercostals, the sternocleidomastoid, the scalenus muscles, the pectoralis muscles, the erector spinae, the serratus anterior, scapular elevators, etc.

4.7. A. The ribs are elevated in inspiration by the sternocleidomastoid, scalenus anterior, external intercostal muscles. The internal intercostal muscles are muscles of expiration and elevate the ribs.

4.8. B. The muscles of expiration include abdominal muscles, internal intercostals, and serratus posterior inferior.

4.9. E. The right ventricular hypertrophy may occur as a result of pulmonary stenosis, pulmonary and tricuspid valve defects, and mitral valve stenosis.

4.10. E. The superior mediastinum contains the brachiocephalic vein, the trachea, part of the left common carotid artery, the arch of the aorta, etc.

4.11. C. The first posterior intercostal vein drains into the corresponding brachiocephalic vein. The second, third, and fourth posterior intercostal veins join to form the superior intercostal vein, which drains into the azygos vein on the right and into the brachiocephalic vein on the left. The rest of the posterior intercostal veins drain into the azygos vein on the right and into the hemiazygos or accessory hemiazygos vein on the left.

4.12. C. The greatest area of the sternocostal surface of the thorax is the right ventricle. The anterior ventricular artery of the heart is a branch of the left coronary artery.

4.13. A. The third rib articulates posteriorly with the transverse process and body of the third vertebra and the body of the second vertebra.

4.14. A. The right primary (or main) bronchus is larger in diameter than the left one, receives more foreign bodies through the trachea, gives rise to the eparterial bronchus, and is shorter than the left one.

4.15. C. The left superior intercostal vein drains into the left brachiocephalic vein, whereas the right superior intercostal vein drains into the azygos vein.

4.16. C. The phrenic nerve descends behind the subclavian vein, passes anterior to the root of the lung, and supplies the pericardium and diaphragm. It contains somatic efferent, somatic afferent, and visceral efferent (postganglionic sympathetic) fibers.

4.17. B. The left recurrent laryngeal nerve hooks around the aortic arch lateral to the ligamentum arteriosum, and thus it may be damaged by aneurysm of the aortic arch, resulting in paralysis of the laryngeal muscles. This nerve ascends behind the subclavian artery and lies in a groove between the trachea and the esophagus. The major part of the esophageal plexus if formed by the vagus nerves.

4.18. E. The left vagus nerve enters the thorax in front of the left subclavian artery but behind the left brachiocephalic vein. It passes behind the left bronchus and breaks up into the pulmonary plexus and continues to form an esophageal plexus. The vagus nerves loose their identity in this plexus. At the lower end of the esophagus, branches of the plexus reunite to form an anterior vagal trunk or anterior gastric nerve which can be cut (vagotomy) to reduce gastric secretion.

4.19. B. The tricuspid valve has three cusps: anterior, posterior, and septal. The septal cusp lies on the margin of the orifice adjacent to the interventricular septum. The atrioventricular bundle descends into the interventricular septum. The pulmonary and mitral valves are not closely associated with the interventricular septum.

4.20. E. At or soon after birth, the following changes in the circulation occur. The umbilical arteries, umbilical vein, and ductus venosus become obliterated. Functional closure of the ductus arteriosus and the foramen ovale occur soon after birth but anatomical closure requires weeks or months. Blood flow through the lung as well as left atrial pressure are increased.

4.21. C. Both the oblique and transverse sinuses are subdivisions of the pericardial cavity.

4.22. A. The oblique pericardial sinus is a recess between the visceral pericardium on the dorsal surface of the left atrium and parietal pericardium, and between the right and left pulmonary veins.

4.23. B. The transverse pericardial sinus is a recess posterior to the aorta and pulmonary trunk and anterior to the atria.

4.24. D. The phrenic nerve descends through the thoracic cavity between the mediastinal pleura and the pericardium.

4.25. A. The oblique sinus of pericardium is separated from the esophagus by parietal pericardium.

4.26. A. The right ventricle forms the major portion of the anterior surface of the heart.

4.27. C. The trabeculae carneae are muscular ridges covering the walls of the ventricles of the heart.

4.28. B. The mitral valve is a bicuspid valve located at the left atrioventricular orifice.

4.29. D. The coronary sinus opens into the right atrium.

4.30. B. The left ventricle receives highly oxygenated blood from the lungs.

4.31. A. The gray rami contain postganglionic sympathetic fibers, whose cell bodies are located in the sympathetic chain ganglia.

4.32. B. The white rami are limited to the spinal cord segments between T1 and L2, whereas the gray rami are connected to every spinal nerve.

4.33. B. The white rami contain visceral afferent fibers whose cell bodies are located in the dorsal root ganglia.

4.34. D. The gray and white rami contain no parasympathetic fibers.

4.35. A. The gray rami contain postganglionic sympathetic fibers that innervate the sweat glands, the arrector pilli muscles of the hair follicles, and the smooth muscle of blood vessels.

4.36. B. The maximum blood flow to the myocardium occurs during ventricular diastole.

4.37. B. The atria are contracted during the ventricular diastole.

4.38. A. The pressure in the ventricles is much higher than in the atria during the ventricular systole.

4.39. B. The impulse is transmitted from the sinoatrial node to the atrioventricular node during ventricular diastole.

4.40. A. The papillary muscles are contracted during the ventricular systole.

4.41. D. The pulmonary and aortic valves are semilunar valves, consisting of three cusps.

4.42. A. The pulmonary valve lies behind the medial end of the third left costal cartilage and adjoining part of the sternum, but it is most audible in the second intercostal space at the left border of the sternum.

4.43. B. The aortic valve is the first to close at the end of the ventricular systole.

4.44. A. The pulmonary valve is situated closer to the anterior surface of the heart.

4.45. C. Both the aortic and pulmonary valves lie anterior to the transverse pericardial sinus.

4.46. A. The vagus nerves break up into the esophageal plexus, after they leave the pulmonary plexus.

4.47. D. The left recurrent laryngeal nerve loops inferior to the arch of the aorta to the left of the ligamentum arteriosum.

4.48. E. The greater splanchnic nerve arises from the fifth through ninth thoracic sympathetic ganglia in the posterior mediastinum, pierces the crus of the diaphragm, and ends in the celiac ganglion.

4.49. B. The phrenic nerve descends between the fibrous pericardium and the mediastinal pleura.

4.50. C. The gray rami connect the sympathetic trunk to every spinal nerve, but the white rami are limited to the spinal cord segments between T1 and L2. The intercostal nerves are ventral primary rami of the thoracic nerves.

4.51. D. The marginal branch of the right coronary artery supplies the anterior wall of the right ventricle.

4.52. E. The right coronary artery gives off the sinus node artery to supply the sinoatrial node. The posterior interventricular artery, a branch of the right coronary artery, gives off a branch to supply the atrioventricular node.

4.53. A. The left coronary artery arises from the left aortic sinus.

4.54. A. The left coronary artery provides the anterior interventricular artery.

4.55. B. The mitral valve is best heard through a stethoscope in the left fifth intercostal space at the midclavicular (or nipple) line.

4.56. C. The pulmonary valve, through which blood leaves the right ventricle, can be auscultated (listened to) over the second left intercostal space just lateral to the sternum.

4.57. A. The right atrium receives blood from the anterior cardiac vein.

4.58. D. The apex of the heart is formed by the tip of the left ventricle and located in the left fifth intercostal space.

4.59. D. The left ventricle would initially become enlarged as a result of coarctation of the aorta.

4.60. A. The sinoatrial node lies in the myocardium of the posterior wall, near the opening of the superior vena cava, of the right atrium.

4.61. C. The cordae tendineae are tendinous strands that extend from the papillary muscles to the cusps and contract to maintain constant tension on the cusps during the ventricular contraction.

4.62. E. The anulus fibrosus is a fibrous ring that surrounds the atrioventricular orifice and gives an attachment of the cusps of the atrioventricular valves.

4.63. B. The septomarginal trabecula is a moderator band that extends from the interventricular septum to the base of the anterior papillary muscle of the right ventricle.

4.64. A. The crista terminalis is a muscular ridge, representing the line of junction between the sinus venarum and the remainder of the right atrium. It is indicated externally by the sulcus terminalis.

4.65. B. The septomarginal trabecula carries the right branch of the atrioventricular bundle from the septum to the opposite wall of the ventricle.

4.66. D. The posterior intercostal arteries arise from the abdominal aorta except for the upper two, which arise from the superior intercostal artery of the costocervical trunk. They run between the internal and innermost intercostal muscles in company with the posterior intercostal vein and nerve and anastomose with the anterior intercostal branches of the internal thoracic artery.

4.67. C. The ductus arteriosus connects the aortic arch to the bifurcation of the pulmonary trunk, but the ligamentum arteriosum connects the aortic arch to the left pulmonary artery. The ligamentum venosum is the fibrous remnant of the ductus venosus and is located between the left lobe and the caudate lobe on the ventral surface of the liver. The left umbilical vein becomes the round ligament of the liver in the adult.

4.68. C. The apex of the heart is found in the fifth left intercostal space.

4.69. A. Normal quiet expiration is achieved by contraction of extensible tissue in the lungs and thoracic wall. The posterior superior serratus, pectoralis major, and rhomboid muscles are muscles of inspiration. The abdominal muscles contract in forced expiration.

4.70. C. The greater splanchnic nerve contains visceral afferent and preganglionic sympathetic fibers.

4.71. D. The upper two posterior intercostal arteries are branches of the highest (or superior) posterior intercostal artery of the costocervical trunk. The rest of the posterior intercostal arteries are branches of the aorta. The internal thoracic artery gives rise to anterior intercostal arteries in the first six intercostal spaces and ends at the sixth intercostal space by dividing into the superior epigastric artery and the musculophrenic artery, which gives off anterior intercostal arteries in the seventh, eighth, ninth, and tenth intercostal spaces.

4.72. D. The white rami communicantes contain preganglionic sympathetic fibers and visceral afferent fibers.

4.73. A. The apex beat of the heart is produced by the mitral valve and is most audible over the fifth intercostal space.

4.74. C. The great cardiac vein accompanies the anterior interventricular artery. The middle cardiac vein accompanies the posterior interventricular artery. The anterior cardiac veins drain into the right atrium. The small cardiac vein accompanies the right marginal artery.

4.75. D. The right ventricle forms a large part of the sternocostal surface of the heart.

4.76. D. The opening between the right atrium and ventricle is guarded by the tricuspid valve.

4.77. C. The sinoatrial node initiates the impulse of contraction and is known as the pacemaker of the heart.

4.78. C. The heart is situated in the middle mediastinum.

4.79. A. The right middle lobe bronchus leads to the medial and lateral bronchopulmonary segments.

4.80. C. The eparterial bronchus is the right superior lobar (secondary) bronchus, whereas all others are the hyparterial bronchi.

5
Abdomen

Anterior Abdominal Wall

I. Muscles

Muscle	Origin	Insertion	Nerve	Action
External oblique abdominis	External surface of lower eight ribs	Medial half of iliac crest; anterior superior iliac spine; pubic tubercle; linea alba	Thoracoabdominal and subcostal n. (T7-12)	Compresses abdomen; flexes trunk; active in forced expiration
Internal oblique abdominis	Lateral two-thirds of inguinal ligament; iliac crest; throacolumbar fascia	Lower four costal caritlages; linea alba; pubic crest; pectineal line	Thoracoabdominal and subcostal n. (T7-L1)	Compresses abdomen; flexes trunk; active in forced expiration
Transversus abdominis	Lateral third of inguinal ligament; iliac crest; throacolumbar fascia; lower six costal cartilages	Linea alba; pubic crest; pectineal line	Thoracoabdominal and subcostal n. (T7-L1)	Compresses abdomen; depresses ribs
Rectus abdominis	Pubic crest and symphysis pubis	Xiphoid process and five to seven costal cartilages	Thoracoabdominal and subcostal n. (T7-L1)	Depresses ribs; flexes trunk
Pyramidalis	Body of pubis	Linea alba	Subcostal n. (T12)	Tenses linea alba
Cremaster	Middle of inguinal ligament; lower margin of internal oblique muscle	Tubercle and crest of pubis	Genitofemoral n.	Retracts testis

II. Fasciae

A. Camper's Fascia (Superficial Layer of Superficial Fascia)

    —is a superficial layer of the subcutaneous tissue of the lower abdomen, which is predominantly a fatty layer.

    —continues over the inguinal ligament as the superficial fascia of the thigh.

    —continues over the pubis and perineum as the superficial layer of the superficial perineal fascia.

B. Scarpa's Fascia (Deep Layer of Superficial Fascia)

    –is a membranous layer of the subcutaneous tissue of the lower abdomen.
    –is attached to the fascia lata just below the inguinal ligament.
    –continues over the pubis and perineum as the membranous layer (Colles')
    of the superficial perineal fascia.
    –continues over the penis as the superficial fascia of the penis.
    –continues over the scrotum as the Dartos tunic, which contains smooth
    muscle.

C. Deep Fascia

    –is the fascia covering the muscles.
    –continues over the spermatic cord at the superficial inguinal ring as the
    external spermatic fascia.
    –continues over the penis as the deep fascia of the penis (Buck's fascia).
    –continues over the pubis and perineum as the deep perineal fascia.

D. Linea Alba

    –is the tendinous medial margin of the rectus abdominis, extending from
    the xiphoid process to the pubic symphysis.
    –gives attachment to the oblique and transverse abdominal muscles.

E. Linea Semilunaris

    –marks the lateral border of the rectus abdominis muscle.

F. Linea Semicircularis (Arcuate Line)

    –is a crescent-shaped line marking the termination of the posterior sheath
    of the rectus abdominis muscle just below the level of the iliac crest.

G. Lacunar Ligament

    –represents the medial triangular expansion of the inguinal ligament to
    the pecten pubis.
    –is continuous with the inguinal ligament from the pubic tubercle along
    the pecten of the pubis.
    –forms the medial border of the femoral ring.
    –extends laterally along the pecten to form the pectineal ligament.

H. Pectineal Ligament (Cooper's)

    –is a strong fibrous band that extends laterally from the lacunar ligament
    along the pectineal line of the pubis.
    –is fused with the periosteum of the superior ramus of the pubis.

I. Inguinal Ligament

    –is the folded lower border of the aponeurosis of the external oblique mus-
    cle.
    –extends between the anterior superior iliac spine and the pubic tubercle.

J. Reflected Inguinal Ligament

    –is formed by certain fibers of the inguinal ligament reflected from the
    pubic tubercle upward toward the linea alba.
    –also has some reflection from the lacunar ligament.

K. Conjoint Tendon (Falx Inguinalis)

    –is formed by the aponeuroses of the internal oblique and transverse ab-
    dominis muscles.
    –strengthens the posterior wall of the medial half of the inguinal canal.

L. Rectus Sheath

–is formed by the fusion of the aponeuroses of the external oblique, internal oblique, and transversus abdominis muscles.
–encloses the rectus abdominis and sometimes the pyramidalis.
–also contains the superior and inferior epigastric vessels and the ventral primary rami of the thoracic nerves 17–12.
–consists of an anterior and a posterior sheath.

1. Anterior Layer

a. above the arcuate line—aponeuroses of the external and internal oblique abdominis muscles.
b. below the arcuate line—aponeuroses of the external oblique, internal oblique, and transversus abdominis muscles.

2. Posterior Layer

a. at the level of the xiphoid—aponeuroses of the transversus abdominis muscle.
b. below this level to the arcuate line—aponeuroses of the internal oblique and transversus abdominis muscles.
c. below the arcuate line—transversalis fascia.

III. Inguinal Region

A. Inguinal Triangle (of Hesselbach)

–is bounded

a. medially by the lateral edge of the rectus abdominis (the linea semilunaris).
b. laterally by the inferior epigastric vessels.
c. inferiorly by the inguinal ligament.
   –is an area of potential weakness and thus often the site of a direct inguinal hernia.

B. Inguinal Rings

1. Superficial Inguinal Ring

–is a triangular opening in the aponeurosis of the external oblique abdominis muscle.
–lies just lateral to the pubic tubercle.
–transmits the spermatic cord in the male and the round ligament of the uterus in the female.

2. Deep Inguinal Ring

–lies in the transversalis fascia, just lateral to the inferior epigastric vessels.
–is formed by the embryonic extension of the processus vaginalis through the abdominal wall and subsequent passage of the testes through the transversalis fascia during the descent of the testes into the scrotum.

C. Inguinal Canal

–begins at the deep inguinal ring and ends at the superficial ring.
–its walls

a. *Anterior wall*

–the aponeurosis of the external oblique muscle and the internal oblique muscles, which take origin from the lateral half of the inguinal ligament.

b. *Posterior wall*

–the aponeurosis of the transversus abdominis and tranversalis fascia.

c. *Roof*

–arching fibers of the internal oblique muscle and transversus abdominis.

d. *Floor*

–the inguinal ligament and lacunar ligament.

–is much smaller in the female than in the male.

–transmits the spermatic cord (or round ligament of the uterus and ilioinguinal nerve.

1. Inguinal Canal in Male Fetus

–transmits the ductus deferens, testicular artery and vein, cremaster muscle, processus vaginalis, genital branch of the genitofemoral nerve, ilioinguinal nerve, artery and vein of the ductus deferens, testicular nervous plexus, lymphatics, etc.

D. Inguinal Hernia

–occurs superior to the inguinal ligament, whereas the femoral hernia occurs inferior to the ligament.

–occurs medial to the pubic tubercle, whereas the femoral hernia occurs lateral to the tubercle.

1. Indirect Inguinal Hernia

–passes through the deep inguinal ring, inguinal canal, and superficial inguinal ring and descends into the scrotum.

–has a peritoneal covering.

–lies lateral to the inferior epigastric vessles.

–is associated with congenital factors, the persistence of the processus vaginalis.

–is found more often in men on the right side and is more common than direct.

–its layers are those of the spermatic cord.

2. Direct Inguinal hernia

–occurs through the posterior wall of the inguinal canal (in the region of the inguinal triangle) but does not descend into the scrotum.

–lies medial to the inferior epigastric vessels.

–is associated with weakness in the posterior wall of the inguinal canal lateral to the conjoint tendon.

–protrudes forward to the superficial inguinal ring, but rarely through.

–its sac is formed by the peritoneum.

IV. Spermatic Cord, Scrotum, and Testis

A. Spermatic Cord

−its fascia (or coverings)

    a. External Spermatic Fascia

        −is derived from external oblique aponeurosis.

    b. Cremasteric Fascia

        −cremaster muscle and fascia. This muscle originates from the internal oblique abdominis muscle and is innervated by the genital branch of the genitofemoral nerve.

    c. Internal Spermatic Fascia

        −is derived from the transversalis fascia.

−its contents are the ductus deferens, deferential vessels, testicular artery, pampiniform plexus of veins, lymphatics, and autonomic nerves of the testes.

B. Processus Vaginalis

−extends into the scrotum before the testis descends.
−is a peritoneal diverticulum (outpouching) in the fetus.
−forms the tunica vaginalis testis.
−normally loses it connection with the peritoneal cavity.
−its partial occulsion may cause fluid accumulation, called hydrocele processus vaginalis.

C. Tunica Vaginalis

−is a double serous membrane, a peritoneal sac (a remnant of the processus vaginalis).
−covers the front and sides of the testis and epididymis.
−is derived from the abdominal peritoneum.
−forms the innermost layer of the scrotum.
−its persistence may result in an indirect inguinal hernia.

D. Gubernaculum Testis

−is homologous to the female ovarian ligament and the round ligament of the uterus.
−is the fetal ligamentous cord that connects the bottom of the fetal testis to the developing scrotum.
−appears to play a significant role in testicular descent (pulls the testis down as it migrates).

V. Inner Surface

A. Supravesical Fossa

−is a depression on the anterior abdominal wall between the median and medial umbilical folds of the peritoneum.

B. Medial Inguinal Fossa

−is a depression on the anterior abdominal wall between the medial and lateral umbilical folds of peritoneum.
−lies lateral to the superior vesical fossa.
−is the fossa where most direct inguinal hernias occur.

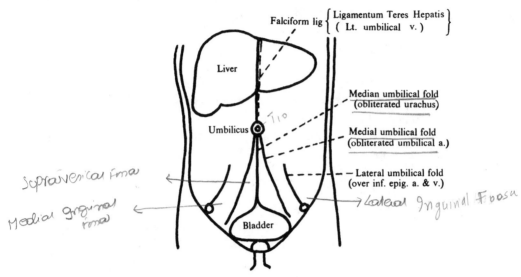

Figure 5.1. Peritoneal folds over the anterior abdominal wall.

C. Lateral Inguinal Fossa

–is a depression on the anterior abdominal wall, lateral to the lateral umbilical fold of peritoneum.

D. Umbilical Folds or Ligaments

1. **Median Umbilical Fold**

   –extends from the apex of the bladder to the umbilicus and contains the urachus, which is the remains of the fetal allantois.

2. **Medial Umbilical Fold**

   –extends from the side of the bladder to the umbilicus and contains the obliterated umbilical artery (a branch of the internal iliac artery).

3. **Lateral Umbilical Fold**

   –extends from the medial side of the deep inguinal ring to the arcuate line and contains inferior epigastric vessels.

E. Transversalis Fascia

–is a layer of connective tissue that lines the abdominal wall and lies between the perietal peritoneum and the muscles.

–continues with the diaphragmatic, psoas, iliac, pelvic, and quadratus lumborum fasciae.

–gives rise to the femoral sheath.

–forms the deep inguinal ring.

–gives rise to the internal spermatic fascia.

–is the principal layer of the posterior sheath of the rectus abdominis muscle, below the arcuate line.

VI. Nerves

A. Thoracoabdominal Nerves

–are the seventh to eleventh intercostal nerves.

–run downward and forward between the internal oblique and transversus abdominis muscles, supplying these and the rectus and the external oblique abdominis muscle.

B. Iliohypogastric Nerve

–runs downward and forward between the internal oblique and transversus abdominis muscles, pierces the internal abdominal oblique muscle, and then continues medially deep to the external abdominal oblique muscle.

–divides into a lateral cutaneous branch to supply the skin of the lateral side of the buttocks, and an anterior cutaneous branch to supply the skin above the pubis.

C. Ilioinguinal Nerve

–pierces the internal oblique muscle near the deep inguinal ring and runs medially through the inguinal canal and then the superficial inguinal ring.

 Anterior part of the scrotum

–gives off the femoral branch, which supplies the upper and medial parts of the thigh, and the anterior scrotal nerve, which supplies the skin of the root of the penis (or the skin of the mons pubis) and the anterior part of the scrotum (or the labium majus).

VII. Lymphatic Drainage

A. Lymphatics in Region Above Umbilicus

–are drained into the axillary lymph nodes.

B. Lymphatics in Region Below Umbilicus

–are drained into the superficial inguinal nodes.

C. Superficial Inguinal Lymph Nodes

–receive lymph from the lower abdominal wall, buttocks, penis, and scrotum (or labium majus). *EXCEPT GLANS PENIS*

VIII. Blood Vessels

A. Superior Epigastric Artery

–arises from the internal thoracic artery, enters the rectus sheath, and descends on the posterior surface of the rectus abdominis muscle.

–anastomoses with the inferior epigastric artery within the rectus abdominis muscle.

B. Inferior Epigastric Artery

–arises from the external iliac artery above the inguinal ligament.

–enters the rectus sheath and ascends between the rectus muscle and the posterior layer of the sheath.

–anastomoses with the superior epigastric and lower posterior intercostal arteries.

–gives off the cremasteric artery, which accompanies the spermatic cord.

C. Deep Circumflex Iliac Artery

–arises from the external iliac artery and runs laterally along the inguinal ligament and the iliac crest between the transversus and the internal oblique.

D. Superficial Epigastric Artery

–arises from the femoral artery and runs superiorly toward the umbilicus over the inguinal ligament.

–anastomoses with branches of the inferior epigastric artery.

E. Superficial Circumflex Iliac Artery

   –arises from the femoral artery and runs laterally upward, parallel to the inguinal ligament.

   –anastomoses with the deep circumflex iliac and lateral femoral circumflex arteries.

F. Superficial External Pudendal Artery

   –arises from the femoral artery, pierces the cribriform fascia that covers the saphenous opening, and runs medially to supply the skin above the pubis.

G. Thoracoepigastric Vein

   –is a longitudinal venous connection between the lateral thoracic vein and the superficial epigastric vein.

   –provides a collateral route for venous return if a caval obstruction occurs.

IX. Abdominal Cavity

   –is tophographically divided into nine regions by two transverse and two longitudinal planes.

   –its subdivisions are right and left hypochondriac, epigastric, right and left lumbar, umbilical, right and left inguinal (iliac), and hypogastric (pubic) regions.

Peritoneum

I. Peritoneum

   –is a serous membrane lined by mesothelial cells.

   –can be thought of as a balloon into which visceral organs are invaginated.

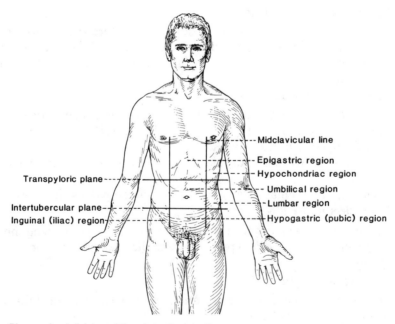

Figure 5.2. Planes of subdivision of the abdominal cavity.

—consists of a **parietal** peritoneum, which lines the abdominal and pelvic walls and the inferior surface of the diaphragm, and a **visceral** peritoneum, which covers the viscera.

—is supplied by the phrenic, thoracoabdominal, subcostal, iliohypogastric, and ilioinguinal nerves; however, the visceral peritoneum is insensitive to pain, tough, and pressure.

II. Peritoneal Reflections

A. Omentum

1. Lesser Omentum

—is a double layer of peritoneum extending from the porta hepatis of the liver to the lesser curvature of the stomach and the beginning of the duodenum.

—consists of the hepatogastric and heptaduodenal ligaments.

—its right free margin contains the hepatic artery, bile duct, and portal vein.

—forms the anterior wall of the lesser sac of the peritoneal cavity.

—contains the left and right gastric vessels, which run between its two layers.

2. Greater Omentum

—hangs down like an apron from the greater curvature of the stomach, covering the transverse colon and other abdominal viscera.

—is often referred to by surgeons as the "abdominal policeman" because it plugs the neck of a hernial sac, preventing the entrance of coils of the small intestine. It also adheres to areas of inflammation and wraps itself around the inflamed organs, thus saving the patient from a serious diffuse peritonitis.

B. Mesenteries

1. Mesentery of Small Intestine (or Mesentery Proper)

—its root extends from the duodenojejunal flexure to the right iliac fossa and is 15 cm (about 6 inches) in length.

—is a double fold of peritoneum that suspends the jejunum and ileum from the posterior abdominal wall.

—its free border encloses the small intestine, which is about 6 m (20 feet) in length.

—transmits the nerves and blood vessels to and from the small intestine.

2. Transverse Mesocolon

—may be considered as an extension of the greater omentum from the posterior surface of the transverse colon to the posterior body wall.

—contains the middle colic vessels, nerves, and lymphatic vessels.

3. Sigmoid Mesocolon

—is an inverted V-shaped peritoneal fold connecting the sigmoid colon to the pelvic wall and contains the sigmoid vessels.

4. Mesoappendix

—connects the appendix to the mesentery of the ileum and contains the appendicular vessels.

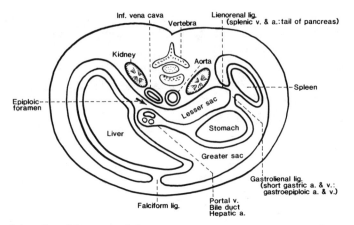

Figure 5.3 Horizontal section of the upper abdomen.

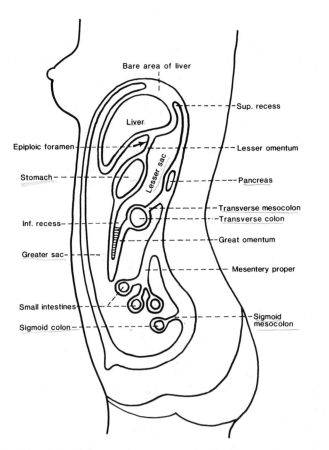

Figure 5.4. Sagittal section of the abdomen.

C. Peritoneal Ligaments

1. **Lienogastric Ligament (Gastrosplenic)**

   —extends from the left portion of the greater curvature of the stomach to the hilus of the spleen.

   —contains the short gastric vessels and the left gastroepiploic vessels.

2. **Lienorenal Ligament**

   —runs from the hilus of the spleen to the left kidney.

   —contains the splenic vessels and the tail of the pancreas.

3. **Gastrophrenic Ligament**

   —runs from he upper part of the greater curvature of the stomach to the diaphragm.

4. **Gastrocolic Ligament**

   —runs from the greater curvature of the stomach to the transverse colon.

5. **Phrenicocolic Ligament**

   —runs from the colic flexure to the diaphragm.

6. **Falciform Ligament**

   —is a sickle-shaped peritoneal fold, connecting the liver to the diaphragm and anterior abdominal wall.

   —demarcates the large right lobe from the small left lobe of the liver on the diaphragmatic surface.

   —contains the ligamentum teres hepatis, which is the fibrous remnant of the left umbilical vein of the fetus.

   —contains the paraumbilical vein, which connects the left branch of the portal vein with the subcutaneous veins in the region of the umbilicus.

7. **Ligamentum Teres Hepatis (Round Ligament of Liver)**

   —lies in the free margin of the falciform ligament.

   —ascends from the umbilicus to the inferior or visceral surface of the liver.

   —is located in the fissure that forms the left boundary of the quadrate lobe of the liver on its inferior surface.

   —is formed after birth from the remnant of the left umbilical vein, which carries oxygenated blood from the placenta to the left branch of the portal vein in the fetus. (The right umbilical vein degenerates during the embryonic period.)

8. **Coronary Ligament**

   —is a peritoneal reflection from the diaphragmatic surface of the liver onto the diaphragm.

   —encloses a triangular area of the right lobe, called the bare area of the liver.

   —forms the **right** and **left triangular ligaments** by its right and left extensions.

9. **Ligamentum Venosum**

   —is the fibrous remnant of the ductus venosus.

   —lies in the fissure on the inferior surface of the liver, forming the left boundary of the caudate lobe of the liver.

D. Peritoneal Folds

–are peritoneal reflections with free edges.

1. Umbilical Folds

–are five folds of peritoneum below the umbilicus, two on each side and one in the median plane.

–include median, medial, and lateral umbilical folds and are described on page 162.

2. Rectouterine Fold

–extends from the cervix to the uterus, along the side of the rectum, to the posterior pelvic wall.

3. Ileocecal Fold

–extends from the terminal ileum to the cecum.

III. Peritoneal Cavity

–is a potential space between the parietal and visceral peritoneum.

–contains a film of fluid that lubricates the surface of the peritoneum and facilitates free movements of the viscera.

–is a completely closed sac in the male, but it has a communication with the exterior through the mouths of the uterine tubes in the female.

–is divided into the lesser and greater sacs.

A. Lesser Sac (Omental Bursa)

–is a closed sac, except for the communication with the greater sac through the epiploic foramen.

–is an irregular space that lies behind the liver, lesser omentum, stomach, and upper anterior part of the greater omentum.

–presents three recesses: superior, inferior, and splenic.

a. Superior Recess

–lies behind the stomach, lesser omentum, and liver.

b. Inferior Recess

–lies behind the stomach, extending into the layers of the greater omentum.

c. Splenic Recess

–extends to the left at the hilus of the spleen.

B. Greater Sac

–extends across the whole breadth of the abdomen and from the diaphragm to the pelvic floor.

C. Epiploic Foramen (Foramen of Winslow)

–is a natural opening between the lesser and greater sacs.

–is bounded superiorly by peritoneum on the caudate lobe of the liver, inferiorly by peritoneum on the first part of the duodenum, anteriorly by the free edge of the lesser omentum, and posteriorly by peritoneum covering the inferior vena cava.

Gastrointestinal Viscera

I. Stomach

–is entirely covered by peritoneum.

–is located in the left hypochondriac and epigastric regions of the abdomen.

–has greater and lesser curvatures, anterior and posterior walls, cardiac and pyloric openings, and cardiac and angular notches.

–is divided into four regions including the cardia, fundus, body, and pylorus. The pylorus divides into the pyloric antrum and canal.

–receives blood from the right and left gastric, right and left gastroepiploic, and short gastric arteries.

–has longitudinal folds of the mucous membrane, the rugae when the organ is contracted.

II. Small Intestine

–extends from the pyloric opening to the ileocecal junction.

–is the place for complete digestion and absorption as well.

–consists of the duodenum, jejunum, and ileum.

A. Duodenum

–is a C-shaped tube, surrounding the head of the pancreas (10 inches or 25 cm long).

–is the shortest but widest part of the small intestine.

–has a mobile or free section at the beginning of the first part, termed the duodenal cap by radiologists, into which the pylorus invaginates. It is covered by peritoneum.

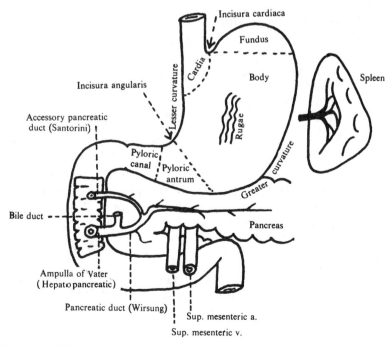

Figure 5.5. Stomach and duodenum.

—is derived from the embryonic foregut and midgut. Its second part has the junction of the foregut and midgut, where the common bile and main pancreatic ducts open.

—is retroperitoneal except for the beginning of the first part, which is connected to the liver by the hepatoduodenal part of the lesser omentum.

—receives blood supply from both the celiac (foregut artery) and superior mesenteric arteries (midgut artery).

—has the greater papilla, on which are terminal openings of the bile and main pancreatic ducts.

—has the lesser papilla, which lies 2 cm above the greater papilla and marks the site of the entry of the accessory pancreatic duct.

B. Jejunum

—makes up the proximal two-fifths of the small intestine, while the ileum comprises the distal three-fifths.

—is more empty, larger in diameter, and thicker walled than the ileum.

—has the plicae circulares, which are tall and closely packed together.

—contains no Peyer's patches, which are aggregations of lymphoid tissue.

—has translucent areas called "windows" between the blood vessels of its mesentery.

—has less prominent arterial arcades in its mesentery than does the ileum.

—has longer vasa recta than the ileum.

C. Ileum

—is longer than the jejunum and occupies the pelvic cavity.

—is characterized by the presence of Peyer's patches (lower portion), shorter plicae circularis and vasa recta, and more mesenteric fat and arterial arcades, when compared to the jejunum.

1. Meckel's Diverticulum

—is an evagination of the terminal part of the ileum.

—is located on the antimesenteric side of the ileum.

—may contain gastric and pancreatic tissues in its wall.

—represents persistent portions of the yolk stalk (vitelline or omphalo-mesenteric duct).

—is clinically important because bleeding may occur from an ulcer in its wall.

—occurs in about 2% of persons.

III. Large Intestine

—extends from the ileocecal junction to the anus and is about 5 feet long.

—consists of cecum, appendix, colon, rectum, and anal canal.

—functions to convert the liquid contents of the ileum into semisolid feces by absorbing fluid and electrolytes.

A. Colon

—consists of the ascending, transverse, descending, and sigmoid parts.

—is characterized by the presence of the

  a. *Teniae coli.*

  b. *Sacculations or haustra.*

  c. *Epiploic appendages.*

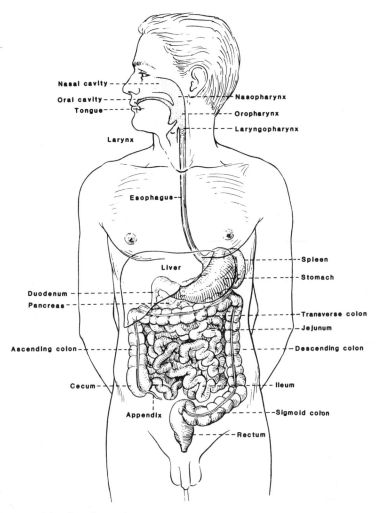

Figure 5.6. Diagram of the digestive system.

—its ascending and descending parts are retroperitoneal in position, and its transverse and sigmoid parts are surrounded by peritoneum (have their own mesenteries called the transverse mesocolon and the sigmoid mesocolon).

—its ascending and transverse parts are supplied by the superior mesenteric artery and the vagus nerve, whereas its descending and sigmoid parts are supplied by the inferior mesenteric artery and the pelvic splanchnic nerve.

B. Cecum

—is the U-shaped blind pouch of the large intestine and lies in the right iliac fossa.

—is usually completely surrounded by peritoneum.

C. Appendix

–is a narrow, hollow, muscular tube containing large aggregations of lymphoid tissue in its wall.

–is suspended from the terminal ileum by a small mesentery, the mesoappendix, that contains the appendicular vessels.

–may have inflammation that causes spasm and distension, resulting in pain that is referred to the epigastrium.

D. Rectum

–is the part of the large intestine that extends from the sigmoid colon to the anal canal.

–follows the curvature of the sacrum and coccyx.

–has a peritoneal covering on its anterior, right, and left sides for the proximal third, only on its front for the middle third, and no covering at all for the distal third.

–its mucous membrane, together with the circular muscle layer, forms three permanent folds, called transverse folds of the rectum (valve of Houston).

–receives blood from the superior, middle, and inferior rectal arteries as well as the middle sacral artery.

–its venous blood returns to the portal venous system by the superior rectal vein, and to the caval (systemic) system by the middle and inferior rectal veins.

–receives parasympathetic nerve fibers by way of the pelvic splanchnic nerve.

E. Anal Canal

–lies below the pelvic diaphragm and ends at the anus.

–is divided into an upper two-thirds (visceral portion), which belongs to the intestine, and a lower third (somatic portion), which belongs to the perineum with respect to the mucosa, blood supply, and nerve supply.

–has the anal columns, which are 5–10 permanent longitudinal folds of mucosa, in its upper half. (Each column contains a small artery and a small vein.)

–has crescent-shaped mucosal folds called anal valves that connect the lower ends of the anal columns.

–has a pouch-like recess at the lower end of the anal columns called the anal sinus, in which the anal gland opens.

–sports the pectinate line, which is a sinuous line following the anal valves and crossing the bases of the anal columns.

a. The epithelium is columnar or cuboidal above the pectinate line and stratified squamous below it.

b. Venous drainage above the pectinate line goes into the portal venous system mainly by the superior rectal vein, and below the pectinate line into the caval system by the inferior rectal vein.

c. Internal hemorrhoids occur above the line and external hemorrhoids below it. (A hemorrhoid is a varicosity of a venous plexus around the rectum and anal canal.)

d. The lymphatic vessels drain into the internal iliac nodes above the line and into the superficial inguinal nodes below it.

e. The sensory innervation above the line is through fibers from the pelvic plexus and thus of the visceral type, but the sensory innervation below it is by somatic nerve fibers of the pudendal nerve (very sensitive).

IV. Accessory Organs of Digestive System

A. Liver

—is the largest visceral organ in the body and surrounded by the peritoneum.

—is attached to the diaphragm by the coronary and the right and left triangular ligaments.

—has a bare area on the diaphragmatic surface, which is limited by layers of the coronary ligament and is devoid of peritoneum.

—is attached to the anterior abdominal wall and the diaphragm by the falciform ligament, which demarcates a large right lobe from a small left lobe on the diaphragmatic surface.

—has an H-shaped group of fissures including a fissure for the **ligamentum teres hepatis** between the left lobe and the quadrate lobe, a fissure for the **ligamentum venosum** between the left lobe and the caudate lobe, a fissure for the **gallbladder** between the quadrate lobe and the major part of the right lobe, a fissure for the **inferior vena cava** between the caudate lobe and the major part of the right lobe, and a cross bar of the H, the **porta hepatis** for the hepatic ducts, the hepatic artery proper and the branches of the portal vein.

—has important roles in bile production, detoxification, blood clotting mechanisms, and glycogen, vitamin, iron, and copper storage, as well as manufacture of red blood cells in the fetus.

—has subdivisions of the right lobe.

a. *Quadrate Lobe of the Liver*

—lies between the gallbladder fossa and the fissure of the ligamentum teres hepatis.

b. *Caudate Lobe of Liver*

—lies between the groove for the inferior vena cava and the fissure of the ligamentum venosum.

—projects into a lesser sac.

B. Gallbladder

—is a pear-shaped sac lying on the inferior surface of the liver in a fossa between the right and quadrate lobes.

—has the fundus (the rounded blind end), the body (the major part), and the neck (the narrow part), which gives rise to the cystic duct with spiral valves.

—has a capacity of about 30 ml.

—receives bile, stores it, and concentrates it by absorbing water and salts.

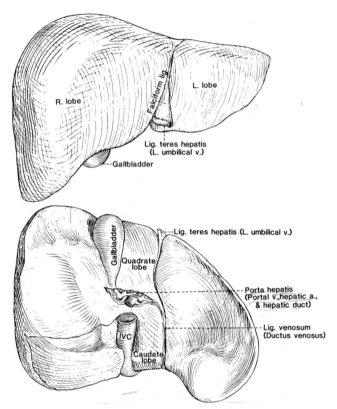

Figure 5.7. Anterior and visceral surfaces of the liver. *IVC*, inferior vena cava.

—is contracted to squeeze bile out by stimulation of a hormone, cholecystokinin, produced by the duodenal mucosa when food arrives in the duodenum.

C. Pancreas

—is an exocrine and endocrine gland.

—is a retroperitoneal organ except for a small portion of its tail, which lies in the lienorenal ligament.

—its head lies within the C-shaped concavity of the duodenum.

—the **uncinate process** is a projection of the lower part of its head to the left behind the superior mesenteric vessels.

—may have tumors in its head that obstruct the bile flow, producing "jaundice."

D. Duct System for Bile Passage

1. Right and Left Hepatic Ducts

—are formed by the union of all of the ducts from each lobe of the liver.

a. *Common Hepatic Duct*

—is formed by the union of the right and left hepatic ducts.

—is accompanied by the proper hepatic artery and the portal vein.

2. Cystic Duct

—has spiral folds (valves) to keep constantly open, and thus bile can pass

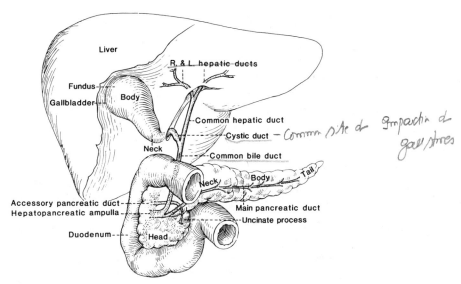

Figure 5.8. Extrahepatic bile passages and pancreatic ducts.

upward into the gallbladder when the bile duct is closed.
—runs alongside the hepatic duct before joining the common hepatic duct.
—is a common site of impaction of gallstones.

3. **Bile Duct (or Ductus Choledochus)**
    —is formed by the union of the common hepatic duct and the cystic duct.
    —lies with the hepatic artery and portal vein in the right free margin of the lesser omentum.
    —descends behind the first part of the duodenum and runs through the head of the pancreas.
    —joins the main pancreatic duct to form the hepatopancreatic duct and/or ampulla, which enters the second part of the duodenum at the greater papilla. (This entrance represents the junction of the embryonic foregut and midgut.)
    —is related medially to the hepatic artery proper and posteriorly to the portal vein.

V. Spleen
    —is a large lymphatic organ lying against the diaphragm and the ninth to eleventh ribs in the left hypogastric region.
    —is developed in the dorsal mesogastrium and supported by the lienogastric and lienorenal ligaments.
    —is composed of **white pulp**, which consists of lymphatic nodules and diffuse lymphatic tissue, and **red pulp**, which consists of venous sinusoids connected by splenic cords.
    —is hematopoietic in early life and later functions in blood destruction.
    —filters blood (removes particulate matter and cellular residue from the blood), stores red corpuscles, and produces lymphocytes and antibodies.

–may be removed surgically with minimal effect on body function.

–is supplied by the splenic artery and is drained by the splenic vein.

VI. Celiac and Mesenteric Arteries

A. Celiac Trunk

–arises from the front of the abdominal aorta immediately below the aortic hiatus of the diaphragm, between the right and left crura.

–divides into the left gastric, splenic, and common hepatic arteries.

1. Left Gastric Artery

Smallest branch

–is the smallest branch of the celiac trunk.

–runs upward and to the left toward the cardia, giving off esophageal and hepatic branches, and then turns to the right and runs along the lesser curvature within the lesser omentum to anastomose with the right gastric artery.

2. Splenic Artery

Largest branch

–is the largest branch of the celiac trunk.

–runs a highly tortuous course along the superior border of the pancreas and enters the lienorenal ligament.

–gives rise to:

a. a number of pancreatic branches including the **dorsal pancreatic artery**.

b. a few **short gastric arteries**, which pass through the lienogastric ligament to reach the fundus of the stomach.

c. the **left gastroepiploic artery**, which reaches the greater omentum through the lienogastric ligament and runs along the greater curvature of the stomach to distribute to the stomach and greater omentum.

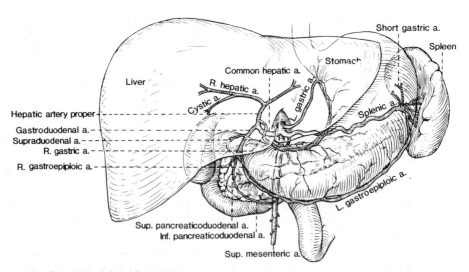

Figure 5.9.   Branches of the celiac trunk.

3. **Common Hepatic Artery**

   –runs to the right along the upper border of the pancreas and divides into the proper hepatic artery, the gastroduodenal artery, and probably the right gastric artery.

   a. *Proper Hepatic Artery*

      –ascends in the free edge of the lesser omentum and divides, near the porta hepatis, into left and right hepatic arteries, the right giving off a cystic artery to the gallbladder.
      –gives off the right gastric artery.

   b. *Right Gastric Artery*

      –runs to the pylorus and then along the lesser curvature of the stomach and anastomoses with the left gastric artery.

   c. *Gastroduodenal Artery*

      –descends behind the first part of the duodenum, giving off the **supraduodenal artery** to its upper aspect and a few **retroduodenal arteries** to its inferior aspect.
      –divides into:

      (1) the **right gastroepiploic artery**, which runs to the left along the greater curvature of the stomach, supplying the stomach and the greater omentum.
      (2) the **superior pancreaticoduodenal artery** which passes between the duodenum and the head of the pancreas and further divides into the anterior superior pancreaticoduodenal and posterior superior pancreaticoduodenal arteries.

B. **Superior Mesenteric Artery**

   –arises from the aorta behind the neck of the pancreas.
   –descends across the uncinate process of the pancreas and the third part of the duodenum and then enters the root of the mesentery behind the transverse colon to run to the right iliac fossa.
   –gives off the following branches:

1. **Inferior Pancreaticoduodenal Artery**

   –passes to the right and divides into anterior inferior pancreaticoduodenal and posterior inferior pancreaticoduodenal arteries that anastomose with the corresponding branches of the superior pancreaticoduodenal arteries.

2. **Middle Colic Artery**

   –enters the transverse mesocolon and divides into the right branch, which anastomoses with the right colic artery, and the left branch, which anastomoses with the left colic artery.

3. **Ileocolic Artery**

   –descends behind the peritoneum toward the right iliac fossa and ends by dividing into:

   a. *an ascending branch that anastomoses with the right colic artery.*
   b. *anterior and posterior cecal branches.*

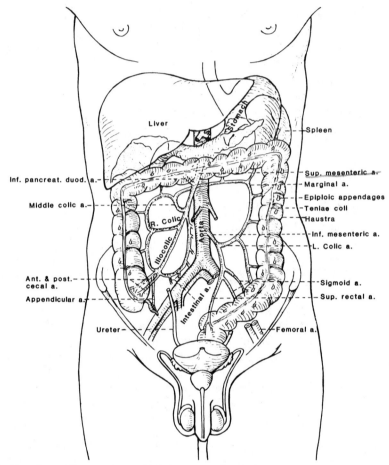

Figure 5.10. Branches of the superior and inferior mesentric arteries.

      c. an appendicular artery.

      d. an ileal branch.

4. Right Colic Artery

    –arises from the superior mesenteric artery or from the ileocolic artery.

    –runs to the right behind the peritoneum and divides into ascending and descending branches, distributing the ascending colon.

5. Intestinal Arteries

    –are 12–15 in number and supply the jejunum and ileum.

    –branch and anastomose to form a series of arcades in the mesentery.

C. Inferior Mesenteric Artery

    –passes to the left behind the peritoneum and distributes to descending and sigmoid colons, and upper portion of the rectum.

    –gives rise to:

1. Left Colic Artery

    –runs to the left behind the peritoneum toward the descending colon and divides into ascending and descending branches.

2. Sigmoid Arteries

–are two to three in number, run toward the sigmoid colon in its mesentery, and divide into ascending and descending branches.

3. Superior Rectal Artery

–is the termination of the inferior mesenteric artery, descends into the pelvis, divides into two branches that follow the sides of the rectum, and anastomoses with the middle and inferior rectal arteries. (The middle and inferior rectal arteries arise from the internal iliac and internal pudendal arteries, respectively.)

VII. Portal Venous System

A. Portal Vein

–drains the abdominal part of the gut, spleen, pancreas, and gallbladder and is 8 cm long.

–is formed by the union of the splenic vein and the superior mesenteric vein behind the neck of the pancreas. The inferior mesenteric vein joins either the splenic, the superior mesenteric, or the junction of these two veins.

–receives the left gastric (or coronary) vein.

–carries deoxygenated blood but contains nutrients.

–carries twice as much blood as the hepatic artery.

–when obstructed, may result in esophageal varices, hemorrhoids, and caput medusa.

–ascends in the free margin of the lesser omentum.

–its tributaries are:

1. Superior Mesenteric Vein

–accompanies the superior mesenteric artery; on its right side in the root of the mesentery.

–crosses the third part of the duodenum and the uncinate process of the pancreas.

–terminates behind the neck of the pancreas by joining the splenic vein, thereby forming the portal vein.

–its tributaries are the veins that accompany the branches of the artery and some that do not.

2. Splenic Vein

–is formed by the union of tributaries from the spleen and receives the short gastric, left gastroepiploic, and pancreatic veins.

3. Inferior Mesenteric Vein

–is formed by the union of the superior rectal and sigmoid veins, receives the left colic vein, and empties into the splenic vein or the superior mesenteric vein or the junction of these two veins.

4. Left Gastric (Coronary) Vein

–drains normally into the portal vein, but the esophageal vein drains into the systemic venous system via the azygos vein.

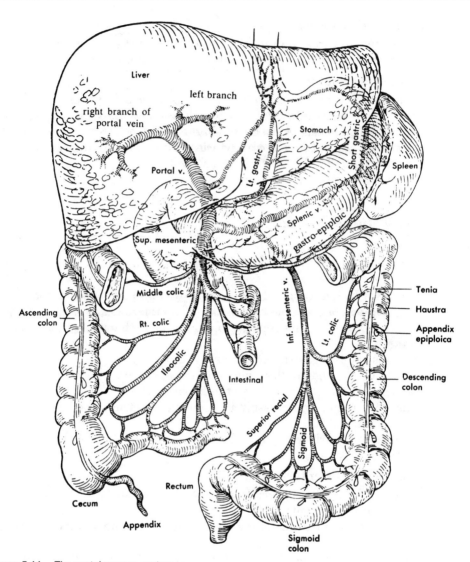

Figure 5.11. The portal venous system.

5. Paraumbilical Veins

–are found in the falciform ligament.

–connect the left branch of the portal vein with the small subcutaneous veins in the region of the umbilicus, which are radicles of the superior epigastric, inferior epigastric, thoracoepigastric, and superficial epigastric veins.

–are virtually closed, but enlarge in portal hypertension.

B. Important Portal-Caval (or Systemic) Anastomoses

–occur between:

  a. the left gastric vein and the esophageal vein of the azygos system.

  b. the superior rectal vein and the middle and inferior rectal veins.

  c. the paraumbilical vein and radicles of epigastric (superficial and inferior) veins.

  d. rectouterine (retroperitoneal) veins and twigs of renal veins.

C. Portal Hypertension

–results from thrombosis of the portal vein or liver cirrhosis.

–causes a dilation of veins in the lower part of the esophagus, forming **esophageal varices**. Their rupture results in vomiting blood (hematemesis).

–results in **caput medusa** (dilated veins radiating from the umbilicus), which occurs because the paraumbilical vein enclosed in the free margin of the falciform ligament anastomoses with branches of the epigastric (superficial and inferior) veins around the umbilicus.

–may result in **hemorrhoids**, which are caused by the enlargement of veins around the anal canal.

–can be reduced by diverting blood from the portal to the caval system by anastomosing the splenic vein to the renal vein or by creating a fistula between the portal vein and the inferior vena cava.

VIII. Clinical Considerations

A. Gastric Ulcer

–erodes the mucosa and penetrates the gastric wall to various depths.

–may perforate into the lesser sac and erode the pancreas and the splenic artery, causing fatal hemorrhage.

B. Duodenal Ulcer

–penetrates the duodenal wall of the first part and erodes the gastroduodenal artery.

–commonly located in the duodenal cap.

C. Liver Cirrhosis

–is a condition in which liver cells are progressively destructed and replaced by fibrous tissue that surrounds the intrahepatic blood vessels and biliary radicles, impeding circulation of blood through the liver.

–causes portal hypertension, resulting in esophageal varices, hemorrhoids, and caput medusa.

D. Gallstones

–are formed by solidifying of bile constituents.

–are composed chiefly of cholesterol crystals.

–may become lodged in the fundus of the gallbladder, which may ulcerate through the wall into the transverse colon or into the duodenum. In the former case, they are passed naturally to the rectum, but in the latter case they may be held up at the ileocolic junction, producing an intestinal obstruction.

–may become lodged in the bile duct, obstructing the bile flow to the duodenum and thus leading to **jaundice**.

–may become lodged in the hepatopancreatic ampulla, blocking both the biliary and the pancreatic duct systems. In this case, bile may enter the pancreatic duct system, causing aseptic or noninfectious **pancreatitis**.

E. Megacolon (Hirschsprung's Disease)

–is caused by the absence of enteric ganglia in the lower part of the colon, which leads to the dilation of the colon proximal to the inactive segment.

–is of congenital origin and is usually found during infancy and childhood, resulting in constipation, abdominal distension, and vomiting.

Retroperitoneal Viscera, Diaphragm, and Posterior Abdominal Wall

I. Kidney, Ureter, and Suprarenal Gland

A. Kidney – *Fim T12 to L4*

–is retroperitoneal and extends from the level of lumbar vertebrae 1–4 in the erect position.

–the right lies a little lower than the left, due to the large size of the right lobe of the liver.

–is invested by a firm fibrous capsule and is surrounded by a mass of fat and fibrous fascia, the renal fascia.

–has an indentation, the hilus on its medial border, through which the ureter, the renal vessels, and the nerves enter or leave the organ.

–**perirenal fat** lies in the perinephric space between the capsule of the kidney and the renal fascia, whereas **pararenal fat** lies external to the renal fascia.

–consists of the medulla and the cortex, containing about a million **nephrons**, which are the functional units of the kidney. (The nephron consists

[handwritten margin note: Left Kidney is bigger than the Rt. Kidney. 2nd portion of the duodenum lies anterior to the Medial border of the Rt. Kidney.]

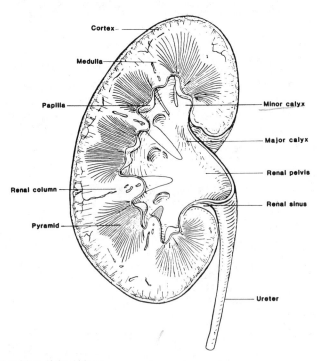

Figure 5.12. Frontal section of the kidney.

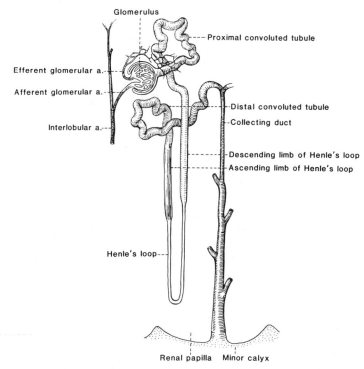

Figure 5.13. The renal tubules.

of a glomerular capsule, a proximal convoluted tubule, Henle's loop, and a distal convoluted tubule.)

1. **Cortex**
    —forms the outer part of the kidney and also projects into the medullary region between the renal pyramids as **renal columns**.
    —contains renal corpuscles and proximal and distal convoluted tubules. (The **renal corpuscle** consists of a **glomerular capsule**, which is the invaginated blind end of the nephron.)

2. **Medulla**
    —forms the inner part of the kidney and consists of 8–12 **renal pyramids**, which contain straight tubules, Henle's loop, and collecting tubules. An apex of the renal pyramid, the **renal papilla**, fits into the cup-shaped **minor calyx** on which open the **collecting tubules**.

3. **Minor Calyces**
    —receive urine from the collecting tubules and empty into two or three **major calyces**, which in turn empty into an upper dilated portion of the ureter, the **renal pelvis**.

B. Ureter
    —is a muscular tube that extends from the kidney to the urinary bladder.
    —is retroperitoneal, descends on the psoas muscle, is crossed by the gonadal vessels, and crosses the bifurcation of the common iliac artery.
    —may be obstructed:

—may be obstructed:

   a. where it joins the renal pelvis (the ureteropelvic junction).

   b. where it crosses the pelvic brim over the distal end of the common iliac artery.

   c. where it enters the wall of the urinary bladder.

—receives blood from the aorta, the renal, gonadal, common and internal iliac, umbilical, superior and inferior vesical, and middle rectal arteries.

C. Suprarenal (Adrenal) Gland   *A I R*

—receives arteries from three sources: the superior suprarenal artery from the inferior phrenic; the middle suprarenal from the abdominal aorta; and the inferior suprarenal from the renal artery.

—is a retroperitoneal organ, lying on the superomedial aspect of the kidney.

—its medulla is the only organ that receives preganglionic sympathetic nerve fibers, whereas the cortex has no nerve supply.

—its vein drains into the inferior vena cava on the right and the renal vein on the left.

Adrenal Cortex has no Nerve supply

II. Blood Vessels

A. Aorta

T12

—passes through the aortic hiatus in the diaphragm at the level of the twelfth thoracic vertebra, descends on the front of the vertebral bodies, and ends by bifurcating into the right and left common iliac arteries in front of the fourth lumbar vertebra. *L4*

—gives rise to:

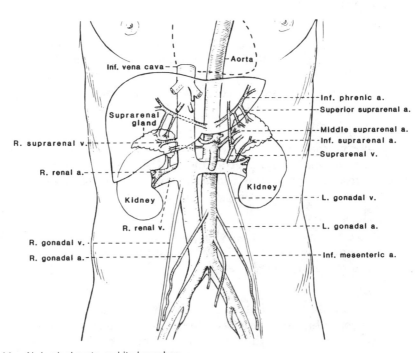

Figure 5.14. Abdominal aorta and its branches.

1. **Inferior Phrenic Arteries**
   –arise from the aorta immediately below the aortic hiatus, and give off superior suprarenal arteries.
   –diverge across the crura of the diaphragm, the left one passing behind the esophagus and the right one passing behind the inferior vena cava.

2. **Middle Suprarenal Arteries**
   –arise from the aorta and run upon the crura of the diaphragm just above the renal arteries.
   * *The **superior suprarenal artery** arises from the inferior phrenic artery.*
   * *The **inferior suprarenal artery** arises from the renal artery.*

3. **Renal Arteries**
   –arise from the aorta below the origin of the superior mesenteric artery. The right one is longer and a little lower than the left and passes behind the inferior vena cava; the left one passes behind the left renal vein.

4. **Testicular or Ovarian Arteries**
   –descend retroperitoneally, laterally on the psoas major muscle, and across the ureter. The testicular artery accompanies the ductus deferens and supplies the spermatic cord, epididymis and the testis, whereas the ovarian artery enters the suspensory ligament of the ovary, supplies the ovary, and anastomoses with the ovarian branch of the uterine artery.

5. **Lumbar Arteries**
   –have four or five pairs.
   –run posterior to the sympathetic trunk and inferior vena cava (on the right side), between the vertebral bodies and the psoas major muscle.

6. **Celiac and Superior and Inferior Mesenteric Arteries**
   –are described on pp. 176–179.

B. Inferior Vena Cava

–is formed on the right side of the fifth lumbar vertebra by the union of the two common iliac veins, below the bifurcation of the aorta.
–is longer than the abdominal aorta and ascends at the right side of the aorta.
–passes through its opening (opening for inferior vena cava) in the central tendon of the diaphragm at the level of the eighth thoracic vertebra and enters the right atrium of the heart.
–receives the right gonadal, suprarenal, and inferior phrenic veins. On the left side these veins usually drain into the left renal veins.

C. Cisterna Chyli

–is the lower dilated end of the thoracic duct.
–lies posterior and a little right of the aorta, usually between two crura of the diaphragm.
–is formed by the intestinal and lumbar lymph trunks.

III. Lumbar Plexus

–is formed by the union of the ventral rami of the first three lumbar nerves and a part of the fourth lumbar nerve.

–lies anterior to the transverse processes of the lumbar vertebrae within the substance of the psoas muscle.

A. Subcostal Nerve

–is the ventral ramus of the twelfth thoracic nerve.

–runs behind the lateral lumbocostal arch and in front of the quadratus lumborum, penetrates the transversus abdominis muscle to run between this muscle and the internal oblique, and supplies the external oblique, internal oblique, and transversus abdominis and pyramidalis.

B. Iliohypogastric Nerve

–arises from the first lumbar nerve, emerges from the lateral border of the psoas, runs in front of the quadratus lumborum, and pierces the transversus abdominis near the iliac crest to run between this muscle and the internal oblique.

–supplies the internal oblique and transversus abdominis muscles and divides into anterior and lateral cutaneous branches to supply the skin above the pubis and the skin of the gluteal region.

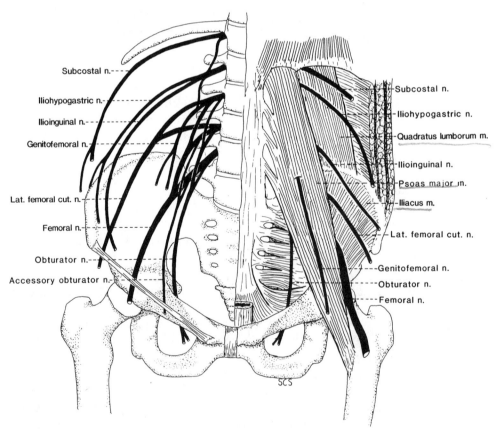

Figure 5.15. The lumbar plexus.

C. **Ilioinguinal Nerve** L1

—arises from the first lumbar nerve, runs in front of the quadratus lumborum, pierces the transversus abdominis and then the internal oblique to run between the internal and external oblique aponeuroses, accompanies the spermatic cord (or the round ligament of the uterus), continues through the inguinal canal, and emerges through the superficial inguinal ring.

—supplies the internal oblique and transversus abdominis muscles and also gives off cutaneous branches to the thigh and anterior scrotal or labial branches.

D. **Lateral Femoral Cutaneous Nerve** L2,3

—arises from the second and third lumbar nerve, emerges from the lateral side of the psoas muscle, runs in front of the iliacus and behind the inguinal ligament, and supplies the skin of the front and side of the thigh.

E. **Genitofemoral Nerve** L1,2

—arises from the first and second lumbar nerves, emerges on the front of the psoas muscle, and descends on its anterior surface.

—divides into a genital branch, which enters the inguinal canal through the deep inguinal ring to supply the cremaster muscle and the scrotum (or labium majus), and a femoral branch, which supplies the skin of the femoral triangle.

F. **Femoral Nerve** L2,3,4

—arises from the second, third, and fourth lumbar nerves, emerges from the lateral border of the psoas major muscle, descends in the groove between the psoas and iliacus muscles, enters the femoral triangle deep to the inguinal ligament, and divides into numerous branches.

G. **Obturator Nerve** L2 3 4

—arises from the second, third, and fourth lumbar nerves, descends along the medial border of the psoas muscle, runs forward on the lateral wall of the pelvis, and enters the thigh through the obturator foramen.

—divides into an anterior and a posterior branch and supplies the adductor group of muscles, the hip and knee joints, and the skin of the medial side of the thigh.

H. **Accessory Obturator Nerve**

—arises from the third and fourth lumbar nerves, descends medial to the psoas muscle, passes over the superior pubic ramus, and supplies the hip joint and the pectineus muscle.

IV. Autonomic Nervous System

—is composed of purely motor or efferent nerves through which cardiac muscle, smooth muscle, and glands are innervated.

—consists of sympathetic (or thoracolumbar outflow) and parasympathetic (or craniosacral outflow) systems.

—involves two neurons: preganglionic and postganglionic.

A. **Parasympathetic Nervous System**

—is also known as the craniosacral division.

—promotes quiet and orderly processes of the body, thereby conserving energy or preserving body tissues.

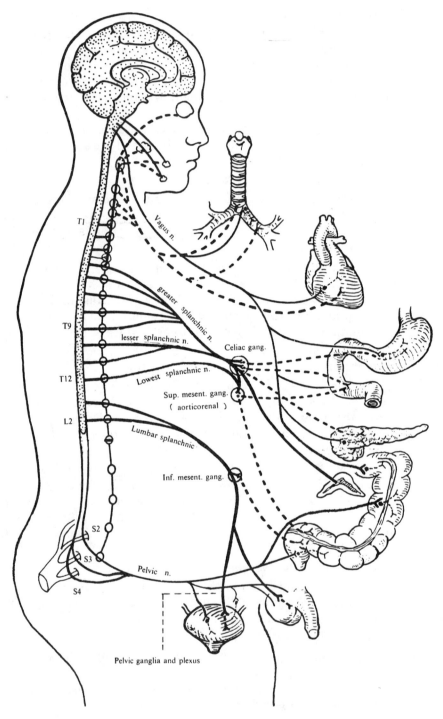

Figure 5.16. The autonomic nervous system.

—is not as widely distributed over the entire body as sympathetic fibers, and the body wall and extremities have no parasympathetic supply.

—preganglionic fibers running in cranial nerves III, VII, and IX pass to cranial autonomic ganglia (namely, the ciliary submandibular and otic ganglia) where they synapse on the postganglionic neurons.

—Preganglionic fibers in cranial nerve X and in pelvic splanchnic nerves (originating from S2,3,4,) pass to terminal ganglia where they synapse.

B. Sympathetic Nervous System

—preganglionic neuron cell bodies are in the lateral horn or intermediolateral cell column of the spinal cord segments between T1 and L2.

—preganglionic fibers pass through the white rami communicantes and enter the sympathetic chain ganglion where they synapse. Postganglionic fibers join each spinal nerve by way of the gray rami and supply the blood vessels, hair follicles (arrector pili muscles), and sweat glands.

—enables the body to cope with various crises or emergencies and thus is often referred to as the fight-or-flight division.

1. Sympathetic Trunk

—is composed primarily of ascending and descending preganglionic sympathetic fibers and visceral afferent fibers.

—also contains cell bodies of the postganglionic sympathetic fibers.

2. White Rami

—contain the preganglionic sympathetic fibers whose cell bodies are located in the lateral horn of the spinal cord.

—contain visceral afferent fibers whose cell bodies are located in the dorsal root ganglia.

—are limited to the spinal cord segments between T1 and L2.

3. Gray Rami

—contain the postganglionic sympathetic fibers whose cell bodies are located in the sympathetic chain ganglia.

—carry the postganglionic sympathetic fibers that supply the blood vessels, hair folliciles, and sweat glands.

—are connected to every spinal nerve.

4. Greater Splanchnic Nerve

—arises from the thoracic ganglia of T5 through T9.

—enters the celiac ganglion, which is formed by the cell bodies of the postganglionic fibers.

—contains the sympathetic preganglionic fibers whose cell bodies are located in the lateral horn of the spinal cord.

—also contains the visceral afferent fibers whose cell bodies are located in the dorsal root ganglia.

—passes through the aortic hiatus.

5. Lesser Splanchnic Nerve

—arises from the thoracic ganglia of T10-11 and enters the aorticorenal ganglion.

—contains the preganglionic sympathetic and visceral afferent fibers.

6. Least Splanchnic Nerve

–arises from the T12 and enters the renal plexus.

–contains the preganglionic sympathetic and visceral afferent fibers.

7. Collateral (Prevertibral) Ganglia

–include the celiac, superior mesenteric, aorticorenal, and inferior mesenteric ganglia, which are usually located near the origin of the arteries.

C. Autonomic Plexuses

1. Celiac Plexus

–is formed by splanchnic nerves and branches from the vagus nerves.

–also contains the celiac ganglia, which receive the greater splanchnic nerves.

–lies on the front of the crura of the diaphragm and on the abdominal aorta at the origins of the celiac trunk and superior mesenteric and renal arteries.

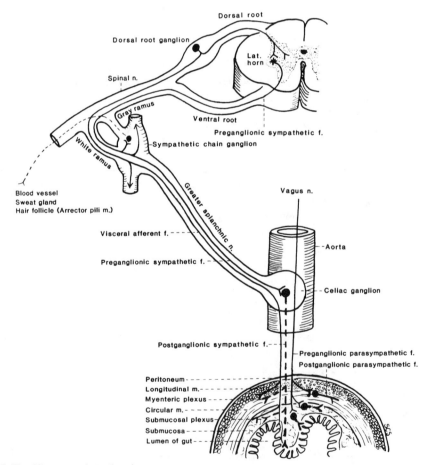

Figure 5.17. Nerve supply to the viscera.

—extends its branches along the branches of the celiac trunk and forms the subsidiary plexuses named according to the arteries along which they pass, such as gastric, splenic, hepatic, suprarenal, and renal plexuses.

2. Aortic Plexus

—is the plexus that is extended from the celiac plexus along the front of the aorta.

—extends its branches along the arteries and forms plexuses that are named accordingly—superior mesenteric, testicular (or ovarian), and inferior mesenteric.

—continues down along the aorta and forms the superior hypogastric plexus just below the bifurcation of the aorta.

IV. Diaphragm and Its Openings

A. Diaphragm

—arises from xiphoid process (sternal part), lower six costal cartilages (costal part), medial and lateral lumbocostal arches (lumbar part), and lumbar vertebrae 1–3 for right crus and lumbar vertebrae 1–2 for left crus.

—inserts into the central tendon.

—is innervated by the phrenic nerve (large central area) and intercostal nerves (peripheral part).

—receives blood from the musculophrenic, pericardiacophrenic, superior phrenic, and inferior phrenic arteries.

—descends when it contracts, causing the increased thoracic volume with a decreased thoracic pressure.

—ascends when it relaxes, causing the decreased thoracic volume with an increased thoracic pressure.

1. Right Crus

—is larger and longer than the left crus.

—originates from the upper three lumbar vertebrae.

—splits to enclose the esophagus.

2. Medial Arcuate Ligament (Medial Lumbocostal Arch)

—extends from the body of the first lumbar vertebra to the transverse process of the first lumbar vertebra.

—passes over the psoas muscle.

3. Lateral Arcuate Ligament (Lateral Lumbocostal Arch)

—extends from the transverse process of the first lumbar vertebra to the twelfth rib.

—passes over the quaratus lumborum.

B. Hiatus or Openings

1. Vena Cava Hiatus

—lies in the diaphragm (central tendon) at the level of the eight thoracic vertebra and transmits the inferior vena cava and the right phrenic nerve.

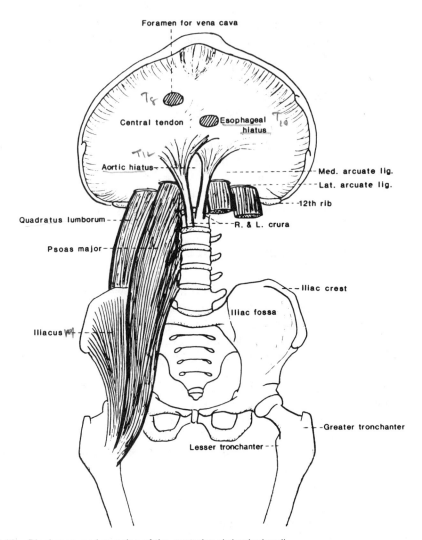

Figure 5.18. Diaphragm and muscles of the posterior abdominal wall.

2. Esophageal Hiatus

—lies in the muscular part of the diaphragm (right crus) at the level of the tenth thoracic vertebra and transmits the esophagus and the vagus nerve.

3. Aortic Hiatus

—lies behind or between two crura at the level of the twelfth thoracic vertebra and transmits the aorta, the thoracic duct, the greater splanchnic nerve, and the azygos vein.

V. Muscles of Posterior Abdominal Wall[a]

Muscle	Origin	Insertion	Nerve	Action
Quadratus lumborum	Transverse processes of LV3-5; iliolumbar ligament; iliac crest	Lower border of last rib; transverse processes of LV1–3	Subcostal n.; L1-3	Depress last rib; flexes trunk laterally
Psoas major	Transverse processes, intervertebral discs and bodies of TV12 to LV5	Lesser trochanter	L2-3	Flexes thigh and trunk
Psoas minor	Bodies and intervertebral discs of TV12 to LV1	Pectineal line; iliopectineal eminence	L1	Flexes trunk

[a]LV, lumbar vertebra; TV, thoracic vertebra.

Review Test

ABDOMEN

DIRECTIONS: For each of the questions or incomplete statements below, *one* or *more* of the answers or completions given are correct. Choose answer:

A. if only **1, 2** and **3** are correct.
B. if only **1** and **3** are correct.
C. if only **2** and **4** are correct.
D. if only **4** is correct.
E. if all are correct.

5.1. The portal-caval anastomosis exists between the following veins:

1. hepatic veins and inferior vena cava.
2. superior rectal vein and middle rectal vein.
3. middle rectal vein and inferior rectal vein.
4. paraumbilical vein and superficial epigastric vein.

5.2. Concerning a splanchnic nerve in the abdomen, it

1. contains only preganglionic sympathetic fibers.
2. is an interconnection between a sympathetic trunk and the abdominal or pelvic parts of the prevertebral plexus.
3. contains only visceral afferent fibers whose cell bodies are in the dorsal root ganglion.
4. contains preganglionic axons whose cell bodies are in the lateral horn of the spinal cord.

5.3 Which of the following statements is (are) correct?

1. Occlusion of the inferior vena cava at L4 may cause the dilation of both right and left thoracoepigastric veins.
2. Occlusion of the portal vein may result in the dilation of the subcutaneous veins in the anterior abdominal wall through which blood flows from the region of the umbilicus toward the inguinal region.
3. Compression of the right brachiocephalic vein may cause dilation of the right thoracoepigastric vein.
4. Compression of the superior vena cava may produce the dilation of the renal vein.

5.4. The suprarenal arteries may arise from the

1. aorta.
2. renal artery.
3. inferior phrenic artery.
4. superior mesenteric artery.

5.5. Unlike the right, the left renal vein receives the

1. suprarenal vein.
2. hepatic vein.
3. testicular (or ovarian) vein.
4. lumbar veins.

194

5.6. The inferior epigastric artery
1. lies medial to a direct inguinal hernia.
2. lies lateral and posterior to an indirect inguinal hernia.
3. is a branch of the internal iliac artery.
4. is a route of collateral circulation in coarctation of the aorta.

5.7. The portal vein
1. is formed by the union of the splenic and superior mesenteric veins.
2. is usually more than 12 cm in length.
3. passes anterior to the epiploic foramen in the free edge of the lesser omentum.
4. has no tributaries cephalad to its beginning.

5.8. A tumor in the uncinate process of the pancreas may compress the
1. common bile duct.
2. superior mesenteric vein.
3. portal vein.
4. duodenojejunal junction.

5.9. The descending colon
1. has teniae coli and appendices epiploicae.
2. is a retroperitoneal organ.
3. is innervated via the sacral parasympathetic system.
4. receives blood mostly from the inferior mesenteric artery.

5.10. Concerning structures that open on the greater duodenal papilla, which of the following are true?
1. The common bile duct traverses the head of the pancreas.
2. Normally, the greater duodenal papilla is in the posterior medial wall of the second part of the duodenum.
3. The common bile duct lies in the free border of the lesser omentum.
4. In most cases, the common bile duct and the main pancreatic duct have separate openings into the duodenum.

5.11. The free edge of the hepatoduodenal ligament
1. forms a boundary of the epiploic foramen.
2. contains the common bile duct, hepatic artery, and portal vein.
3. is part of the lesser omentum.
4. is attached to the second part of the duodenum.

5.12. Of the following structures, which ones are usually described as having a mesentery (suspended from the body wall by a double layer of an extension of peritoneum)?
1. the first inch of first part of duodenum.
2. transverse colon.
3. sigmoid colon.
4. appendix.

5.13. Of the following, which are found in the abdominal cavity (as opposed to being in the peritoneal cavity)?
1. stomach.
2. pancreas.
3. spleen.
4. kidney.

5.14. Of the following arteries, usually, which do *not* give direct branches to the ureter?
1. renal.
2. celiac.
3. middle rectal.
4. inferior phrenic.

5.15. Of the following, which one(s) would most likely contain(s) pain fibers from the abdominal viscera?
1. splanchnic nerves.
2. roots of T5, 6, 7, 8, and 9.
3. sympathetic nerves to viscera.
4. vagal fibers.

DIRECTIONS: For each numbered item, select the *one* numbered heading that is most closely associated with it. Each numbered heading may be selected once, more than once, or not at all.

A. Hepatic vein
B. Portal vein
C. Superior mesenteric vein
D. Coronary vein (left gastric)
E. Inferior mesenteric vein

5.16. Is not part of the portal system.

5.17. Lies in front of the uncinate process of the pancreas.

5.18. Drains blood directly from the lesser curvature of the stomach.

5.19. Usually empties into the splenic vein.

5.20. Lies immediately anterior to the epiploic foramen.

A. Linea alba
B. Linea semilunaris
C. Linea semicircularis
D. Transversalis fascia
E. Conjoint tendon (falx inguinalis)

5.21. Defines the lateral margin of the rectus abdominis muscle.

5.22. Forms the posterior sheath of the rectus abdominis, below the arcuate line.

5.23. Is a tendinous mesial line, extending from the xiphoid process to the public symphysis.

5.24. Is composed of the aponeurosis of the internal oblique and transversus abdominis muscles.

5.25. Is a crescentic line marking the termination of the posterior sheath of the rectus abdominis muscle.

A. Lienorenal ligament
B. Lienogastric ligament
C. Gastrophrenic ligament
D. Falciform ligament
E. Hepatoduodenal ligament

5.26. Contains a bile duct.

5.27. Contains a paraumbilical vein.

5.28. Contains short gastric arteries.

5.29. Contains a small portion of the tail of the pancreas.

5.30. Contains splenic vessels.

A. Right gastric artery
B. Left gastroepiploic artery
C. Splenic artery
D. Gastroduodenal artery
E. Cystic artery

5.31. Is found within the lienogastric ligament.

5.32. Gives rise to the superior pancreaticoduodenal artery.

5.33. Is a direct branch of the celiac artery.

5.34. Runs along the lesser curvature of the stomach.

5.35. Runs along the superior border of the pancreas during its course.

DIRECTIONS: Each set of letters headings below is followed by a list of numbered words or phrases. Choose answer:

A. if the item is associated with **A** only.
B. if the item is associated with **B** only.
C. if the item is associated with both **A** and **B**.
D. if the item is associated with neither **A** nor **B**.

A. Ilioinguinal nerve
B. Genitofemoral nerve
C. Both
D. Neither

5.36. Supplies motor fibers to the cremaster muscle.

5.37. Passes superficial to the inguinal ligament.

5.38. Gives rise to the anterior scrotal (or labial) branches.

5.39. Usually lies on the anterior surface of the psoas muscle.

5.40. Emerges from the superficial inguinal ring.

A. Indirect inguinal hernia
B. Direct inguinal hernia
C. Both
D. Neither

5.46. Has a peritoneal covering.

5.47. May pass through both the deep and superficial inguinal rings.

5.48. Occurs through the posterior wall of the inguinal canal in the region of the inguinal triangle.

5.49. Lies medial to the inferior epigastric vessels.

5.50. May have the same three fascial coverings as the spermatic cord.

A. Anterior rectus sheath
B. Posterior rectus sheath
C. Both
D. Neither

5.41. Between the costal arch and the arcuate line, it is formed by the aponeurosis of the internal oblique abdominis muscle.

5.42. Below the arcuate line, it is formed in part by the transversalis fascia.

5.43. The inferior epigastric artery is in contact with this structure.

5.44. Is formed in part by the aponeurosis of the internal oblique abdominis muscle at all levels.

5.45. Encloses the pyramidalis muscle if present.

A. Ascending colon
B. Descending colon
C. Both
D. Neither

5.51. Is retroperitoneal in position.

5.52. Drains its venous blood directly or indirectly into the portal venous system.

5.53. Receives parasympathetic fibers primarily from the vagus nerve.

5.54. Is characterized by the presence of the teniae coli and haustra or sacculations.

5.55. Receives arterial blood primarily from the inferior mesenteric artery.

DIRECTIONS: Each of the questions or incomplete statements below is followed by five suggested answers or completions. Choose the *one* that is best in each case.

5.56. Find one *incorrect* statement concerning the portal venous system.

A. Normally, the blood pressure in the portal vein is maintained at a higher pressure than that found in the inferior vena cava.
B. The injurious effects of abnormally high pressures in the portal vein are due to valves in the portal vein that permit distension of the portal vein.
C. The most potentially dangerous area where varices or venous dilations occur as a result of portal hypertension is the lower end of the esophagus.
D. Portal hypertension may cause caput medusae.
E. The volume of blood carried to the liver by the portal vein is at least twice the volume delivered by the hepatic artery.

5.57. Concerning the lower end of the ileum:

A. The plicae circularis (circular folds) are more prominent and numerous here than in the upper part of the jejunum.
B. The mesenteric arterial arcades are more numerous here than in the upper part of the jejunum.
C. Maximum digestion and absorption of nutrients occur here.
D. The vasa recta is longer than that of the jejunum.
E. Its mesentery contains less fat than the jejunal mesentery.

5.58. One of the following fetal vessels becomes the round ligament of the liver after birth.

A. ductus venosus.
B. vitelline vein.
C. umbilical artery.
D. ductus ateriosus.
E. umbilical vein.

5.59. Of the following veins, which one does *not* belong to the portal system?

A. veins from sigmoid mesocolon.
B. superior rectal.
C. splenic.
D. gastroepiploic.
E. suprarenal.

5.60. On either side of the body

A. the conjoined tendon (falx inguinalis) includes fibers of the aponeurosis of the transversus abdominis and internal oblique abdominis muscles.
B. the lacunar ligament is a triangular expansion of the lateral end of the inguinal ligament.
C. the inguinal ligament is formed by the aponeuroses of the external and internal oblique abdominis muscles.
D. the inferior epigastric vessels course between the superficial inguinal ring and the medial umbilical ligament (a ligament formed by the obliterated umbilical artery).

5.61. Because of the anatomic relations of the pancreas, which of the following would most likely result in obstructive jaundice?

A. aneurysm of the splenic artery.
B. perforated ulcer of the stomach.
C. damage to the pancreas during splenectomy.
D. cancer of the head of the pancreas.
E. tumor in the body of the pancreas.

5.62. Of the following arteries, which one (branches included) would not follow a mesentery in order to reach the organ that it supplies?

A. hepatic.
B. mesenteric.
C. middle colic.
D. sigmoid branch of left colic.
E. dorsal pancreatic.

5.63. Which of the following structures are not related to embryonic or fetal blood vessels?

A. median umbilical ligament.
B. medial umbilical ligament.
C. ligamentum venosum.
D. ligamentum teres hepatis.
E. ligamentum arteriosum.

5.64. Select the correct statement(s).

A. Between the costal margin and the umbilicus the posterior layer of the sheath of the rectus abdominis muscle is formed by the aponeuroses of the internal oblique and transversus abdominis muscles.
B. Normally the deep inguinal ring is in the aponeurosis of the transversus abdominis muscle.
C. The external spermatic fascia is continuous with the transversalis fascia.
D. The pyramidalis muscle, when present, is attached to the xiphoid process.

5.65. Normally, which one of the following veins is *not* a direct tributary to the superior mesenteric vein?

A. middle colic.
B. right colic.
C. pancreaticoduodenal.
D. iliocolic.
E. lower left colic.

5.66. Normally, structures that do not directly enter or leave the liver by way of the porta hepatis are

A. right hepatic artery.
B. branches of the anterior gastric nerves.
C. common hepatic artery.
D. hepatic ducts.
E. portal vein.

5.67. Preganglionic parasympathetic fibers of the liver travel in

A. sympathetic trunks.
B. visceral branches of sympathetic trunks.
C. pelvic splanchnic nerves.
D. vagus nerves.
E. splanchnic branches of sympathetic trunks.

5.68. The cell bodies of both afferent and efferent nerve fibers in visceral branches of the sympathetic trunk are located in

A. collateral ganglia, ventral horn of spinal cord, and terminal ganglia only.
B. intermediolateral cell column of spinal cord and dorsal root ganglia.
C. dorsal root ganglia only.
D. sympathetic chain ganglia only.
E. intermediolateral cell column of spinal cord and sympathetic chain ganglia only.

5.69. Normally, of the following structures, which one is a retroperitoneal organ?

A. stomach.
B. transverse colon.
C. jejunum.
D. descending colon.
E. spleen.

5.70. Nerve fibers innervating cells in the adrenal medulla responsible for secreting noradrenaline are

A. preganglionic sympathetic.
B. postganglionic sympathetic.
C. somatic motor.
D. postganglionic parasympathetic.
E. preganglionic parasympathetic.

5.71. The internal oblique muscle is considered to be part of, or contributing to the formation of the

A. cremaster muscle.
B. lacunar ligament.
C. floor of the inguinal canal.
D. external spermatic fascia.
E. internal spermatic fascia.

5.72. Normally, of the following arteries, which one would *least* likely give off direct branches to the pancreas?

A. middle colic.
B. splenic.
C. gastroduodenal.
D. superior mesenteric.

5.73. In the adult, remnants of the embryonic urachus forms a structure called the

A. medial umbilical fold.
B. round ligament of the uterus.
C. inguinal ligament.
D. median umbilical ligament.
E. lateral umbilical fold.

5.74. Of the following arteries, which would be most likely *not* to send branches to the ureter?

A. superior mesenteric.
B. testicular (ovarian).
C. renal.
D. superior vesical.
E. aorta.

5.75. Select the *incorrect* statement regarding the adrenal glands.

A. Usually, there are more arteries than veins associated with each adrenal gland.
B. The thoracic splanchnic nerves bring postganglionic sympathetic fibers to the medulla of each gland.
C. Each gland is surrounded by an extension of the renal fascia.
D. Part of the left adrenal lies posterior to the lesser peritoneal sac.
E. Normally most or all of each adrenal gland lies on the diaphragm.

5.76. One member of each of the three pairs of veins listed below terminates in a vein on one side of the body, which is a different vein from the one that the other member of the pair terminates in on the other side of the body. From the four pairs listed, choose the pair of which both members terminate in the same vein.

A. ovarians.
B. testiculars.
C. inferior phrenics.
D. adrenals (suprarenals).
E. third lumbars.

5.77. Select the *incorrect* statement regarding the jejunum.

A. The veins draining this organ are direct or indirect tributaries of the portal vein.
B. It receives blood from branches of the superior mesenteric artery.
C. It is commonly affected by cancer of the head of the pancreas.
D. It is surrounded by the peritoneum throughout its length.
E. It has no teniae coli in its wall.

5.78. Which one of the following structures crosses or lies anterior to the inferior vena cava?

A. right sympathetic trunk.
B. third right lumbar vein.
C. third part of the duodenum.
D. right renal artery.
E. cisternal chyli.

5.79. Which one of the following structures lies posterior to the aorta?

A. third left lumbar vein.
B. left renal vein.
C. fourth part of the duodenum
D. root of the mesentery.
E. uncinate process of the pancreas.

5.80. The white rami communicantes

A. contain preganglionic sympathetic fibers whose cell bodies are in the anterior horn of the spinal cord.
B. contain preganglionic sympathetic fibers whose cell bodies are in the lateral horn of the spinal cord.
C. contain postganglionic sympathetic fibers whose cell bodies are in the sympathetic chain ganglion.
D. contain postganglionic sympathetic fibers that supply the blood vessels and sweat gland.
E. contain somatic afferent fibers whose cell bodies are in the dorsal root ganglia.

Answers and Explanations

ABDOMEN

5.1. C. Both the hepatic veins and inferior vena cava are systemic (caval) veins. Both the middle and inferior rectal veins also belong to the caval system.

5.2. C. The splanchnic nerve in the abdomen extends from the sympathetic trunk to the abdominal parts of the prevertebral plexuses. It contains preganglionic sympathetic axons whose cell bodies are in the lateral horn of the spinal cord.

5.3. A. The thoracoepigastric vein can be dilated by occulusion of the superior vena cava, or brachiocephalic vein, or lower part of the inferior vena cava. The dilation of subcutaneous veins around the umbilicus results from the obstruction of the portal vein and this condition is called "caput medusa." This is because the paraumbilical vein connects the left branch of the portal vein to subcutaneous veins around the umbilicus.

5.4. A. The suprarenal gland receives arteries from three sources: the superior suprarenal artery from the inferior phrenic; the middle suprarenal from the abdominal aorta; and the inferior suprarenal from the renal artery.

5.5. B. The adrenal, inferior phrenic and testicular or ovarian veins drain into the renal vein on the left and into the inferior vena cava on the right.

5.6. D. The inferior epigastric artery is a branch of the external iliac artery and lies lateral to the direct inguinal hernia but medial to the indirect inguinal hernia. This artery provides a route of collateral circulation in coarctation of the aorta by anastomosing with the superior epigastric branch of the internal throacic artery.

5.7. B. The portal vein is formed by the union of the splenic and superior mesenteric veins and is about 8 cm long. It passes anterior to the epiploic foramen in the free edge of the lesser omentum and has tributaries such as the left and right gastric veins and the posterior superior pancreaticoduodenal vein.

5.8. C. The head of the pancreas is surrounded by the C-shaped duodenum. The common bile duct traverses the head of the pancreas. The superior mesenteric vein crosses the uncinate process of the pancreas and joins, behind the neck of the pancreas, the splenic vein to form the portal vein.

5.9. E. The descending colon is retroperitoneal in position and has external characteristics such as teniae coli, epiploic appendices, and haustra. It receives blood mostly from the inferior mesenteric artery and parasympathetic fibers from the pelvic splanchnic nerve, which arises from the sacral segments of the spinal cord (S2-4).

5.10. A. The common bile duct traverses the head of the pancreas and is joined by the main pancreatic duct to form the hepatopancreatic duct and/or ampulla, which opens into the greater papilla in the posterior medial wall of the second part of the duodenum.

5.11. A. The hepatoduodenal ligament is attached to the beginning of the first part of the duodenum.

5.12. E. The first inch of the first part of the duodenum is surrounded by peritoneum (hepatoduodenal ligament). The transverse and sigmoid colons and the appendix have their own mesenteries, such as the transverse and sigmoid mesocolons and the mesoappendix.

5.13. E. The peritoneal cavity contains nothing but a film of fluid that lubricates the surface of the peritoneum.

5.14. C. The ureter receives blood from the aorta, the renal, gonadal, common iliac, internal iliac, umbilical, superior and inferior vesical, and middle rectal arteries.

5.15. A. The vagus nerve contains sensory fibers associated with reflexes but no pain fibers.

5.16. A. The hepatic vein belongs to the systemic (caval) venous system.

5.17. C. The superior mesenteric vessels lie in front of the uncinate process of the pancreas.

5.18. D. The coronary (left gastric) vein drains blood from the lesser curvature of the stomach into the portal vein.

5.19. E. The inferior mesenteric vein usually empties into the splenic vein, but it may join the superior mesenteric vein or the junction of the superior mesenteric and splenic veins.

5.20. B. The portal vein lies immediately anterior to the epiploic foramen in the free margin of the lesser omentum.

5.21. B. The linea semilunaris is the lateral margin of the rectus abdominis muscle.

5.22. D. The transversalis fascia forms the posterior layer of the rectus sheath, below the arcuate line.

5.23. A. The linea alba is a tendinous medial line, extending from the xiphoid process to the symphysis pubis.

5.24. E. The conjoint tendon (falx inguinalis) is formed by the aponeuroses of the internal oblique and transversus abdominis muscles.

5.25. C. The linea semicircularis is a crescentic line marking the termination of the posterior layer of the rectus sheath.

5.26. E. The hepatoduodenal ligament is a part of the lesser omentum and contains the bile duct, the hepatic artery, and the portal vein.

5.27. D. The falciform ligament contains a paraumbilical vein that connects the left branch of the portal vein with subcutaneous veins around the umbilicus.

5.28. B. The lienogastric (or gastrosplenic) ligament contains several short gastric and left gastroepiploic vessels.

5.29. A. The lienorenal ligament contains a small portion of the tail of the pancreas and the splenic vessels.

5.30. A. See 5.29.

5.31. B. The lienogastric ligament contains the left gastroepiploic and short gastric vessels.

5.32. D. The gastroduodenal artery is divided into the superior pancreaticoduodenal and right gastroepiploic arteries.

5.33. C. The direct branches of the celiac trunk are the left gastric, splenic, and common hepatic arteries.

5.34. A. The right gastric artery arises from either the hepatic artery proper or the common hepatic artery and runs between layers of the lesser omentum along the lesser curvature of the stomach.

5.35. C. The splenic artery takes the tortuous course along the superior border of the pancreas.

5.36. B. The genitofemoral nerve descends in front of the psoas muscle and superficial to the inguinal ligament. It divides into a genital branch, which supplies the cremaster muscle, and a femoral branch, which supplies the skin of the femoral triangle.

5.37. C. See 5.36 and 5.38.

5.38. A. The ilioinguinal nerve passes through the inguinal canal, emerges through the superficial inguinal ring, and runs superficial to the inguinal ligament. It gives rise to the anterior scrotal (or labial) nerve. The posterior scrotal (or labial) nerve arises from the perineal nerve.

5.39. B. See 5.36.

5.40. A. See 5.38.

5.41. C. Above the arcuate line, the anterior rectus sheath is formed by the aponeuroses of the external and internal oblique abdominis muscles, whereas the posterior rectus sheath is formed by the aponeuroses of the internal oblique and transversus abdominis muscles.

5.42. B. Below the arcuate line, the posterior rectus sheath is formed by the transversalis fascia, whereas the anterior rectus sheath is formed by the aponeuroses of the external oblique, internal oblique, and transversus abdominis muscles.

5.43. B. The inferior epigastric artery is in contact with the posterior rectus sheath.

5.44. A. The anterior rectus sheath is formed in part by the aponeurosis of the internal oblique abdominis muscle at all levels.

5.45. A. The anterior rectus sheath splits and encloses the pyramidalis muscle if present.

5.46. C. Both direct and indirect herniae have peritoneal coverings.

5.47. A. The indirect hernia passes through the deep inguinal ring, inguinal canal, and superficial inguinal ring and descends into the scrotum.

5.48. A. The direct hernia occurs through the posterior wall of the inguinal canal in the inguinal triangle and does not usually descend into the scrotum.

5.49. B. The direct inguinal hernia lies medial to the inferior epigastric vessels, whereas the indirect hernia lies lateral to these vessels.

5.50. A. The indirect hernia may have the same three facial coverings as the spermatic cord.

5.51. C. Both the ascending and descending colons are retroperitoneal in position.

5.52. C. Both the ascending and descending colons drain their venous blood directly or indirectly into the portal venous system.

5.53. A. The ascending colon receives parasympathetic fibers from the vagus nerve, whereas the descending colon receives them from the pelvic splanchnic nerve.

5.54. C. The colon consists of the ascending, transverse, descending, and sigmoid parts, which are characterized by the presence of the teniae coli, haustra (or succulations), and epiploic appendages.

5.55. B. The ascending colon receives blood primarily from the superior mesenteric artery, whereas the descending colon receives it from the inferior mesenteric artery.

5.56. B. The portal vein and its tributaries have no valves or, if present, they are insignificant.

5.57. B. When compared to the jejunum, the ileum has less prominent (shorter) plicae circularis, more numerous mesenteric arterial arcades, more mesenteric fat, and shorter vasa recta. Digestion and absorption of nutrients occur less in the lower end of the ileum.

5.58. E. The left umbilical vein becomes the round ligament of the liver after birth.

5.59. E. The suprarenal vein belongs to the systemic (or caval) venous system and drains into the inferior vena cava on the right and into the renal vein on the left.

5.60. A. The lacunar ligament is a triangular expansion of the medial end of the inguinal ligament. The inguinal ligament is the folded lower border of the aponeurosis of the external oblique abdominis. The inferior epigastric vessels run from the deep inguinal ring toward the umbilicus, forming the lateral umbilical fold (or ligament).

5.61. D. The bile duct traverses the head of the pancreas and thus cancer in this are obstructs the bile duct, resulting in jaundice.

5.62. E. The pancreas is a retroperitoneal organ except for a small portion of its tail, and thus the dorsal pancreatic artery arising from the splenic artery runs behind peritoneum.

5.63. A. The median umbilical ligament contains the urachus, which is the fibrous remains of the fetal allantois.

5.64. A. The deep inguinal ring is in the transversalis fascia. The external spermatic fascia is continuous with the aponeurosis of the external oblique abdominis. The pyramidalis arises from the body of the pubis and inserts on the linea alba.

5.65. E. The lower left colic vein is a tributary to the inferior mesenteric vein.

5.66. C. The common hepatic artery gives off the gastroduodenal artery and the hepatic artery proper, which divides into the right and left hepatic arteries.

5.67. D. Preganglionic parasympathetic fibers of the liver travel in the vagus nerve.

5.68. B. The cell bodies of the visceral efferent fibers are located in the intermediolateral cell column (or lateral horn) of the spinal cord, whereas those of the visceral afferent fibers are in the dorsal root ganglia.

5.69. D. The descending colon is a retroperitoneal organ.

5.70. A. The adrenal medulla is the only organ that receives preganglionic sympathetic fibers.

5.71. A. The cremaster muscle and fascia arise from the internal oblique abdominis muscle.

5.72. A. The middle colic artery does not supply the pancreas. The splenic artery gives off a number of pancreatic branches, including the dorsal pancreatic artery. The superior pancreaticoduodenal artery arises from the gastroduodenal artery, whereas the inferior pancreaticoduodenal artery arises from the superior mesenteric artery.

5.73. D. The median umbilical fold contains remnants of the embryonic urachus.

5.74. A. The superior mesenteric artery does not send branches to the ureter.

5.75. B. The chromaffin cells in the adrenal medulla may be considered as modified postganglionic sympathetic neurons.

5.76. E. The third lumbar veins drain into the inferior vena cava on both sides.

5.77. C. The duodenum is a C-shaped tube, surrounding the head of the pancreas.

5.78. C. The third part of the duodenum crosses anterior to the inferior vena cava.

5.79. A. The left third lumbar vein runs posterior to the abdominal aorta.

5.80. B. The white rami commuicantes contain preganglionic sympathetic and visceral afferent fibers whose cell bodies are located in the lateral horn of the spinal cord and the dorsal root ganglia, respectively.

6
Perineum and Pelvis

Perineal Region

I. Perineum

–is a diamond-shaped space that has the same boundaries as the inferior aperture of the pelvis:

  a. *Anterior*

   –the arcuate pubic ligament and the inferior rami of the pubis and ischium.

  b. *Posterior*

   –the tip of the coccyx.

  c. *Lateral*

   –the sacrotuberous ligaments and ischial tuberosities.

–its floor is skin and fascia.

–its roof is formed by the pelvic diaphragm with its fascial covering.

–divides into an anterior urogenital triangle and a posterior anal triangle by a line connecting the two ischial tuberosities.

II. Urogenital Triangle

A. Superficial Perineal Pouch or Space

–lies between the inferior fascia of the urogenital diaphragm (the perineal membrane) and the membranous layer of the superficial perineal fascia (Colles' fascia).

–contains the superficial transverse perineal muscle, ischiocavernosus muscle and crura of the penis, bulbospongiosus muscle and bulb of the penis, and central tendon of the perineum.

1. Colles' Fascia

–is the deep membranous layer of the superficial perineal fascia.

–is continuous with the Dartos tunic in the male.

–passes over the penis as the superficial fascia of the penis.

205

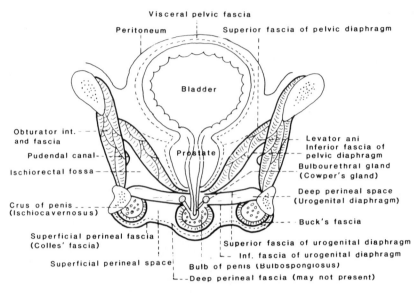

Figure 6.1. Frontal section of the male perineum and pelvis.

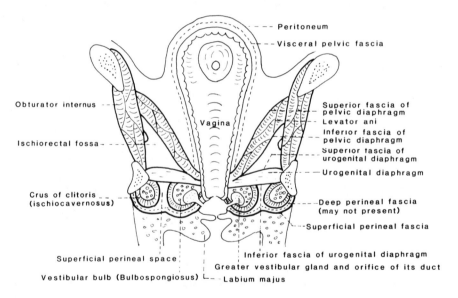

Figure 6.2. Frontal section of the female perineum and pelvis.

—is continuous with Scarpa's fascia.

—forms the lower boundary of the superficial perineal pouch.

2. Perineal Membrane

—is the inferior fascia of the urogenital diaphragm.

—forms the inferior boundary of the deep perineal pouch and the superior boundary of the superficial pouch.

3. Muscles

a. *Ischiocavernosus Muscle*

–arises from the lower part of the inner surface of the ischiopubic ramus.

–inserts into the corpus cavernosum (the crus of the penis or clitoris).

–is innervated by the perineal branch of the pudendal nerve.

–maintains erection of the penis by compressing the crus and thereby retarding the venous return.

b. *Bulbospongiosus Muscle*

–arises from the perineal body and the fibrous raphe of the bulb of the penis.

–inserts into the corpus spongiosum.

–is innervated by the perineal branch of the pudendal nerve.

–its contraction (along with ischiocavernous) constricts the corpus spongiosum, expelling the last drops of urine or semen in ejaculation.

–in the male, compresses the bulb, impeding venous return from the penis and thereby maintains erection. It expells the last drop of urine.

–in the female compresses the erectile tissue of the bulb of the vestibule and constricts the vaginal orifice.

c. *Transversus Perinei Superficialis Muscle*

–arises from the ischial ramus and tuberosity.

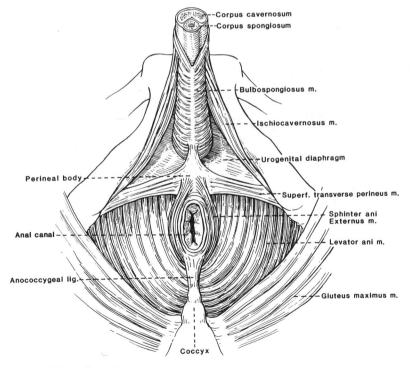

Figure 6.3. Muscles of the male perineum.

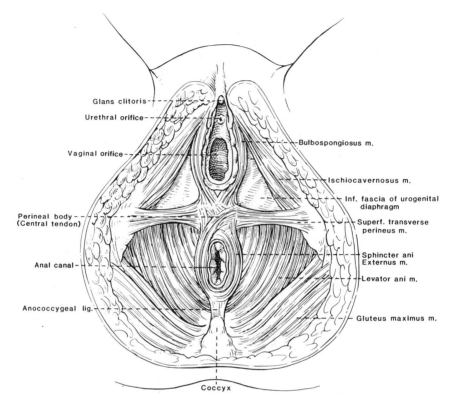

Figure 6.4. Muscles of the female perineum.

—inserts into the central tendon.
—is supplied by the perineal branch of the pudendal nerve.
—fixes the central tendon in place.

4. **Perineal Body or Central Tendon of Perineum**
   —is a fibromuscular mass located in the center of the perineum between the anal canal and the vagina (or the bulb of the penis).
   —serves as a site of attachment for the superficial and deep transversus perinei, bulbospongiosus, levator ani, and external anal sphincter.
   —is especially important in the female, because it may be torn during parturition. To prevent uncontrolled tearing, the birth canal is enlarged by making an incision through the posterior vaginal wall and the perineal body (posterior episiotomy).

5. **Greater Vestibular Gland (Bartholin's)**
   —lies in the superficial perineal pouch, under cover of and/or behind the bulb of the vestibule.
   —is the homolog of the bulbourethral gland of the male.
   —is compressed during coitus and secretes mucus that lubricates the vagina.
   —its duct opens into the vestibule between the labium minus and the hymen.

B. Deep Perineal Pouch or Space
–lies between the superior and inferior fasciae of the urogenital diaphragm.
–contains the deep transversus perineal muscle, sphincter urethrae, membranous part of urethra, bulbourethral glands, branches of the internal pudendal vessels, and perineal nerve.

1. Muscles
a. *Transversus Perinei Profundus Muscle*
–arises from the inner surface of the inferior ischial ramus.
–inserts into the medial tendinous raphe and the side of the vagina in the female, and the perineal body.
–is supplied by the perineal branches of the pudendal nerve.
–fixes the perineal body and supports the prostate or the vagina.

b. *Sphincter Urethrae Muscle*
–arises from the inferior pubic ramus.
–inserts into the median raphe and the perineal body.
–is supplied by the perineal branch of the pudendal nerve.
–compresses the urethra.

2. Urogenital Diaphragm
–consists of the deep transverse perinei and the sphincter urethrae, invested by the superior and inferior fasciae.
–stretches between the two pubic rami and ischial rami.
–has the crura of the penis attached to the inferior surface of its inferior fascia.
–is pierced by the urethra and the vagina.
–is innervated by the deep branches of the perineal nerve.
–does not reach the pubic symphysis anteriorly.

3. Bulbourethral Gland (Cowper's Gland)
–lies among the fibers of the sphincter urethrae in the deep perineal pouch.
–its ducts open into the bulbous portion of the spongy (penile) urethra.
–lies on both sides of the membranous portion of the urethra.

III. Anal Triangle
A. Ischiorectal Fossa
–its boundaries:
a. *Anterior*
–the superficial and deep transverse perineal muscles and the perineal line.
b. *Posterior*
–the gluteus maximus and sacrotuberous ligament.
c. *Superomedial*
–the sphincter ani externus and levator ani muscles.
d. *Lateral*
–the obturator fascia covering the obturator internus.

e. Floor

   —the skin over the anal triangle

—is located in the anal triangle.

—contains fat and the inferior rectal nerve and vessels.

B. Muscles

1. Obturator Internus Muscle

—arises from the inner surface of the obturator membrane.

—its tendon passes around the lesser sciatic notch to insert into the medial surface of the greater trochanter of the femur.

—is innervated by the nerve to the obturator internus.

—laterally rotates the thigh.

2. Sphincter Ani Externus Muscle

—arises from the tip of the coccyx and the anococcygeal ligament.

—inserts into the central tendon of the perineum.

—is supplied by the inferior rectal nerve.

—closes the anus.

3. Levator Ani Muscle

—arises from the body of the pubis, the arcus tendineus, and the ischial spine.

—inserts into the coccyx and anococcygeal raphe.

—is supplied by the branches of the anterior rami of the third and fourth sacral nerves and the perineal branch of the pudendal nerve.

—supports and raises the pelvic floor.

—consists of the puborectalis, pubococcygeus, and ilicoccygeus.

4. Coccygeus Muscle

—arises from the ischial spine and the sacrospinous ligament.

—inserts into the coccyx and the lower part of the sacrum.

—is supplied by the branches of the third and fourth sacral nerves.

—supports and raises the pelvic floor.

IV. Male External Genitalia and Associated Structures

A. Fascia and Ligaments

1. Fundiform Ligaments of Penis

—arise from the linea alba and the membranous layer of the superficial fascia of the abdomen.

—split into left and right parts, encircle the body of the penis, and blend with the superficial penile fascia.

—enter the septum of the scrotum.

2. Suspensory Ligament of Penis (or Clitoris)

—arises from the pubic symphysis and the arcuate pubic ligament.

—inserts into the deep fascia of the penis (or clitoris).

—lies deep to the fundiform ligaments.

3. Buck's Fascia

—is the continuation of Colles' fascia upon the penis.

—is the deep fascia of the penis.

4. Tunica Albuginea

−is a fibrous connective tissue layer that envelopes both the corpora cavernosa and the corpus spongiosum.

−is very dense surrounding the corpora cavernosa, thereby greatly impeding venous return and resulting in the extreme turgidity of these structures when the erectile tissue becomes engorged with blood.

−is more elastic surrounding the corpus spongiosum, which therefore does *not* become excessively turgid on erection and permits the passage of the ejaculate.

5. Tunica Vaginalis

−is a double serous membrane; a peritoneal sac on the end of the processus vaginalis.

−covers the front and sides of the testis and epididymis.

−is derived from the abdominal peritoneum.

−forms the innermost layer of the scrotum.

−is a closed sac.

−consists of a parietal layer, which is adjacent to the internal spermatic fascia, and a visceral layer, which is adherent to the testis and epididymis.

6. Processus Vaginalis

−is a peritoneal diverticulum in the fetus.

−forms the visceral and parietal layers of the tunica vaginalis.

−its neck normally fuses at birth or shortly thereafter.

−normally loses its connection with the peritoneal cavity.

7. Gubernaculum Testis

−its homologs in the female are the ovarian and round ligaments.

−is the fetal cord that connects the fetal testis to the developing scrotum.

−appears to play a significant role in testicular descent (by pulling the testis down as it migrates).

B. Scrotum

−is the cutaneous pouch, consisting of the skin and the underlying dartos.

−its skin is relatively thin with little or no fat, which is important to maintain a temperature lower than the rest of the body.

−contains the testis and its covering and the epididymis which are described on page 219.

−its dartos tunic:

    a. is continuous with the superficial penile fascia and the superficial perineal fascia.

    b. is formed by the fusion of the superficial and deep layers of superficial fascia.

    c. consists largely of smooth muscle fibers, contains no fat, and functions in temperature regulation.

−is contracted and wrinkled under the influence of cold (or sexual stimulation), bringing the testis into close contact with the body to conserve heat.

—is relaxed under the influence of warmth, causing it to be flaccid and distended to dissipate heat.

—is supplied by:

a. the anterior scrotal branch of the ilioinguinal nerve.

b. the genital branch of the genitofemoral nerve.

c. the posterior scrotal branch of the perineal branch of the pudendal nerve.

d. the perineal branch of the posterior femoral cutaneous nerve.

C. Penis

—consists of three masses of a vascular erectile tissue, the paired corpora cavernosa and the midline corpus spongiosum, which are bounded by tunica albuginea.

—has a root, which includes two crura and the bulb of the penis, and the body, which contains the single corpus spongiosum and the paired corpora cavernosa.

—the glans is formed by the terminal part of the corpus spongiosum and covered by a double fold of skin, the **prepuce**. The frenulum of the prepuce is a median ventral fold that is attached to the external urethral orifice.

V. Female External Genitalia

A. Labia Majora

—are two longitudinal folds of skin that run downward and backward from the mons pubis.

—meet in front in the anterior commisure.

—their outer surfaces are covered by pigmented skin with sebaceous and sweat glands and covered with hairs after puberty.

—are homologus to the scrotum of the male.

—contain the terminations of the round ligaments of the uterus.

B. Labia Minora

—unlike the labia majora, they are hairless and contain no fat.

—divide into two parts, upper (superolateral) and lower (superomedial).

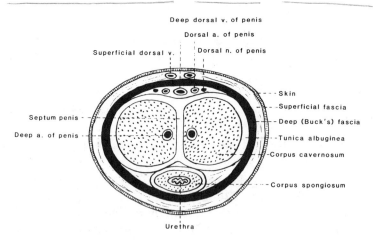

Figure 6.5. Cross-section of the penis.

      a. The lateral parts, above the clitoris, fuse to form the prepuce of the clitoris.

      b. The medial parts, below the clitoris, fuse to form the frenulum of the clitoris.

C. Vestibule of Vagina

–is the space or cleft between the labia minora.

–has the openings of the urethra, the vagina, and the ducts of the greater vestibular glands in its floor.

D. Clitoris

–is homologous with the penis in the male.

–consists of erectile tissue and is enlarged as a result of engorgement with blood.

–consists of two crura, two corpora cavernosa, and a glans but has no corpus spongiosum. The glans is covered by a very sensitive epithelium.

VI. Nerve Supply

A. Pudendal Nerve

–passes through the greater sciatic foramen between the piriformis and coccygeus.

–crosses the ischial spine and enters the perineum with the internal pudendal artery through the lesser sciatic foramen.

–enters the pudendal canal, gives off the inferior rectal nerve and the perineal nerve, and terminates as the dorsal nerve of the penis (or clitoris).

1. Inferior Rectal Nerve

–arises within the pudendal canal, breaks up into several branches, crosses the ischiorectal fossa, and supplies the sphincter ani externus and the skin around the anus.

2. Perineal Nerve

–arises within the pudendal canal and divides into the deep branch, which supplies all of the perineal muscles, and the superficial (posterior scrotal or labial) branch, which in turn divides into two branches to supply the scrotum.

3. Dorsal Nerve of Penis or Clitoris

–pierces the perineal membrane, runs between the two layers of the suspensory ligament, and runs deep to the deep fascia on the dorsum of the penis or clitoris to supply the skin, prepuce, and glans.

VII. Blood Supply

A. Internal Pudendal Artery

–arises from the internal iliac artery.

–leaves the pelvis by way of the greater sciatic foramen below the piriformis and coccygeus muscles and immediately enters the perineum through the lesser sciatic foramen by hooking around the ischial spine.

–enters the ischiorectal fossa via the lesser sciatic foramen.

–is accompanied by the pudendal nerve.

–passes along the lateral wall of the ischiorectal fossa in the pudendal canal.

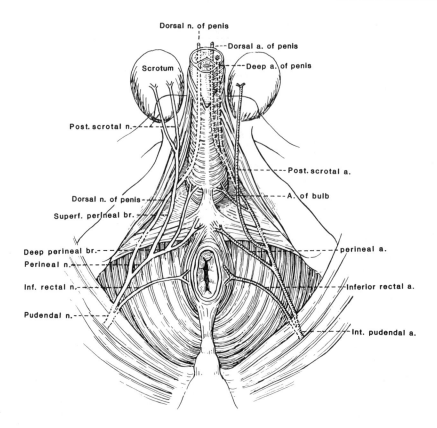

Figure 6.6. Internal pudendal artery and pudendal nerve and their branches.

1. Inferior Rectal Artery

—arises within the pudendal canal, pierces the wall of the pudendal canal, breaks into several branches which cross the ischiorectal fossa to muscles and skin around the anal canal.

2. Perineal Artery

—supplies the superficial perineal muscles and gives rise to a transverse perineal branch and a posterior scrotal branch.

3. Artery of Bulb

—arises within the deep perineal space, pierces the perineal membrane, and supplies the bulb of the penis or vestibule, and the bulbourethral gland or the greater vestibular gland.

4. Urethral Artery

—pierces the perineal membrane, enters the corpus spongiosum penis or clitoris, and continues to the glans penis or clitoris.

5. Deep Artery of Penis or Clitoris

—pierces the perineal membrane and enters the corpus cavernosum penis or clitoris to run in its center.

6. Dorsal Artery of Penis or Clitoris

–is a paired artery on each side of the deep dorsal vein and runs deep to the deep fascia (Buck's) and superficial to the tunica albuginea to supply the glans and the prepuce.

–pierces the perineal membrane and passes through the suspensory ligament of the penis or clitoris.

B. External Pudendal Artery

–arises from the femoral artery, emerges through the saphenous ring, and passes medially over the spermatic cord or the round ligament of the uterus to supply the skin above the pubis, the penis, and the scrotum or the labium majus.

C. Some Veins

1. Deep Dorsal Vein of Penis

–is an unpaired vein and lies in the dorsal midline deep to the deep fascia and superficial to the tunica albuginea.

–leaves the perineum through the gap between the arcuate pubic ligament and transverse perineal ligament.

–passes through the suspensory ligament of the penis below the infrapubic ligament.

–drains into the prostatic and pelvic venous plexuses.

2. Superficial Dorsal Vein of Penis

–runs toward the symphysis pubis between the superficial and deep fasciae on the dorsum of the penis and divides into the right and left branches, which end in the superficial external pudendal veins. (These veins drain into the greater saphenous vein.)

VIII. Clinical Consideration

A. Extravasated Urine

–may result from rupture of the urethra below the urogenital diaphragm.

–may remain in the perineum.

–can escape into the superficial perineal space but cannot spread backward or laterally.

–does spread down into the scrotum and upward on the abdominal wall.

Pelvis

I. Bony Pelvis

A. Pelvis

–is the basin-shaped ring of bone formed by the hip bones, sacrum, and coccyx. (The hip or "coxal" bone consists of the ilium, ischium, and pubis.)

–is divided by the iliopectineal line or pelvic brim into the pelvis major (false pelvis) above and the pelvis minor (true pelvis) below.

–its outlet is closed by the coccygeus and levator ani, which form the floor of the pelvis.

–is tilted in anatomical position, so that:

a. anterior superior iliac spine and the pubic tubercles are in the same vertical plane.

b. the coccyx is in the same horizontal plane as the upper margin of the symphysis pubis.

c. the axis of the pelvic cavity running through the central point of the inlet and the outlet almost parallels the curvature of the sacrum.

B. Female Pelvis

−usually has smaller, lighter, and thinner bones compared to the male.

−its inlet is usually oval; its outlet is larger than in the male because of the everted ischial tuberosities.

−the false pelvis is deeper, the greater sciatic notch wider, and the subpubic angle greater than in the male.

−the obturator foramen is oval in the female but round in the male.

C. Upper Pelvic Aperture (Pelvic Inlet or Pelvic Brim or Linea Terminalis)

−is the superior rim of the pelvic cavity.

−is bounded posteriorly by the promontory of the sacrum; laterally by the arcuate line of the ilium, the pectineal line; and anteriorly by the pubic crest and the superior margin of the symphysis pubis.

−has transverse, oblique, and anteroposterior (conjugate) diameters.

D. Lower Pelvic Aperture (Pelvic Outlet)

−is a diamond-shaped aperture.

−is bounded posteriorly by the sacrum and coccyx, laterally by the ischial tuberosities and sacrotuberous ligaments, and anteriorly by the symphysis pubis, the arcuate ligament, and the rami of the pubis and ischium.

−is closed by the pelvic and urogenital diaphragms.

E. Pelvis Major (False Pelvis)

−is the expanded portion of the pelvis above the pelvic brim.

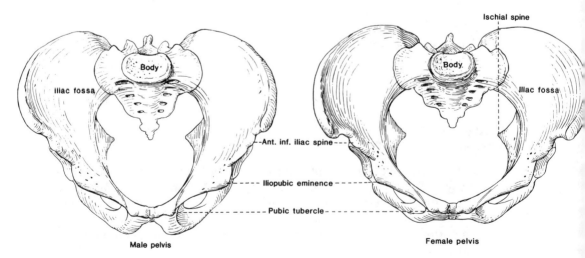

Figure 6.7. Male and female pelvic bones.

F. Pelvis Minor (True Pelvis)

–is the cavity of the pelvis below the pelvic brim or superior aperture.

–is limited below by the inferior aperture; and is formed anteriorly by the sacrum and coccyx, laterally by the ischial tuberosities and sacrotuberous ligaments, and anteriorly by the symphysis pubis and rami of the pubis and ischium.

–its outlet is closed by the coccygeus, levator ani, and perineal fascia, which form the floor of the pelvis.

–has an upper pelvic aperture (pelvic inlet or pelvic brim), a cavity, and a lower aperture (pelvic outlet).

G. Linea Terminalis

–is an oblique ridge on the inner surface of the ilium and the pubis, forming the lower boundary of the iliac fossa.

–consists of the iliopectineal line (pecten pubis) and the arcuate line on the ilium.

–separates the pelvis minor (true pelvis) from the pelvis major (false pelvis).

II. Ligaments

A. Broad Ligament

–is the two layers of peritoneum that extends from the lateral margin of the uterus to the lateral pelvic wall.

–contains the uterine tube, uterine vessels, round ligament of the uterus, ovarian ligament, ureter, uterovaginal nerve plexus, and lymphatic vessels.

–its posterior layer curves from the cervix of the uterus as the rectouterine fold, to the posterior wall of the pelvis alongside of the rectum.

1. Mesovarium

–is a fold of peritoneum that connects the anterior surface of the ovary with the posterior layer of the broad ligament.

2. Mesosalpinx

–is a fold of the broad ligament that suspends the uterine tube.

3. Mesometrium

–is a major part of the broad ligament below the mesosalpinx and mesovarium.

B. Round Ligament of Uterus

–is attached to the uterus on the front of the attachment of the ovarian ligament.

–contains smooth muscle fibers and holds the fundus forward.

–enters the inguinal canal at the deep inguinal ring, emerges from the superficial inguinal ring, and becomes lost in the subcutaneous tissue of the labium majus.

C. Ovarian Ligament

–is a fibromuscular cord that extends from the uterine end of the ovary to the side of the uterus through the broad ligament.

D. Suspensory Ligament of Ovary
—is a band of peritoneum that extends upward from the ovary to the pelvic wall.
—transmits the ovarian vessels, nerves, and lymphatics.

E. Cardinal Ligaments
—consist of tissue extending laterally below the base of the broad ligament.
—contain smooth muscle.
—are considered to be the chief ligaments that hold the uterus.
—the ureter and uterine artery runs on its upper aspect.

III. Ureter and Urinary Bladder

A. Ureter
—is a muscular tube, transmitting urine by peristaltic waves.
—has three constrictions along its course:

    a. at its origin where the pelvis of the ureter joins the ureter.
    b. where it crosses the pelvic brim.
    c. at its junction with the bladder.

—crosses the pelvic brim in front of the bifurcation of the common iliac artery.
—descends retroperitoneally on the lateral pelvic wall.
—passes in front of and below the internal iliac artery, and runs medially to the umbilical artery and the obturator vessels and nerve.
—lies 1–2 cm lateral to the cervix of the uterus in the female.
—passes posterior and medial to the ductus deferens and lies in front of the seminal vesicle in the male.
—in the female, is accompanied in its course by the uterine artery, which runs above and anterior to it—"water runs under the bridge."
—is sometimes injured by a clamp; may be ligated and sectioned to control uterine bleeding in the process of a hysterectomy.
—receives blood from the aorta, the renal, gonadal, common and internal iliac, umbilical, superior and inferior vesical, and middle recta arteries.

B. Urinary Bladder
—is situated below the peritoneum and slightly lower in the female than in the male.
—has a section where the mucous membrane is firmly bound to the muscular coat and is always smooth, called the trigone.
—its trigone is bounded by the two orifices of the ureters and the internal urethral orifice.
—its musculature (bundles of smooth muscle fibers) as a whole is known as the detrusor urinae muscle.
—extends up above the pelvic brim as it fills and may reach as high as the umbilicus if fully distended.
—receives blood from the superior and inferior vesical arteries, and also from the vaginal artery in the female.
—its venous blood is drained by the prostatic (or vesical) plexus of veins, which empties into the internal iliac vein.
—is supplied by nerve fibers from the vesical and prostatic plexuses, which

[handwritten margin note:] —the Serous Coat or Completely Surrounds the Urinary bladder. Non Keratanized transitional Epithelim.

are extensions from the inferior hypogastric plexuses. The parasympathetic nerve originating from the cord segment, S2-4, causes the musculature of the bladder wall to contract, relaxes the internal sphincter, and promotes emptying.

IV. Male Genital Organ

A. Testis

–develops retroperitoneally and descends into the scrotum retroperitoneally.
–its outer covering is the tunica albuginea, which lies beneath the visceral layer of the tunica vaginalis.
–produces spermatozoa and secretes sex hormones.
–is supplied by the testicular artery from the abdominal aorta and is drained by veins of the pampiniform plexus.

B. Epididymis

–consists of the head, body, and tail, containing a convoluted duct about 20 feet long.

C. Ductus Deferens

–is a thick-walled tube with a relatively small lumen.
–enters the pelvis at the deep inguinal ring at the lateral side of the inferior epigastric artery.
–crosses the medial side of the umbilical artery, ureter, and obturator nerve and vessels during its course.
–its dilated part is termed the ampulla.
–receives innervation mainly from sympathetics of the hypogastric plexus.

D. Ejaculatory Duct

–is formed by the union of the ductus deferens with the duct of the seminal vesicle.

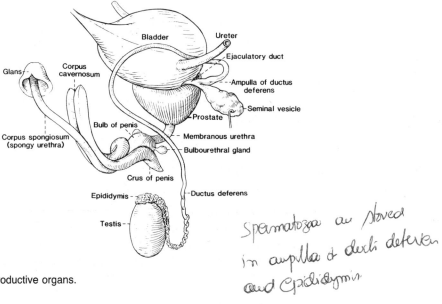

Spermatozoa are stored in ampulla of ducti deferens and epididymis.

Figure 6.8. Male reproductive organs.

—opens into the prostatic urethra on the **seminal colliculus** just lateral to the blind prostatic utricle.

E. Seminal Vesicles

—are enclosed by dense endopelvic fascia.
—are lobulated glandular structures, which are diverticula of the ductus deferens.
—lie lateral to the ampullae of the ductus deferens against the fundus (base) of the bladder.
—produce an alkaline constituent of the seminal fluid.
—its lower end becomes narrow to form a duct that joins the ampulla of the ductus deferens to form the ejaculatory duct.
—normally do not store spermatozoa. (Spermatozoa are stored in the ampulla of the ductus deferens and in the epididymis.)

F. Prostate Gland

—consists chiefly of glandular tissue, mixed with smooth muscle and fibrous tissue.
—secretes a fluid that causes the characteristic odor of semen and, together with the secretion of the seminal vesicles, forms the seminal fluid.
—its ducts open into the **prostatic sinus**, which is a groove on each side of the **urethral crest**.
—receives the ejaculatory duct, which opens into the urethra on the **seminal colliculus** just lateral to the blind **prostatic utricle**.
—the portion below the ejaculatory ducts is the posterior lobe, which is the most frequent site of cancer of the prostate.

G. Urethral Crest

—is located on the posterior wall of the prostatic urethra.
—has numerous openings for the prostatic ducts on either side.
—has an ovoid enlargement called the **seminal colliculus**.
—at the summit of the colliculus is the **prostatic utricle**, which is an invagination (a blind pouch) about 5 mm deep.

H. Prostatic Sinus

—is a groove between the urethral crest and the wall of the prostatic urethra.
—receives the ducts of the prostate gland.

I. Seminal Colliculus is a small elevated portion of the urethral crest upon which open the two ejaculatory ducts and the prostatic utricle.

J. Prostatic Utricle

—is a minute pouch on the summit of the seminal colliculus.
—is an analog of the uterus and vagina in the female.

V. Female Genital Organ

A. Ovary

—lies on the posterior aspect of the broad ligament on the side wall of the pelvic minor and is bounded by the external and internal iliac vessels.
—is not covered by peritoneum, and thus the ovum or oocyte is expelled into the peritoneal cavity and then into the uterine tube.
—is not enclosed in broad ligament but its anterior surface is attached to the posterior surface of the broad ligament by the mesovarium.

Female pudendum → Mons pubis, clituin, Bulb of the vestibule, Greater vestibular gland.

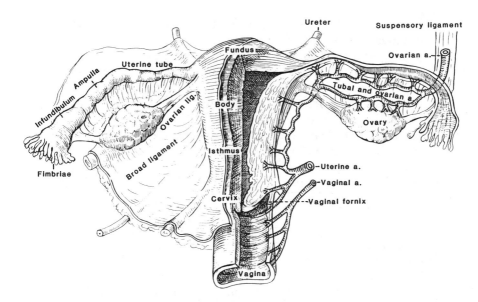

Figure 6.9. Female reproductive organs.

—is supplied primarily by the ovarian artery, which is contained in the suspensory ligament and anastomoses with branches of the uterine artery.

—is drained by the ovarian vein, which joins the inferior vena cava on the right and the left renal vein on the left.

B. Uterine Tube

—extends from the uterus to the uterine end of the ovary and connects the uterine cavity to the peritoneal cavity.

—is subdivided into four parts: the uterine part, **isthmus, ampulla** (the longest and widest part), and infundibulum (the funnel-shaped termination formed of **fimbriae**).

—conveys the fertilized or unfertilized oocytes to the uterus by its ciliary action and muscular contraction, which takes 3–4 days.

—transports spermatozoa in the opposite direction; fertilization takes place within the tube, usually in the infundibulum or ampulla.

C. Uterus

—is divided into the fundus, body, isthmus and cervix.

—is normally **anteverted** in respect to the vagina and **anteflexed** at the junction of its cervix and body.

—is supported by the pelvic diaphragm, as well as by the round, broad, transverse cervical, pubocervical, and sacrocervical ligaments.

—is supplied primarily by the uterine artery and less by the ovarian artery.

—its anterior surface rests upon the posterosuperior surface of the bladder.

D. Vagina

—extends between the vestibule and the cervix of the uterus.

—is the female genital canal and the lower end of the birth canal, serving as the excretory duct for the products of menstruation.

—has a subdivision called the fornix, which is the recess between the cervix and the wall of the vagina.

Internal female genital organ include ovary, Uterine tube, Uterus and the vagina.

–in the virgin, its opening into the vestibule is partially closed by a membranous crescentic fold, the hymen.

–is supported by the levator ani muscles; the transverse cervical, pubo-cervical, and sacrocervical ligaments (upper part): urogenital diaphragm (middle part); and perineal body (lower part).

–receives blood from the vaginal branches of the uterine artery and of the internal iliac artery.

–has lymphatic drainage in two directions: the lymphatics from the upper three-fourths drain into the internal iliac nodes, whereas those from the lower fourth below the hymen drain downward to the perineum and thus into the superficial inguinal nodes.

VI. Rectum and Anal Canal

A. Rectum

–is the part of the large intestine that extends from the sigmoid colon to the anal canal.

–follows the curvature of the sacrum and coccyx.

–has a peritoneal covering on its anterior, right, and left sides for the proximal third; only on its front for the middle third; and no covering at all for the distal third.

–its mucous membrane, together with the circular muscle layer, forms three permanent folds, called transverse folds of the rectum (valve of Houston).

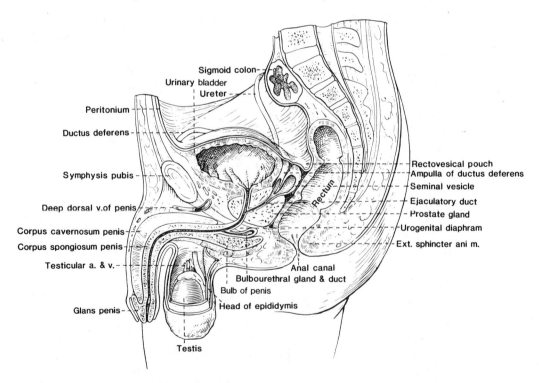

Figure 6.10. Sagittal section of the male pelvis.

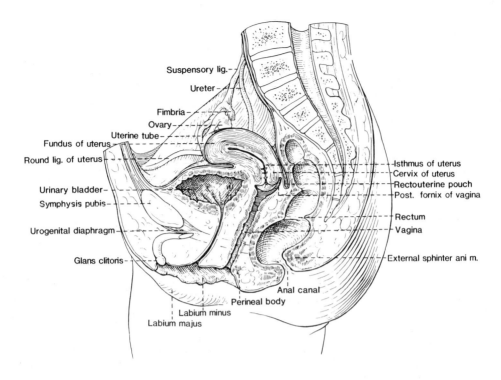

Figure 6.11. Sagittal section of the female pelvis.

—receives blood from the superior, middle, and inferior rectal arteries as well as the middle sacral artery.

—its venous blood returns to the portal venous system by the superior rectal vein, and to the caval (systemic) system by the middle and inferior rectal veins.

—receives parasympathetic nerve fibers by way of the pelvic splanchnic nerve.

B. Anal Canal

—lies below the pelvic diaphragm and ends at the anus.

—is divided into an upper two-thirds (visceral portion), which belongs to the intestine, and a lower third (somatic portion), which belongs to the perineum with respect to the mucosa, blood supply, and nerve supply.

—the **anal columns**, are 5–10 permanent longitudinal folds of mucosa in its upper half. (Each column contains a small artery and a small vein.)

—has crescent-shaped mucosal folds called **anal valves** that connect the lower ends of the anal columns.

—has a pouch-like recesses at the lower end of the anal column called the **anal sinus** in which the anal gland opens.

—the **internal anal sphincter** is a thickening of the circular smooth muscle in the lower part of rectum and is separated from the external anal sphincter (skeletal muscle) by **Hilton's white line**.

—sports the **pectinate line**, which is a sinuous line following the anal valves and crossing the bases of the anal columns.

a. The epithelium is columnar or cuboidal above the pectinate line and stratified squamous below it.

b. Venous drainage above the pectinate line goes into the portal venous system mainly by the superior rectal vein, and below the pectinate line into the caval system by the inferior rectal vein.

c. **Internal hemorrhoids** occur above the pectinate line, and **external hemorrhoids** below it. (A hemorrhoid is a varicosity of a venous plexus around the rectum and anal canal.)

d. The lymphatic vessels drain into the internal iliac nodes above the line and into the superficial inguinal nodes below it.

e. The sensory innervation above the line is through fibers from the pelvic plexus and thus of the visceral type, but the sensory innervation below it is by somatic nerve fibers of the pudendal nerve (very sensitive).

VII. Other Features

A. Pelvic Diaphragm

–forms the pelvic floor and supports all of the pelvic viscerae.

–is formed by the levator ani and coccygeus muscles and their fascial coverings.

–lies posterior and deep to the urogenital diaphragm as well as medial and deep to the ischiorectal fossa.

–upon contraction, raises the entire pelvic floor.

–flexes the anorectal canal during defecation and helps the voluntary control of micturition.

–helps to direct the fetal head toward the birth canal during parturition.

B. Female Hormones during Parturition

–cause relaxation of the ligaments that support the pubic symphysis, sacroiliac and sacrococcygeal joints.

–soften the interpubic disc of the pubic symphysis, increasing in pelvic dimensions to facilitate the passage of the fetus through the birth canal.

C. Emptying of Bowel

–results from activity of the pelvic splanchnic nerves, which increase peristaltic action of the rectum, and increased abdominal pressure, which helps to move the feces through the anal canal.

D. Prolapse of Uterus

–causes a bearing-down sensation in the womb.

–causes increased frequency of and burning on urination.

–results in the cervix of the uterus dropping down into the vagina close to the vestibule.

–occurs as a result of increased relaxation and loss of tonus of the muscular and fascial structures that constitute the support of the pelvic viscera, due to advancing age.

–may be surgically corrected; however, during prolapse surgery, the ureter may be mistaken for the uterine artery and erroneously ligated in surgical removal of the uterus. Remember—"water runs under the bridge," which is to say that the uterine artery crosses cranially and anterior to the ureter.

E. Lymph from Anal Canal

–above the pectinate line drains into the internal iliac nodes, whereas the lymph from the anal canal below the pectinate line, as well as from the scrotum and lower part of the vagina, drains into the superficial inguinal nodes.

VIII. Blood Vessels

A. Internal Iliac Artery

–arises from the bifurcation of the common iliac artery, in front of the sacroiliac joint.

–is crossed in front by the ureter at the pelvic brim.

–is commonly divided into a posterior division, which gives off the iliolumbar, lateral sacral, and superior gluteal arteries, and an anterior division, which gives off the umbilical, obturator, inferior vesical, uterine, middle rectal, internal pudendal, and inferior gluteal arteries.

1. Iliolumbar Artery

–runs superolaterally to the iliac fossa, passing deep to the psoas major muscle.

–divides into an iliac branch supplying the iliacus muscle and the ilium, and a lumbar branch supplying the psoas major and the quadratus lumborum.

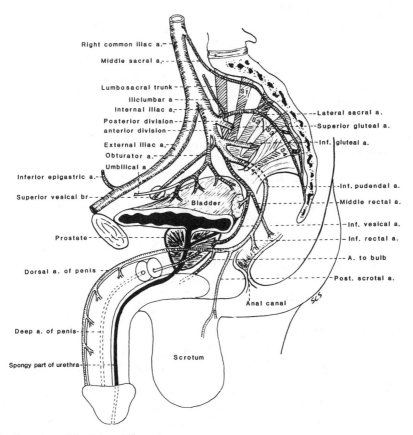

Figure 6.12. Branches of the internal iliac artery.

2. **Lateral Sacral Arteries**

   –are usually two, a superior and an inferior, which may arise from a common trunk. The superior artery enters the first or second pelvic sacral foramen. The inferior artery descends in front of the piriformis and the sacral nerves and then on the pelvic surface of the sacrum between the sacral sympathetic trunk and the sacral foramina. It anastomoses with the median sacral artery.

3. **Superior Gluteal Artery**

   –usually runs between the lumbosacral trunk and the first sacral nerve.
   –leaves the pelvis through the greater sciatic foramen above the piriformis muscle to supply muscles in the buttocks.

4. **Inferior Gluteal Artery**

   –runs between the first and second, or second and third sacral nerves.
   –leaves the pelvis through the greater sciatic foramen, distal to the piriformis.

5. **Internal Pudendal Artery**

   –leaves the pelvis through the greater sciatic foramen, passing between the piriformis and the coccygeus.
   –enters the perineum through the lesser sciatic foramen.
   –its further course is described on page 213.

6. **Umbilical Artery**

   –runs forward along the lateral pelvic wall and along the side of the bladder.
   –gives off the **superior vesical artery** to the superior part of the bladder, and the **artery of the ductus deferens**, which supplies the ductus deferens, the seminal vesicles, the lower part of the ureter, and the bladder.

7. **Obturator Artery**

   –usually arises from the internal iliac artery, but it may arise from the inferior epigastric artery.
   –runs through the upper part of the obturator foramen, divides into the anterior and posterior branches, and supplies the muscles of the thigh. Its posterior branch gives rise to an acetabular branch that enters the joint through the acetabular notch and reaches the head of the femur by way of the ligamentum capitis femoris.

8. **Inferior Vesical Artery**

   –corresponds to the vaginal artery in the female.
   –supplies the fundus of the bladder, the prostate, the seminal vesicles, the ductus deferens, and the lower part of the ureter.

9. **Middle Rectal Artery**

   –runs medially to the middle portion of the rectum.
   –also supplies the prostate, seminal vesicles, ureter, and vagina.

10. **Uterine Artery**

    –is homologous with the artery of the ductus deferens in the male.
    –arises from the internal iliac, or in common with the vaginal or middle rectal artery.

—runs medially in the base of the broad ligament to reach the junction of the cervix and body of the uterus.

—runs in front of and above the ureter near the lateral fornix of the vagina.

—divides into a large superior branch supplying the body and fundus of the uterus, and a smaller vaginal branch supplying the cervix and vagina.

—takes a tortuous course along the lateral margin of the uterus and ends by anastomosing with the ovarian artery.

11. Vaginal Artery

—arises from the uterine, or internal iliac artery.

—gives rise to numerous branches to the anterior and posterior wall of the vagina, and makes longitudinal anastomoses in the median plane to form the anterior and posterior azygos arteries of the vagina.

B. Median Sacral Artery

—is an unpaired artery, arising from the posterior aspect of the abdominal aorta just before its bifurcation.

—descends in front of the sacrum and ends in the coccygeal body, which is a small cellular and vascular mass located in front of the tip of the coccyx.

C. Superior Rectal Artery

—is the direct continuation of the inferior mesenteric artery.

D. Ovarian Artery

—arises from the abdominal aorta.

—crosses the proximal end of the external iliac artery to enter the pelvic minor and reaches the ovary through the suspensory ligament of the ovary.

IX. Sacral Plexus

—is formed by the fourth and fifth lumbar ventral rami (the lumbosacral trunk) and the first four sacral ventral rami.

—lies largely in front of the piriformis in the pelvis.

A. Superior Gluteal Nerve (L4–S1)

—leaves the pelvis through the greater sciatic foramen, above the piriformis.

—supplies the gluteus medius and minimus and the tensor fascia lata.

B. Inferior Gluteal Nerve (L5–S2)

—leaves the pelvis through the greater sciatic foramen, below the piriformis.

—supplies the gluteus maximus.

C. Sciatic Nerve (L4–S3)

—is the largest nerve in the body and composed of the peroneal and tibial parts.

—leaves the pelvis through the greater sciatic foramen below the piriformis.

—enters the thigh in the hollow between the ischial tuberosity and the greater trochanter of the femur.

D. Nerve to Obturator Internus (L5–S2)

—leaves the pelvis through the greater sciatic foramen below the piriformis.

—enters the perineum through the lesser sciatic foramen.

–supplies the obturator internus and the superior gemellus.

E. Nerve to Quadratus Femoris (L5–S2)

–leaves the pelvis through the greater sciatic foramen, below the piriformis.

–descends deep to the gemelli and obturator internus and ends in the deep surface of the quadratus femoris, supplying this muscle and the inferior gemellus.

F. Posterior Femoral Cutaneous Nerve (S1,2,3)

–leaves the pelvis through the greater sciatic foramen below the piriformis.

–lies alongside the sciatic nerve and descends on the back of the knee.

–gives off several inferior cluneal nerves and perineal branches.

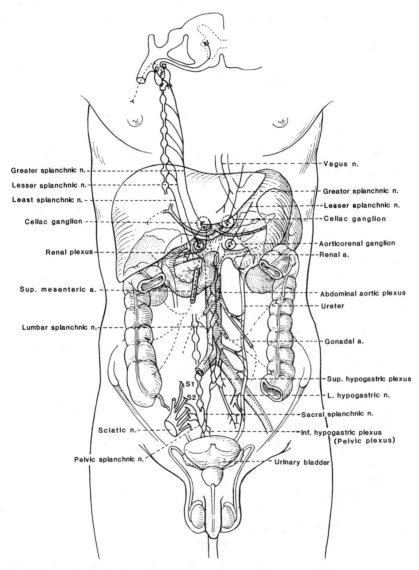

Figure 6.13. The autonomic ganglia and plexuses.

G. Pudendal Nerve (S2,3,4)

–leaves the pelvis through the greater sciatic nerve below the piriformis.
–enters the perineum through the lesser sciatic foramen.
–enters the pudendal canal in the lateral wall of the ischiorectal fossa.

H. Branches Distributed to Pelvis

–include the nerve to the piriformis (S1,2), the nerves to the levator ani and coccygeus (S3,4), the nerve to the sphincter ani externus, and the pelvic splanchnic nerves (S2,3,4).

X. Autonomic Nerves

A. Superior Hypogastric Plexus

–is the continuation of the aortic plexus below the aortic bifurcation and receives the lower two lumbar splanchnic nerves.
–lies behind the peritoneum and descends in front of the fifth lumbar vertebra.
–contains preganglionic and postganglionic sympathetic fibers and visceral afferent fibers.
–ends by bifurcation into right and left hypogastric nerves in front of the sacrum.
–apparently does not contain any parasympathetic fibers.

B. Hypogastric Nerve

–is the lateral extension of the superior hypogastric plexus.
–lies in the extraperitoneal connective tissue lateral to the rectum.
–provides branches to the sigmoid colon and the descending colon.
–is joined by the pelvic splanchnic nerve to form the inferior hypogastric or pelvic plexus.

C. Inferior Hypogastric Plexus (or Pelvic Plexus)

–is formed by the union of hypogastric, pelvic splanchnic, and sacral splanchnic nerves.
–lies against the posterolateral pelvic wall, lateral to the rectum, vagina, and base of the bladder.
–contains pelvic ganglia, in which both sympathetic and parasympathetic preganglionic fibers synapse. Hence, it consists of preganglionic and postganglionic sympathetic fibers, preganglionic and postganglionic parasympathetic fibers, and visceral afferent fibers.
–gives rise to subsidiary plexuses including the middle rectal plexus, uterovaginal plexus, vesical plexus, differential plexus, prostatic plexus, etc.

D. Sacral Splanchnic Nerve

–consists primarily of preganglionic sympathetic fibers that join the inferior hypogastric plexus.

E. Pelvic Splanchnic Nerve

–is the only splanchnic nerve that carries parasympathetic fibers. (All other splanchnic nerves are sympathetic.)
–arises from the sacral segment of the spinal cord (S2,3,4).
–contributes to the formation of the pelvic (or inferior hypogastric) plexus and supplies the descending colon, sigmoid colon, and other viscera in the pelvis and perineum.

Review Test

PERINEUM AND PELVIS

DIRECTIONS: For each of the questions or incomplete statements below, *one* or *more* of the answers or completions given are correct. Choose answer:

A. if only **1, 2,** and **3** are correct.
B. if only **1** and **3** are correct.
C. if only **2** and **4** are correct.
D. if only **4** is correct.
E. if all are correct.

6.1. The round ligament of the uterus
1. contains smooth muscle fibers.
2. inserts into the pecten of the pubic bone.
3. traverses the inguinal canal.
4. contains the uterine artery.

6.2. The superficial inguinal lymph nodes drain the
1. perineum.
2. lower end of the anal canal.
3. external genitalia.
4. lower part of the anterior abdominal wall.

6.3. Ejaculation involves
1. closure of the urethral sphincters at the neck of the bladder.
2. contractions of the prostate, the seminal vesicles and the bulbourethral glands.
3. contractions of smooth muscle of the efferent ducts and the vas deferens.
4. delivery of semen into the urethra.

6.4. The bulbourethral (Cowper's) gland
1. lies in the superficial perineal pouch.
2. lies in the deep perineal pouch.
3. its duct opens into the membranous part of the urethra.
4. its duct opens into the bulbous portion of the penile urethra.

6.5. The external sphincter urethrae is
1. striated muscle.
2. innervated by the perineal nerve.
3. supplied by spinal cord segments S2–S4.
4. enclosed in the pelvic fascia.

6.6. Muscles in the urogenital diaphragm include the
1. sphincter urethrae.
2. coccygeus.
3. transversus perinei profundus.
4. levator ani.

6.7. The ejaculatory duct
1. is formed by the union of the excretory ducts of the bulbourethral (Cowper's) gland and ductus deferens.
2. passes through part of the prostate gland.
3. opens into the membranous urethra.
4. is formed by the union of the ampulla of the ductus deferens and the excretory duct of the seminal vesicle.

6.8. Superficial inguinal nodes receive lymph from the following organs and structures:
1. lower part of the anal canal.
2. labium majus.
3. clitoris.
4. testis.

6.9. Concerning the inguinal canal, it
1. extends from the anterior superior iliac spine to the pubic tubercle.
2. begins at the deep inguinal ring.
3. has an anterior wall primarily formed by external oblique muscles, including aponeurosis and fascia.
4. transmits the round ligament of the uterus or spermatic cord.

6.10. Which of the following structures pass(es) through a gap between the arcuate pubic ligament and the transverse perineal ligament?

1. dorsal nerve of the penis.
2. superficial dorsal vein of the penis.
3. dorsal artery of the penis.
4. deep dorsal vein of the penis.

6.11. Usually a direct inguinal hernia

1. enters the inguinal canal through its posterior wall.
2. lies medial to the inferior epigastric artery.
3. pushes the transversalis fascia ahead of it.
4. pushes a layer of peritoneum ahead of it.

6.12. Of the following structures, which form boundaries of the pelvic outlet?

1. sacrotuberous ligament.
2. coccyx.
3. ischiopubic ramus.
4. pecten pubis.

6.13. Muscles, that find attachment to the perineal body (central tendon of the perineum) are:

1. ischiocavernosus and sphincter urethrae.
2. transversus perinei profundus and obturator internus.
3. superficial sphincter of anus and sphincter urethrae.
4. bulbospongiosus and transversus perinei superficialis.

6.14. Which of the statements concerning the prostate gland are true?

1. The prostatic utricle opens at the apex of the seminal colliculus.
2. The middle lobe of the prostate is posterior to the urethra.
3. The uvula of the male bladder is often accentuated (made larger) by the hypertrophy of the middle lobe of the prostate.
4. The prostatic utricle is the terminal end of the duct of the prostate.

6.15. Which of the following perineal structures would be found between the inferior fascia of the urogenital diaphragm and the superficial perineal (Colles') fascia?

1. prostate gland.
2. bulbourethral (Cowper's) gland.
3. membranous part of male urethra.
4. transversus perinei superficialis muscle.

6.16. The following structures open onto the urethral crest of the prostatic urethra.

1. the ureter.
2. the ducts from the prostate gland.
3. the ejaculatory ducts.
4. the bulbourethral glands.

6.17. The inguinal ligament

1. is formed by the inferior free edge of the internal abdominal oblique muscle.
2. extends between the anterior inferior iliac spine and the ischial tuberosity.
3. forms the roof of the inguinal canal.
4. forms the floor of the inguinal canal.

6.18. Which of the following structures lie in the broad ligament in all or part of their course?

1. ovarian ligament.
2. uterine artery.
3. round ligament of the uterus.
4. uterine tube.

6.19. The normal position of the uterus is

1. anteflexed.
2. retroflexed.
3. anteverted.
4. retroverted.

6.20. The pelvic splanchnic nerves consist primarily of

1. postganglionic parasympathetic neurons.
2. postganglionic sympathetic neurons.
3. preganglionic sympathetic neurons.
4. preganglionic parasympathetic neurons.

6.21. The following structures form part of the pelvic inlet:

1. promontory of the sacrum.
2. ischiopubic rami.
3. pectineal line.
4. iliac crest.

6.22. The pudendal nerve

1. passes through the lesser sciatic foramen.
2. provides sensory innervation to the scrotum.
3. gives off branches that provide sensory innervation to the labia majora.
4. may be blocked by injection of an anesthetic near the inferior margin of the ischial spine.

6.23. The urinary bladder
1. Although it is always a pelvic organ, it may become an abdominal organ.
2. The motor nerve supply to the muscle of the bladder wall is the pudendal nerve.
3. If the spinal cord is cut transversely at the level of the fifth lumbar segment, the motor supply to the bladder wall muscle (detrusor) would still be intact.
4. Entrance of sperm into the urinary bladder during ejaculation is prevented by pelvic splanchnic nerves.

6.24. Concerning the ureter
1. Three areas where normal constriction of the ureter may impede passage of a stone are: (*a*) junction of the ureter with renal pelvis, (*b*) as it passes over the brim of the pelvis, and (*c*) its junction with the bladder.
2. Urine is propelled along the ureter by peristaltic waves.
3. In the female it lies about 1–2 cm lateral to the cervix of the uterus and the lateral fornix of the vagina.
4. It is supplied by the common iliac and superior vesical arteries.

6.25. Concerning the levator ani muscle
1. The "puborectal sling" (puborectalis) relaxes during defecation.
2. The iliococcygeus muscle is usually the most well-developed portion of the levator ani.
3. The pubococcygeus may be torn or damaged during parturition and thereby may allow the descent of the pelvic viscera.
4. It forms the lateral wall of the ischiorectal fossa.

DIRECTIONS: Each set of lettered headings below is followed by a list of numbered words or phrases. Choose answer.
   A. if the item is associated with **A** only.
   B. if the item is associated with **B** only.
   C. if the item is associated with both **A** and **B**.
   D. if the item is associated with neither **A** nor **B**.

A. Direct inguinal hernia
B. Indirect inguinal hernia
C. Both
D. Neither

6.26. Enters the deep inguinal ring to gain access to the inguinal canal.

6.27. Pushes through some part of the posterior wall of the inguinal canal medial to the inferior epigastric artery.

6.28. The herniated gut has as its first covering a layer of parietal peritoneum or its derivative.

6.29. If it passes through the superficial ring it has the same three fascial coverings as the spermatic cord.

6.30. The hernia passes posterior (deep) to the inguinal ligament.

A. Pelvic diaphragm
B. Urogenital diaphragm
C. Both
D. Neither

6.31. The major vestibular glands lie within this structure.

6.32. The sphincter urethrae muscle forms part of this structure.

6.33. Is a major support of the uterus.

6.34. Forms the floor of the pelvis minor.

6.35. Forms the medial wall of the ischiorectal fossa.

A. Superficial perineal pouch
B. Deep perineal pouch
C. Both
D. Neither

6.36. Contains the prostatic portion of the urethra.

6.37. Contains the bulb of the vestibule.

6.38. Contains the greater vestibular glands.

6.39. Contains the bulbourethral (Cowper's) glands.

6.40. Its roof or superior boundary is formed by the inferior fascia of the urogenital diaphragm (perineal membrane).

A. Pelvic splanchnic nerve
B. Sacral splanchnic nerve
C. Both
D. Neither

6.41. Contributes to the formation of the inferior hypogastric (pelvic) plexus.

6.42. Transmits parasympathetic preganglionic fibers to the autonomic plexus.

6.43. Arises from second, third, and fourth sacral spinal nerves.

6.44. Transmits sympathetic preganglionic fibers.

6.45. Transmits parasympathetic postganglionic fibers to the autonomic plexus.

A. Internal hemorrhoids
B. External hemorrhoids
C. Both
D. Neither

6.46. Are enlargements of small veins located inferior to the pectinate line.

6.47. Are enlargements of small veins located primarily within the anal columns.

6.48. Are located in an area from which the lymphatic vessels drain into the superficial inguinal lymph nodes.

6.49. Are located in an area supplied by visceral afferent nerve fibers.

6.50. Veins associated with these hemorrhoids drain primarily into the portal venous system via the superior rectal vein.

DIRECTIONS: Select the *one* numbered heading that is most closely associated with a question. Each numbered heading may be selected once, more than once, or not at all.

A. Bulbospongiosus muscle
B. Ischiocavernosus muscle
C. Sphincter urethrae muscle
D. Levator ani muscle
E. Obturator internus muscle

6.51. Is a major support of the uterus.

6.52. Covers or is in close proximity to the major vestibular glands.

6.53. Lies on the surface of the crura.

6.54. The pudendal canal lies on its medial surface.

6.55. An accessory gland of reproduction is embedded in this muscle in the male.

A. Prostate gland
B. Seminal vesicle
C. Great vestibular gland
D. Bulbourethral gland
E. Anal gland

6.56. Lies on the posterolateral aspect of the bladder.

6.57. Lies in the superficial perineal pouch.

6.58. Opens by numerous ducts into the urethra.

6.59. Lies lateral to the membranous urethra.

6.60. Its ducts empty into the bulb of the penis.

A. Ovary
B. Uterus
C. Uterine tube
D. Vagina
E. Clitoris

6.61. Fertilization of the ova takes place in this structure.

6.62. Opens into the peritoneal cavity.

6.63. Is supported by the cardinal ligaments.

6.64. Is not enclosed in the broad ligament and is bounded by the external and internal iliac vessels.

6.65. Is attached to the pubic symphysis by the suspensory ligament.

DIRECTIONS: Each of the questions or incomplete statements below is followed by suggested answers or completions. Select the *one* that is *best* in each case.

6.66. The processus vaginalis is an extension of the

A. external spermatic fascia.
B. internal spermatic fascia.
C. extraperitoneal connective tissue.
D. peritoneum.
E. mucosa of the vagina.

6.67. In order to anesthetize the skin of the urogenital triangle completely it would be necessary to block sensation carried by

A. pudendal and ilioinguinal nerves.
B. pudendal and perineal branch of posterior cutaneous nerve of the thigh.
C. pudendal, perineal branch of posterior cutaneous nerve of the thigh and ilioinguinal nerves.
D. perineal branch of posterior cutaneous nerve of thigh and ilioinguinal nerves.

6.68. Carcinoma of the uterus can spread directly to the labia majora by traveling in lymphatics that follow the

A. ligament of the ovary.
B. suspensory ligament of the ovary.
C. round ligament of the uterus.
D. suspensory ligament of clitoris.
E. cardinal ligament (transverse cervical ligament).

6.69. A left testicle exhibits tenderness and swelling which may be produced by thrombosis in one of the following veins:

A. internal pudendal vein.
B. inferior epigastric vein.
C. internal iliac vein.
D. left renal vein.
E. external pudendal vein.

6.70. Of the following listing of structures usually seen leaving the pelvis, which is to be found leaving *above* the piriformis muscle?

A. sciatic nerve.
B. internal pudendal artery.
C. superior gluteal nerve.
D. inferior gluteal artery.
E. posterior cutaneous nerve of the thigh (posterior femoral cutaneous).

6.71. Which of the following is *not* a boundary of the perineum?

A. pubic arcuate ligament.
B. tip of the coccyx.
C. ischial tuberosities.
D. sacrospinous ligament.
E. sacrotuberous ligament.

6.72. Which of the following statements concerning the scrotum is incorrect?

A. It is innervated anteriorly by the ilioinguinal nerve.
B. It is partitioned into two sacs by a septum of superficial fascia.
C. It receives its blood supply from the testicular artery.
D. It has lymphatic drainage primarily into superficial inguinal lymph nodes.
E. It has a dartos layer of fascia and muscle that is continuous with Colles' layer of superficial fascia in the perineum.

6.73. A structure that does not contribute to the support of the uterus is the

A. sacrogenital folds.
B. round ligament of the uterus.
C. lateral cervical (cardinal) ligaments.
D. pelvic diaphragm.
E. uterosacral (rectouterine) ligaments.

6.74. Which one of the following does not constitute a part of the boundary of the inferior pelvic aperature?

A. sacrospinous ligament.
B. ischial tuberosities.
C. inferior rami of the pubis.
D. rami of the ischium.
E. arcuate ligament of the pubis.

6.75. Normally, part of which of the following ligaments would be found in the inguinal canal?

A. suspensory ligaments of the ovary.
B. ovarian ligaments.
C. broad ligament.
D. round ligaments of the uterus.
E. pubovesical ligaments.

6.76. Which of the following arteries would be most likely *not* to send branches (direct or indirect) to the labia majora?

A. internal iliac.
B. obturator.
C. inferior gluteal.
D. internal pudendal.
E. external pudendal.

6.77. The perineal membrane is a connective tissue layer

A. on the superior surface of the urogenital diaphragm.
B. on the inferior surface of the levator ani muscle.
C. which is part of the deep layer of the superficial fascia covering the body.
D. covering the inferior surface of the urogenital diaphragm.
E. on the superior surface of the pelvic diaphragm.

6.78. Of the following components of the lumbosacral plexus, which one does *not* leave the abdominal or pelvic cavity?

A. ilioinguinal.
B. genitofemoral.
C. lumbosacral trunk.
D. femoral.
E. lateral femoral cutaneous.

6.79. Pelvic splanchnic nerves carry preganglionic efferent fibers that synapse in

A. terminal ganglia near or on the viscera.
B. sympathetic chain (paravertebral) ganglia.
C. collateral (preaortic) ganglia.
D. dorsal root ganglia.
E. the ganglion impar.

6.80. On either side of the body, the uterine artery on its way from the anterior division of the internal iliac artery to the uterus crosses a structure that is sometimes mistakenly ligated during pelvic surgery. This structure is the

A. ovarian artery.
B. ovarian ligament.
C. mesovarium.
D. ureter.
E. vaginal artery.

6.81. Select the correct statement.

A. Branches of the uterine artery usually anastomose with branches of the ovarian artery.
B. The inferior gluteal artery is usually a branch of the superior gluteal artery.
C. The prostatic plexus of veins is *not* either directly or indirectly connected with veins outside of the pelvis (i.e., veins on the external part of the body).
D. The inferior vesical arteries are usually branches of the obturator artery.
E. Normally, the internal pudendal artery is a branch of the posterior division of the internal iliac artery.

6.82. Select the incorrect statement.

A. The dorsal artery of the penis in the male lies deep to the penile (Buck's) fascia.
B. Penile (Buck's) fascia intervenes between the bulb of the penis and Colles' fascia.
C. The terminal branches of the internal pudendal artery are the deep artery of the penis and the dorsal artery of the penis.
D. The superficial perineal pouch lies between the pelvic fascia and the perineal membrane.
E. The perineal branch of the pudendal nerve gives branches to the cavernous urethra.

6.83. The ischiorectal fossa

A. is bounded anteriorly by the transverse ligament of the urogenital diaphragm.
B. is bounded posteriorly in part by the gluteus maximus muscle.
C. contains the pudendal canal along its medial wall.
D. is separated from the urogenital triangle by the levator ani muscle.
E. contains a perineal branch of the fifth lumbar nerve.

6.84. The superior (deep) boundary of the superficial perineal space is the

A. pelvic diaphragm.
B. perineal membrane.
C. superficial layer of the superficial fascia.
D. deep layer of the superficial fascia.
E. Colles' fascia.

6.85. The following structures are found in the urogenital diaphragm (deep pouch or space) of the male:

A. transversus perinei profundus muscles, bulbourethral (Cowper's) glands, and the membranous urethra.
B. transversus perinei profundus muscles, bulbospongiosus muscles, and part of the spongy urethra.
C. arteries to the bulb, ischiocavernosus muscles, and bulbourethral glands.
D. transversus perinei superficialis muscles, prostatic urethra, and sphincter urethrae muscles.
E. sphincter urethrae muscles, bulbourethral glands, and great vestibular glands.

6.86. Which of the following structures do *not* lie in the superficial perineal space?

A. ischiocavernosus muscles.
B. transversus perinei superficialis muscles.
C. greater vestibular glands of the female.
D. Cowper's (bulbourethral) gland of the male.
E. bulb of the vestibule.

6.87. The external anal sphincter

A. is primarily innervated and controlled by autonomic nerves.
B. contains mostly smooth muscle.
C. is usually described as having deep, superficial, and subcutaneous components.
D. has some lateral fibers that interdigitate with those of the obturator internus muscle.
E. extends superiorly as far as the lower end of the sigmoid colon.

6.88. Ducts from the prostate gland open

A. into the membranous part of the urethra.
B. onto the seminal colliculus.
C. by several openings onto the cavernous urethra.
D. on either side of the urethral crest.
E. into the prostatic utricle on a given side of the body.

6.89. On a given side of the body, a duct from a seminal vesicle

A. joins the duct of a bulbourethral gland to form the ejaculatory duct.
B. opens into the membranous urethra.
C. becomes wider just before it opens into the urinary bladder to form the ejaculatory duct.
D. forms a widened portion called the ampulla of the ductus deferens.
E. unites with the ductus deferens to form a single duct.

6.90. Of the following, which is *not* considered to be a part of the broad ligament?

A. ovarian ligament.
B. mesometrium.
C. mesosalpinx.
D. peritoneum and underlying connective tissues covering the oviducts.
E. peritoneum and underlying connective tissues on the posterior surface of the uterus.

Answers and Explanations

PERINEUM AND PELVIS

6.1. B. The round ligament of the uterus enters the inguinal canal through the deep inguinal ring, emerges through the superficial inguinal ring, and becomes lost in the subcutaneous tissue of the labium majus. It contains smooth muscle fibers.

6.2. E. The superficial inguinal lymph nodes drain the perineum, lower end of the anal canal, external genitalia, and lower part of the anterior abdominal wall.

6.3. E. Ejaculation occurs with the contraction of smooth muscle of the epididymal ducts and ductus deferens. During ejaculation a sphincter at the neck of the bladder contracts, and thus prevents sperm entering the bladder and urine leaving it. Also, the seminal vesicles, prostate gland, and bulbourethral glands contract to pump their secretions into the urethra. The semen is propelled through the ducts and out the external urethral opening.

6.4. C. The bulbourethral (Cowper's) gland lies on the side of the membranous portion of the urethra in the deep perineal pouch and its duct opens into the bulbous portion of the spongy (penile) urethra.

6.5. A. The external urethral sphincter consists of skeletal muscle and forms a part of the urogenital diaphragm. It is innervated by the perineal branch of the pudendal nerve that originated from spinal cord segments. S2–4.

6.6. B. The urogenital diaphragm consists of the sphincter urethrae and transversus perinei profundus muscles.

6.7. C. The ejaculatory duct is formed by the ampulla of the ductus deferens and duct of the seminal vesicle, passes through the prostate gland, and opens into the prostatic urethra on the seminal colliculus.

6.8. A. The lymphatic vessels from the testis and epididymis ascend along the testicular vessels in the spermatic cord through the inguinal canal and run upward in the abdomen to drain into the upper lumbar nodes.

6.9. E. The inguinal canal extends from the anterior superior iliac spine to the pubic tubercle. It begins at the deep inguinal ring in the transversalis fascia and ends at the superficial inguinal ring in the external oblique abdominis aponeurosis.

6.10. D. The deep dorsal vein of the penis enters the pelvis through a gap between the arcuate pubic ligament and the transverse perineal ligament.

6.11. E. The direct inguinal hernia occurs through the posterior wall of the inguinal canal and thus it lies medial to the inferior epigastric vessels. It pushes a layer of peritoneum and transversalis fascia within the region of the inguinal triangle.

6.12. A. The pecten pubis (or pectineal line) forms a boundary of the pelvic inlet (or pelvic brim).

6.13. D. The perineal body is a fibromuscular node at the center of the perineum and gives attachment for the bulbospongiosus, the transversus perinei superficialis, etc.

6.14. A. The prostatic utricle is a minute pouch on the summit of the seminal colliculus.

6.15. D. The transversus perinei superficialis muscle is found in a space between the inferior fascia of the urogenital diaphragm and the superficial perineal (Colles') fascia, which is the superficial perineal pouch. The bulbourethral (Cowper's) gland and the membranous urethra are found in the deep perineal pouch.

6.16. B. The ducts of the prostate gland open into the prostatic sinus, which is a groove on each side of the urethral crest. The ejaculatory duct opens into the prostatic urethra on the seminal colliculus. The duct of the bulbourethral gland opens into the lumen of the bulbous portion of the penile urethra.

6.17. D. The inguinal ligament extends from the anterior superior iliac spine to the pubic tubercle and forms the floor of the inguinal canal.

6.18. E. The broad ligament contains the ovarian ligament, uterine artery, round ligament of the uterus, uterine tube, ureter, etc.

6.19. B. The normal position of the uterus is anteflexed and anteverted.

6.20. D. The pelvic splanchnic nerve consists primarily of preganglionic parasympathetic neurons.

6.21. B. The pelvic inlet (or pelvic brim) is bounded by the promontory of the sacrum, the arcuate line of the ilium, the pectineal line, the pubic crest, and the superior margin of the symphysis pubis.

6.22. E. The pudendal nerve leaves the pelvis through the greater sciatic foramen and enters the perineum through the lesser sciatic foramen near the inferior margin of the ischial spine. It provides sensory innervation to the scrotum or labium majus.

6.23. B. The autonomic nerves from the pelvic plexus supply the musculature of the bladder wall. The sympathetic fibers reaching the bladder are from spinal cord segments T12–L2, whereas the parasympathetic fibers originating from cord segments S2–4, cause the bladder wall to contract, relax the internal sphincter, and promote emptying.

6.24. E. The ureter has three constrictions at its origin, at the pelvic brim and near the bladder. It is a muscular tube and transmits urine by peristaltic waves. It lies 1–2 cm lateral to the cervix of the uterus and the lateral fornix of the vagina and is supplied by the aorta, the renal, gonadal, common and internal iliac, umbilical, superior and inferior vesical, and middle rectal arteries.

6.25. A. The lateral wall of the ischiorectal fossa is formed by the obturator internus muscle.

6.26. A. The sphincter urethrae and the transversus perinei profundus form the urogenital diaphragm.

6.27. C. The sphincter urethrae is innervated by the perineal branch of the pudendal nerve, and the sphincter ani externus is innervated by the inferior rectal branch of the pudendal nerve, which enters the perineum through the lesser sciatic foramen.

6.28. A. The bulbourethral glands are embedded in the substance of the sphincter urethrae.

6.29. D. The obturator internus forms the lateral wall of the ischiorectal fossa.

6.30. B. The sphincter urethrae is attached to the perineal body, which is located in the center of the perineum.

6.31. D. The major vestibular glands lie in the superficial perineal pouch.

6.32. B. The sphincter urethrae and transversus perinei profundus muscles form the urogenital diaphragm.

6.33. A. The pelvic diaphragm consists of the levator ani and coccygeus muscles, is a major support of the uterus, and forms the floor of the pelvic minor and medial wall of the ischiorectal fossa.

6.34. A. See 6.33.

6.35. A. See 6.33.

6.36. D. The prostatic portion of the urethra is in the pelvic cavity.

6.37. A. The superficial perineal pouch contains the bulb of the vestibule and the greater vestibular glands.

6.38. A. The greater vestibular glands are located in the superficial pouch.

6.39. B. The bulbourethral glands are found in the deep perineal pouch.

6.40. A. The inferior fascia of the urogenital diaphragm (perineal membrane) forms the floor or inferior boundary of the deep perineal pouch, and also forms the roof or superior boundary of the superficial perineal pouch.

6.41. C. Both the pelvic and sacral splanchnic nerves as well as the hypogastric nerve contribute to the formation of the inferior hypogastric (pelvic) plexus.

6.42. A. The pelvic splanchnic nerve transmits parasympathetic preganglionic fibers to the autonomic plexus.

6.43. A. The pelvic splanchnic nerve arises from the second, third, and fourth sacral spinal nerves.

6.44. B. The sacral splanchnic nerve transmits sympathetic preganglionic fibers to the autonomic plexus.

6.45. D. The pelvic and sacral splanchnic nerves transmit parasympathetic and sympathetic preganglionic fibers to the autonomic plexuses, respectively. See 6.42 and 6.44.

6.46. B. External hemorrhoids are enlargements of veins around the anal canal inferior to the pectinate line.

6.47. A. Internal hemorrhoids are enlargements of veins around the rectum and anal canal above the pectinate line.

6.48. B. The lymphatic vessels above the pectinate line drain into the internal iliac nodes, but the lymphatic vessels below it drain into the superficial inguinal nodes.

6.49. A. The sensory innervation above the pectinate line is through fibers from the pelvic plexus and thus of the visceral type, but the sensory innervation below it is by somatic nerve fibers of the pudendal nerve (very sensitive).

6.50. A. Veins draining the rectum and anal canal above the pectinate line empty primarily into the portal venous system via the superior rectal vein.

6.51. D. The levator ani and coccygeus muscles form the pelvic diaphragm, which is a major support of the uterus.

6.52. A. The bulbospongiosus covers or is in close proximity to the major vestibular glands.

6.53. B. The ischiocavernosus lies on the surface of the crus of the penis (or clitoris).

6.54. E. The pudendal (Alcock's) canal is the fascial space within the obturator fascia lining the lateral wall of the ischiorectal fossa and transmits the pudendal nerve and the internal pudendal vessels.

6.55. C. The bulbourethral gland is embedded in the sphincter urethrae.

6.56. B. The seminal vesicles are lobulated glandular structures and lie lateral to the ampullae of the ductus deferens, against the posterolateral aspect of the bladder.

6.57. C. The greater vestibular glands are found in the superficial perineal pouch.

6.58. A. The prostate gland opens its ducts into the prostatic sinus, which is a groove on each side of the urethral crest.

6.59. D. The bulbourethral glands lie lateral to the membranous urethra in the deep perineal pouch and open their ducts into the bulb of the penis.

6.60. D. See 6.59.

6.61. C. Fertilization of the ova takes place in the uterine tube, usually in the infundibulum or ampulla.

6.62. C. The uterine tube opens into the peritoneal cavity.

6.63. B. The uterus is also supported by the cardinal ligaments.

6.64. A. The ovary is not enclosed by peritoneum (broad ligament) but is attached along its posterior surface by the mesovarium. It is bounded by the external and internal iliac vessels.

6.65. E. The clitoris is attached to the symphysis pubis by the suspensory ligament.

6.66. D. The processus vaginalis is an extension of the peritoneum.

6.67. C. The skin of the urogenital triangle is innervated by the pudendal nerve and perineal branches of the posterior femoral cutaneous nerve.

6.68. C. The round ligament of the uterus runs laterally from the uterus through the deep inguinal ring, inguinal canal, and superficial inguinal ring and becomes lost in the subcutaneous tissues of the labium majus. Thus carcinoma of the uterus can spread directly to the labium majus by traveling in lymphatics that follow the ligament.

6.69. D. A tender swollen left testis could be produced by thrombosis in the left renal vein because the left testicular vein drains into the left renal vein.

6.70. C. The superior gluteal nerve and vessels leave the pelvis above the piriformis muscle, whereas the sciatic nerve, the internal pudendal vessels, the inferior gluteal vessels and nerve, and the posterior femoral cutaneous nerve leave the pelvis below the piriformis muscle.

6.71. D. The sacrospinous ligament does not form a boundary of the perineum but forms a boundary of the lesser sciatic foramen.

6.72. C. The testis has lymphatic drainage primarily into the upper lumbar lymph nodes.

6.73. A. The uterus is supported by the pelvic diaphragm and the round ligament of the uterus as well as the lateral cervical (cardinal), rectouterine, transverse cervical, pubocervical, and sacrocervical ligaments.

6.74. A. The inferior pelvic aperture (pelvic outlet) is formed by the ischial tuberosities, rami of the pubis and ischium, the arcuate ligament of the pubis, and the symphysis pubis.

6.75. D. The round ligament of the uterus is found in the inguinal canal during its course.

6.76. C. The uterine artery remains within the pelvic cavity. It does not enter or leave the pelvic cavity.

6.77. D. The perineal membrane is a connective tissue covering the inferior surface of the urogenital diaphragm.

6.78. C. The lumbosacral trunk is formed by part of the ventral ramus of the fourth lumbar nerve and the ventral ramus of the fifth lumbar nerve. This trunk contributes to the formation of the sacral plexus by joining the ventral ramus of the first sacral nerve in the pelvic cavity.

6.79. A. The pelvic splanchnic nerves carry preganglionic efferent fibers that synapse in the ganglia of the inferior hypogastric plexus and in minute ganglia in the muscular walls of the pelvic organs.

6.80. D. The ureter runs under the uterine artery near the cervix, and thus the ureter is sometimes mistakenly ligated during pelvic surgery.

6.81. A. Branches of the uterine artery usually anastomose with branches of the ovarian artery. The prostatic plexus of veins is connected with the external pudendal vein and the superficial and deep dorsal veins of the penis. The inferior vesical artery is a branch of the internal iliac artery. The internal pudendal artery is a branch of the posterior division of the internal iliac artery.

6.82. D. The superficial perineal pouch lies between the membranous layer of the superficial perineal (Colles') fascia and the perineal membrane.

6.83. B. The ischiorectal fossa is bounded anteriorly by the transversus perinei superficialis and profundus muscles and posteriorly by the gluteus maximus and the sacrotuberous ligament. It contains the inferior rectal nerve and vessels. It also contains the pudendal canal along its lateral wall.

6.84. B. The lymph vessels from the scrotum drain into the superficial inguinal nodes, whereas the lymph vessels from the testis drain into the upper lumbar nodes.

6.85. A. The urogenital diaphragm (deep perineal space) contains the transversus perinei profundus, the sphincter urethrae, the membranous urethra, and the bulbourethral (Cowper's) glands.

6.86. D. The superficial perineal space contains the ischiocavernosus, the transversus perinei superficial is, the greater vestibular gland, and the bulb of the vestibule covered with the bulbospongiosus.

6.87. C. The external anal sphincter has deep, superficial, and subcutaneous components.

6.88. D. Ducts from the prostate gland open on either side of the urethral crest.

6.89. E. A duct from a seminal vesicle joins the ductus deferens to form an ejaculatory duct.

6.90. A. An ovarian ligament is not considered to be part of the broad ligament.

Proctodeum: It's a pit or depression created by the proliferation of mesenchymal tissue surrounding the anal membrane. This pit is covered by epithelium of ectodermal origin and takes the form of stratified squamous epithelium. The proctodeal portion of the definitive anal canal is the area external to the pectinate junction.

7

Back

Back

I. Superficial Back

A. Superficial Muscles

Muscle	Origin	Insertion	Nerve	Action
Trapezius	External occipital protuberance, superior nuchal line, ligamentum nuchae, spines of C7–T12	Spine of scapula, acromion, and lateral third of clavicle	Spinal accessory n., C3–C4	Adducts, rotates, elevates, and depresses scapula
Levator scapulae	Transverse processes of C1–C4	Medical border of scapula	Dorsal scapular n., C3–C4	Elevates scapula
Rhomboid minor	Spines of C7–T1	Root of spine of scapula	Dorsal scapular n.	Adducts scapula
Rhomboid major	Spines of T2–T5	Medical border of scapula	Dorsal scapular n.	Adducts scapula
Latissimus dorsi	Spines of T7–T12, lumbodorsal fascia, iliac crest, 9–12 ribs	Floor of bicipital groove of humerus	Thoracodorsal n.	Adducts, extends, and rotates arm medially
Serratus posterior superior	Ligamentum nuchae, supraspinal ligament, and spines of C7–T3	Upper border of ribs 2–5	Intercostal n., T1–4	Elevates ribs
Serratus posterior inferior	Supraspinous ligament and spines of T11–L3	Lower border of ribs 9–12	Intercostal n., T9–11	Depresses ribs

B. Triangle of Auscultation
- is bounded by upper border of the latissimus dorsi, lateral border of the trapezius, medial border of the scapula.
- its floor is formed by the rhomboid major.
- is the site to hear breathing sounds most clearly.

C. Lumbar Triangle
- is formed by the iliac crest, latissimus dorsi, and posterior free border of the external oblique abdominis muscle.

D. Thoracolumbar (Lumbar) Fascia
- invests the deep muscles of the back.

243

—its anterior layer lies anterior to the erector spinae muscle and attaches to the vertebral transverse process.

—its posterior layer lies posterior to the erector spinae and attaches to the spinous processes.

II. Deep Back

A. Deep or Intrinsic Muscles

1. Superficial Layer: Spinotransverse Group

—originates from the spinous processes and inserts into the transverse processes (or the mastoid process and the superior nuchal line).

—consists of:

a. Splenius capitis.

b. Splenius cervicis.

—acts to rotate the head and neck toward the same side, extend the head and the trunk.

2. Intermediate Layer: Sacrospinalis Group (Erector Spinae)

—originates from the sacrum, the ilium, and the lumbar spines.

—divides into three columns:

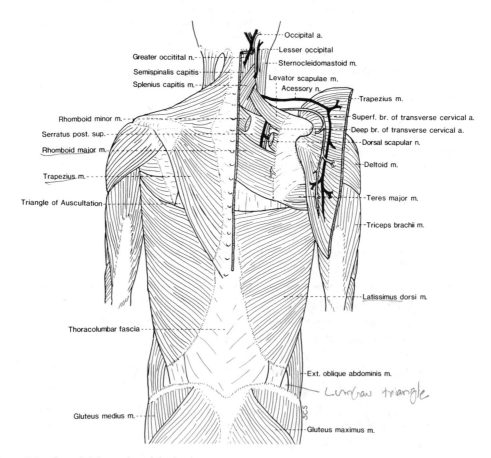

Figure 7.1. Superficial muscles of the back.

    a. Iliocostalis (lateral column).

       –inserts on angles of the ribs and cervical transverse processes.

    b. Longissimus (medial column).

       –inserts into transverse processes and the mastoid process.

    c. Spinalis (most medial column).

       –arises from spinous processes and inserts into spinous processes.

   –acts to flex the vertebral column to the same side and extend and rotate the vertebral column.

3. Deep Layer: Transversospinalis Group

–originates from the transverse processes and inserts into the spinous processes.

–consists of

    a. Semispinalis capitis, cervicis, and thoracis

    b. Multifidus (deep to semispinalis)

    c. Rotators

       (1). Long Rotators

          –run from transverse processes to spinous processes two vertebrae above.

       (2). Short Rotators

          –run from transverse processes to spinous processes of adjacent vertebrae.

–acts to rotate the neck and trunk to the opposite side and extend the neck and vertebral column.

B. Segmental Muscles

–extend from one vertebra to the next.

–consists of

1. Interspinales

–run between adjacent spinous processes.

–aid in extension of the vertebral column.

2. Intertransversarii

–run between adjacent transverse processes.

–aid in lateral flexion of the vertebral column.

III. Suboccipital Area

A. Suboccipital Triangle

–is bound medially by the rectus capitis posterior major, laterally by the oblique capitis superior, and inferiorly by the oblique capitis inferior.

–its roof is formed by the semispinalis capitis and longissimus capitis muscles.

–its floor is formed by the posterior arch of the atlas and posterior atlanto-occipital membrane.

–contains the vertebral artery and suboccipital nerve and vessels.

B. Suboccipital Nerve

–is derived from the dorsal ramus of C1.

–is located within the suboccipital triangle.

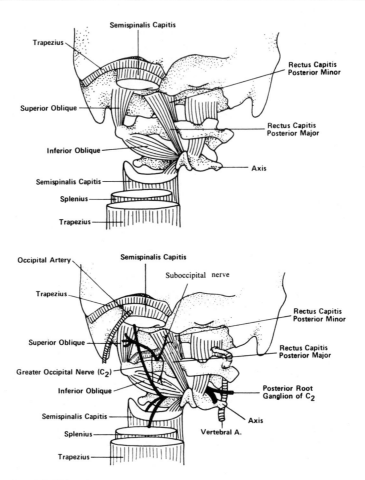

Figure 7.2. The suboccipital triangle.

–emerges between the vertebral artery above and the posterior arch of the atlas below.

–supplies the muscles of the suboccipital triangle and semispinalis capitis.

C. Suboccipital Muscles

Muscle	Origin	Insertion	Nerve	Action
Rectus capitis posterior major	Spine of axis	Lateral portion of inferior nuchal line	Suboccipital n.	Extends, rotates, and flexes head laterally
Rectus capitis posterior minor	Posterior tubercle of atlas	Occipital bone below inferior nuchal line	Suboccipital n.	Extends and flexes head laterally
Obliquus capitis superior	Transverse process of atlas	Occipital bone above inferior nuchal lines	Suboccipital n.	Extends, rotates, and flexes head laterally
Obliquus capitis inferior	Spine of axis	Transverse process of atlas	Suboccipital n.	Extends head and rotates it laterally

D. Joints

1. Atlanto-Occipital Joint

–is ellipsoid in shape.

–is between the superior articular facets of the atlas and the occipital condyles.

–is primarily involved in flexion and extension.

2. Atlanto-Axial Joints

–are synovial.

–are three in number: two planes that are between the superior and inferior articular facets of the atlas and axis, and one pivot that is the median joint between the dens of the axis and the anterior arch and transverse ligament of the atlas.

–are involved in rotation of the head.

E. Occipito-Axial Ligament Includes Four Ligaments

1. Cruciform Ligament

a. *Transverse Ligament*

–runs between the lateral masses of the atlas, arching around the dens of the axis.

b. *Longitudinal Ligament*

–extends from the dens of the axis to the anterior aspect of the foramen magnum and to body of axis.

2. Apical Ligament

–extends from the apex of the dens to the anterior aspect of the foramen magnum (of the occipital bone).

3. Alar Ligament

–extends from the apex of the dens to the medial side of the occipital bone.

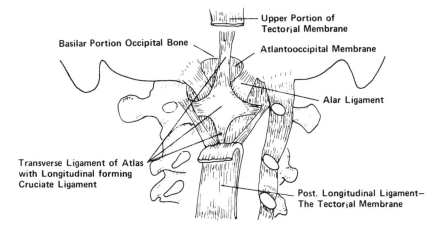

Figure 7.3. Ligaments of the atlas and the axis.

4. Membrana Tectoria

—is an upward extension of the posterior longitudinal ligament from the body of the axis to the basilar part of the occipital bone.

—lies external to the dura mater of the spinal cord.

IV. Vertebral Column

—consists of 33 vertebrae, which include 7 cervical, 12 thoracic, 5 lumbar, 5 fused sacral, and 4 fused coccygeal vertebrae.

—presents the **primary curvatures**, which are located in the thoracic and sacral regions, and the **secondary curvatures**, which are in the cervical and lumbar regions.

—may have abnormal curvature such as:

1. Kyphosis (Hunch Back)

—is an abnormal exaggerated primary curvature of the vertebral column.

2. Lordosis (Sway Back)

—is an abnormal accentuation of secondary curvature.

3. Scoliosis

—is a condition of a lateral deviation due to unequal growth of the spinal column.

A. Typical Vertebra

—consists of a body and a vertebral arch with several processes for muscular and articular attachments.

1. Body

—is a short cylinder.

—functions to support weight.

—is separated and also bound together by the intervertebral discs.

2. Vertebral Arch

—consists of paired **pedicles** laterally and paired **laminae** posteriorly.

—gives rise to seven processes: one spinous, two transverse, and four articular.

a. Spina Bifida

—results from the failure of the fusion of the vertebral arches.

—is classified as follows:

(1). Spina Bifida Occulta

—bony defect only.

(2). Meningocele

—protrusion of the meninges through the unfused arch of the vertebra.

(3). Meningomyelocele

—protrusion of the spinal cord as well as the meninges.

3. Foramina

a. Vertebral Foramina

—are formed by the vertebral bodies and vertebral arches (pedicles and laminae). A series of vertebral foramina forms the **vertebral canal**.

–transmit the spinal cord with its meningeal coverings and associated vessels.

b. *Intervertebral Foramina*

–are located between the inferior and superior surfaces of the pedicles of the adjacent vertebrae.

–transmit the spinal nerves and accompanying vessels as they exit the vertebral canal.

c. *Transverse Foramina*

–are present in each transverse process of the cervical vertebra.

–transmit the vertebral artery (except for seventh cervical vertebra), the vertebral vein, and autonomic nerves.

4. Processes

a. *Spinous Process*

–projects posteriorly from the vertebral arch.

b. *Transverse Processes*

–project on each side from the junction of the pedicle and the lamina.

c. *Costal Facets (Processes)*

–arise on the sides of a vertebral body anterior to the pedicle.

–articulate with the heads of the ribs, whereas facets on the transverse processes articulate with the tubercles of the ribs.

B. Intervertebral Disc

–lies between the bodies of two vertebrae.

–consists of a central mucoid substance, the **nucleus pulposus**, and a surrounding fibrocartilaginous lamina, the **anulus fibrosus**.

–plays an important role in movements between the vertebrae and in absorbing shocks.

1. Anulus Fibrosus

–consists of fibrous tissue and fibrocartilage in concentric layers around the circumference of the intervertebral disc.

–functions in the shock-absorbing mechanism.

–binds the vertebral column together, retains the nucleus, and permits a small amount of movement.

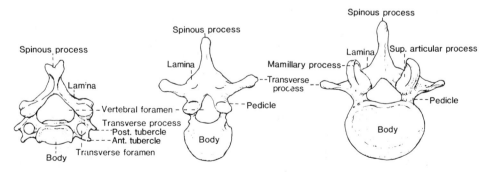

Figure 7.4. Cervical and lumbar vertebrae.

2. Nucleus Pulposus

–is situated in the central portion of the intervertebral disc.

–is composed of fibrocartilage of a semisolid nature.

–can be extruded out of its confinement in the direction of least resistance.

–may protrude or extrude (herniate) through the anulus fibrosus, thereby compressing the spinal nerve.

–also functions in the shock-absorbing mechanism, like the anulus fibrosus.

–is involved in equalizing pressure and exchanging fluids between the disc and the capillaries of the vertebrae.

C. Regional Characteristics of Vertebrae

1. First Cervical Vertebra (Atlas)

–supports the skull, and thus it was named after Atlas, who, according to Greek mythology, was known to support the heavens.

–has no body and no spinous process.

–consists of anterior and posterior arches and paired transverse processes.

–articulates superiorly with the occipital condyles of the skull, forming the atlanto-occipital joints, and inferiorly with the axis, forming the atlanto-axial joints.

2. Second Cervical Vertebra (Axis)

–has the smallest transverse process.

–is characterized by the presence of the dens or odontoid process.

Smallest transverse process

a. Dens of Axis

–projects superiorly from the body of the axis.

–articulates with the anterior arch of the atlas.

–forms the pivot around which the atlas rotates.

–is supported by the cruciform, apical, and alar ligaments and the membrana tectoria.

3. Seventh Cervical Vertebra

–is called the vertebra prominens due to its long spinous process, which is visible through the skin and gives attachment of the ligamentum nuchae.

Longest Spinous process

4. Fifth Lumbar Vertebra

–has the largest body of the vertebrae.

–is characterized by a strong, massive transverse process.

Largest body massive transverse process

5. Sacrum

–is a large, triangular, wedge-shaped bone.

–is composed of five fused sacral vertebrae.

–has four pairs of foramina for the exit of the ventral and dorsal primary rami of the first four sacral nerves.

–forms the posterior part of the pelvis and provides strength and stability of the pelvis.

–exhibits its promontory, that is the prominent anterior lip of its base.

6. Coccyx

–is a single bone formed by the union of the four coccygeal vertebrae.
–provides attachment for the coccygeus and the levator ani.

D. Ligaments

1. Anterior Longitudinal Ligament

–interconnects the vertebral bodies and intervertebral discs anteriorly.
–extends between the bodies of vertebrae on their anterior and anterolateral surfaces.
–is a very broad band and extends from the base of the skull to the sacrum.
–limits extension (dorsiflexion) of the vertebral column.
–supports the anulus fibrosus anteriorly.
–resists the gravitational pull, preventing lordosis.

2. Posterior Longitudinal Ligament

–interconnects the vertebral bodies and intervertebral discs posteriorly.
–supports the posterior aspect of the vertebral column.
–limits flexion of the vertebral column.
–supports the anulus fibrosus posteriorly.
–resists the gravitational pull, preventing kyphosis.

3. Ligamentum Flavum

–connects the laminae of two adjacent vertebrae.
–is thickest and strongest in the lumbar region; narrow but strong in the thoracic; and thinnest and broadest in the cervical region.
–may be pierced during lumbar (spinal) puncture.

4. Ligamentum Nuchae

–is a triangular fibrous membrane that forms a septum between the muscles on the two sides of the neck.
–is an upward extension of the supraspinal ligament that extends from the seventh cervical vertebra to the external occipital protuberance and crest.
–is attached to the posterior tubercle of the atlas and to the spinous processes of the cervical vertebrae.

E. Vertebral Venosus System

–is a valveless plexiform consisting of three interconnecting channels:

1. Internal Vertebral Venous Plexus

–lies in the epidural space between the wall of the vertebral canal and the dura mater and consists of four vertically arranged longitudinal veins (two anterior and two posterior) that drain into segmental veins.

2. Venous Plexus in Marrow Space

–is found in the body of the vertebra.

3. External Vertebral Venous Plexus

a. Anterior Part

–consists of longitudinal veins, lying in front of vertebral body; transverse vein, extending laterally from longitudinal veins. These veins communicate with the intervertebral and basivertebral veins.

    b. Posterior Part

       —lies on the vertebral arch.

—communicates above with the cranial dural sinus, below with the pelvic vein, and in the thorax-abdomen with both the azygos and caval systems.

—is thought to be the route of early metastasis of carcinoma of the lung, breast, and prostate to bones and the central nervous system.

[handwritten note: Route of Early Metastasis]

V. Spinal cord and Associated Structures

A. Spinal Cord

—is cylindrical in shape and occupies about the upper two-thirds of the vertebral canal.

—has cervical and lumbar enlargements for nerve supply of upper and lower limbs respectively.

—its gray matter is found in the interior (in contrast to the cerebral hemispheres), surrounded by white matter.

—its conical end is known as the **conus medullaris**.

—grows much more slowly than the bony vertebral column during the intrauterine development, and thus its terminal end gradually shifts to a higher level.

—ends at the level of L2 in the adult and at the level of L3 in the newborn.

—receives blood from the anterior spinal artery and two posterior spinal arteries as well as anterior and posterior radicular branches of spinal branches of the vertebral, cervical, and posterior intercostal and lumbar arteries.

—is enveloped by the three meninges.

B. Spinal Nerves

—have 31 pairs of nerves, including 8 cervical, 12 thoracic, 5 lumbar, 5 sacral, and 1 coccygeal (through their 33 vertebrae).

—are divided into the ventral and dorsal primary rami.

—are connected with the sympathetic chain ganglia by rami communicantes.

—are mixed nerves, containing motor fibers and sensory fibers.

—contain fibers whose cell bodies are in the dorsal root ganglion (general somatic afferent and general visceral afferent).

—contain fibers whose cell bodies are in the anterior horn of the spinal cord (general somatic efferent).

—contain fibers (general visceral efferent) whose cell bodies are in the lateral horn of the spinal cord (segments between T1-L2).

C. Meninges and Spinal Cord

1. Pia Mater

—is closely applied to the spinal cord, and thus it cannot be dissected from it.

—has lateral extensions between nerve roots of spinal nerves, known as denticulate (dentate) ligaments.

—enmeshes blood vessels on the surfaces of the spinal cord.

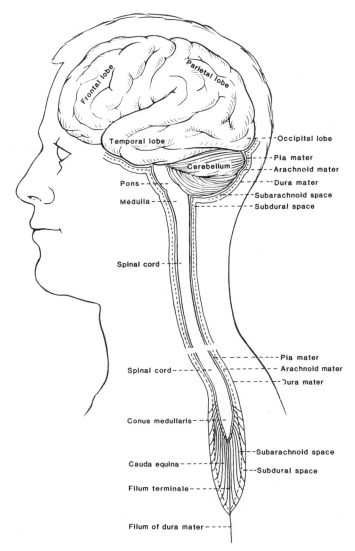

Figure 7.5. The meninges.

2. Arachnoid

– is a filmy, transparent, spidery layer and is connected to the pia mater by web-like trabeculations.

– is separated from the pia mater by the **subarachnoid space**, which is filled with cerebrospinal fluid.

3. Dura Mater

– is the tough, fibrous, outermost layer of the meninges.

– the **subdural space** is internal to it (between the arachnoid and dura).

– the **epidural space** is external to it, which contains the internal vertebral venous plexus.

D. Cauda Equina ("Horse's Tail")

—is formed by a great lash of dorsal and ventral roots that surround the filum terminale.

—is located within the subarachnoid space, below the level of the conus medullaris.

—is free to float in the cerebrospinal fluid.

E. Denticulate Ligament

—is a lateral extension of the pia through the arachnoid, attaching to the inner surface of the dura.

—presents a free lateral border and consists of 21 pairs of tooth-like processes that attache to the dura mater between nerve roots.

—helps to suspend the spinal cord within the subarachnoid space.

F. Filum Terminale of Spinal Cord

Pia matter ←

—is a prolongation of the pia mater from the tip (conus medularis) of the spinal cord.

—begins where the spinal cord ends at the level of L2.

—lies in the midst of the cauda equina and ends at the level of S2 by attaching to the apex of the dural sac.

—blends with the dura at the apex of the dural sac and then the dura continues downward as the **filum of the dura mater** (or **coccygeal ligament**), which is attached to the dorsum of the coccyx.

G. Cerebrospinal Fluid

—is contained in the subarachnoid space between the arachnoid and pia mater.

—is formed by vascular choroid plexuses in the ventricles of the brain.

—circulates through the ventricles, enters the subarachnoid space, and eventually filters into the venous system.

H. Lumbar Puncture (Spinal Tap)

—is the tapping of the subarachnoid space in the lumbar region, usually between the laminae of the third and fourth or fourth and fifth lumbar vertebrae.

—allows measurement of the pressure of the cerebrospinal fluid; withdrawal of some of it for bacteriological and chemical examinations; or introduction of anesthesia, drugs, or radiopaque material into the subarachnoid space.

Compare to serum CSF. Contains light amat of Cl⁻. pH
and Lactate

Review Test

BACK

DIRECTIONS: For each of the questions or incomplete statements in this section, *one* or *more* of the answers or completions given are correct. Choose answer:

A. if only **1**, **2**, and **3** are correct.
B. if only **1** and **3** are correct.
C. if only **2** and **4** are correct.
D. if only **4** is correct.
E. if all are correct.

7.1. In order to withdraw cerebrospinal fluid by lumbar puncture, a needle should penetrate the
1. dura mater.
2. anulus fibrosus.
3. outer arachnoid layer.
4. pia mater.

7.2. The spinal epidural space
1. may be entered via the sacral hiatus.
2. is continuous from the sacrum to the base of the skull.
3. contains a venous plexus, sometimes injured during lumbar puncture.
4. contains cerebrospinal fluid.

7.3. The vertebral venous plexus
1. communicates with the cranial venous sinuses.
2. is formed by thin-walled veins with many valves.
3. communicates with veins of thorax, abdomen, and pelvis.
4. is located in the subdural space.

7.4. The anterior longitudinal ligament
1. lies between the intervertebral disc and the dura.
2. extends from the sacrum to the atlas.
3. ends superiorly as the tectorial membrane.
4. limits dorsiflexion of the vertebral column.

7.5. The suboccipital nerve (dorsal primary ramus of C1) supplies the following muscles:
1. rectus capitis posterior major.
2. rectus capitis lateralis.
3. semispinalis capitis.
4. rectus capitis anterior.

DIRECTIONS: For each numbered item, select the *one* lettered heading that is most closely associated with it. Each lettered heading may be selected once, more than once, or not at all.

A. Conus medularis
B. Dorsal root ganglion
C. Cauda equina
D. Internal vertebral venous plexus
E. Arachnoid layer of the meninges

7.6. Is found within the vertebral canal but external to the dura mater of the spinal cord.

7.7. The cerebrospinal fluid is enclosed by this structure.

7.8. The inferior limit is usually the lower border of the first lumbar vertebra.

7.9. Contains the cell bodies of sensory nerve fibers.

7.10. Is formed by the root of the lumbar and sacral nerves.

A. Nucleus pulposus
B. Scoliosis
C. Anulus fibrosus
D. Intervertebral disc
E. Lordosis (sway back)

7.11. Binds the vertebral column together, retains the nucleus, and permits a small amount of movement.

7.12. Is situated in the central portion of the intervertebral disc.

7.13. Lies between the bodies of two vertebrae.

7.14. Is abnormal accentuation of secondary curvature.

7.15. Is a condition of a lateral deviation due to unequal growth of the spinal column.

A. Longitudinal ligament of the cruciform ligament
B. Apical ligament
C. Alar ligament
D. Ligamentum flavum
E. Denticulate ligament

7.16. Extends from the apex of the dens to the anterior aspect of the foramen magnum.

7.17. Extends from dens of axis to anterior aspect of the foramen magnum and the body of the axis.

7.18. Extends from the apex of the dens to the medial side of the occipital bone.

7.19. Is a lateral extension of the pia mater and helps to anchor the spinal cord within the vertebral canal.

7.20. Connects the laminae of two adjacent vertebrae.

DIRECTIONS: Each of the questions or incomplete statements below is followed by suggested answers or completions. Choose the *one* that is *best* in each case.

7.21. Choose the incorrect statement.

A. The rectus capitis posterior major participates in bounding the suboccipital triangle.
B. The rectus capitis posterior minor does not participate in bounding the suboccipital triangle.
C. Both obliquus capitis superior and obliquus capitis inferior are boundaries of the triangle.
D. All of the previously mentioned are supplied by the greater occipital nerve.
E. Within the floor of the triangle, the vertebral artery occupies the groove on the superior surface of the posterior arch of the atlas.

7.22. With regard to relationship of ligaments to spinal cord in the cervical and thoracic region, identify the correct statement.

A. The anterior longitudinal, but not the posterior longitudinal, ligament is anterior to the spinal cord.
B. Both anterior and posterior longitudinal ligaments are anterior to the cord.
C. Both anterior longitudinal ligament and ligamentum flavum are anterior to the cord.
D. Only the ligamentum flavum is anterior to the cord.
E. The supraspinal and interspinal ligaments are anterior to the cord.

7.23. Because of its common innervation by dorsal (posterior) rami, one of the following muscles does *not* belong in this listing. Identify it.

A. semispinalis capitis.
B. splenius.
C. serratus posterior superior.
D. iliocostalis.
E. spinalis.

7.24. In the spinal region, cerebrospinal fluid is found

A. in the epidural space.
B. in the subdural space.
C. between the pia mater and the spinal cord.
D. in the subarachnoid space.
E. between the arachnoid and dura mater.

7.25. Choose the incorrect statement. The multifidus muscle

A. is a transversospinalis muscle.
B. is the deepest muscle of the back.
C. is attached to the spinous processes.
D. is innervated by the ventral primary rami of the spinal nerve.
E. lies deep to the semispinalis muscle.

DIRECTIONS: Each set of lettered headings below is followed by a list of numbered words or phrases. Choose answer.

        A. if the item is associated with **A** only.
        B. if the item is associated with **B** only.
        C. if the item is associated with both **A** and **B**.
        D. if the item is associated with neither **A** nor **B**.

A. Semispinalis capitis
B. Splenius capitis
C. Both
D. Neither

7.26. Originates from the transverse processes of the upper thoracic vertebrae.

7.27. Originates from the spinous processes of the lower cervical vertebrae.

7.28. Inserts on the transverse processes of the upper cervical vertebrae.

7.29. Is innervated by the dorsal primary rami of the cervical nerve.

7.30. Is supplied by the branches of the occipital artery.

Answers and Explanations

BACK

7.1. B. The cerebrospinal fluid is located in the subarachnoid space between the arachnoid and pia mater. The anulus fibrosus is the fibrocartilaginous ring forming the circumference of the intervertebral disc.

7.2. A. The spinal epidural space is the space external to the dura mater and contains the internal vertebral venous plexus. It extends from the base of the skull to the sacrum and can be entered through the sacral hiatus for caudal (extradural) anesthesia.

7.3. B. The vertebral venous system consists of thin-walled, valveless veins, lies in the epidural space, and communicates with the cranial venous sinuses and paravertebral veins in the thorax, abdomen, and pelvis.

7.4. C. The anterior longitudinal ligament extends from the base of the skull to the sacrum and limits extension (dorsiflexion) of the vertebral column.

7.5. B. The suboccipital nerve (dorsal primary ramus of C1) supplies the muscles of the suboccipital area and the semispinalis capitis.

7.6. D. The internal vertebral venous plexus is found in the epidural space.

7.7. E. The cerebrospinal fluid is found in the subarachnoid space between the pia mater and the arachnoid mater.

7.8. A. The conus medularis is a conical end of the spinal cord at the level of the first or second lumbar vertebra.

7.9. B. The dorsal root ganglion contains the cell bodies of the visceral and somatic sensory nerve fibers.

7.10. C. The cauda equina is formed by the dorsal and ventral roots of the lumbar and sacral nerves.

7.11. C. The anulus fibrosus is the fibrocartilaginous ring forming the circumference of the intervertebral disc and thus retains the nucleus pulposus. It binds the vertebral column together and permits a small amount of movement.

7.12. A. The nucleus pulposus is the soft fibrocartilage central portion of the intervertebral disc, surrounded by the anulus fibrosus.

7.13. D. The intervertebral disc consists of the nucleus pulposus and the anulus fibrosus and lies between the bodies of two vertebra.

7.14. E. Lordosis (sway back) is an abnormal accentuation of the secondary curvature.

7.15. B. Scoliosis is a condition of a lateral deviation due to unequal growth of the spinal column.

7.16. B. The apical ligament of the dens extends from the tip of the dens to the anterior margin of the foramen magnum of the occipital bone.

7.17. A. The longitudinal ligament of the cruciform ligament extends from the body of the axis, over the dens, to the occipital bone (or anterior margin of the foramen magnum).

7.18. C. The alar ligament extends from the side of the apex of the dens to the medial side of the occipital condyle (or the lateral margin of the foramen magnum).

7.19. E. The denticulate ligament is a lateral extension of the pia mater and helps to anchor the spinal cord within the vertebral canal.

7.20. D. The ligamentum flavum extends between the laminae of two adjacent vertebrae.

7.21. D. The suboccipital triangle is bounded by the rectus capitis posterior major and the obliquus capitis superior and inferior muscles.

7.22. D. The ligamentum flavum connects the laminae of the two adjacent vertebrae and lies in front of the spinal cord. The anterior and posterior longitudinal ligaments as well as the supraspinal and interspinal ligaments are posterior to the spinal cord.

7.23. B. The serratus posterior superior is innervated by the anterior primary rami of the upper four thoracic nerves. The deep muscles of the back are innervated by the posterior primary rami of the spinal nerves.

7.24. D. The cerebrospinal fluid is found in the subarachnoid space.

7.25. D. The multifidus muscle is innervated by the posterior primary rami of the spinal nerves.

7.26. A. The semispinalis capitis muscle originates from the transverse processes of the upper six thoracic vertebrae and the articular processes of the lower four cervical ones.

7.27. B. The splenius capitis muscle originates from the lower half of the ligamentum nuchae and the spinous processes of the seventh cervical and upper four to six cervical vertebrae.

7.28. D. Both the semispinalis capitis and splenius capitis muscles are inserted on the skull, innervated by posterior primary rami of the spinal nerves, and supplied by branches of the occipital artery.

7.29. C. See 7.28.

7.30. C. See 7.28.

8

Head and Neck

Cervical Triangles and Deep Structures of Neck

I. Cervical Triangles

A. Posterior Cervical Triangle

—is bounded by the superior border of the sternomastoid, anterior border of the trapezius, and superior border of the clavicle.

—Its roof is formed by the platysma and the deep cervical fascia.

—its floor is formed by the splenius capitis, levator scapulae, and scalenus anterior, medius, and posterior.

—contains the accessory nerve, cutaneous branches of the cervical plexus, external jugular vein, posterior belly of the omohyoid, roots and trunks of the brachial plexus, and transverse cervical and suprascapular vessels.

—is further divided into the occipital and subclavian triangles by the omohyoid posterior belly.

B. Anterior Triangle

—is bounded by the anterior border of the sternomastoid, the anteromedian line of the neck, and the inferior border of the mandible and an extension of this line to the mastoid process.

—its roof is formed by the platysma and the deep cervical fascia.

—is further divided by the omohyoid anterior belly and the digastric anterior and posterior bellies into the digastric (submandibular), submental (suprahyoid), carotid, and muscular (inferior carotid) triangles.

II. Muscles

Muscle	Origin	Insertion	Nerve	Action
Cervical Muscles				
Platysma	Superficial fascia over upper part of deltoid and pectoralis major	Mandible; skin and muscles over mandible and angle of mouth	Facial n.	Depresses lower jaw and lip; tenses and ridges skin of neck
Sternocleidomastoid	Manubrium sterni and medial third of clavicle	Mastoid process and laterial half of superior nuchal line	Spinal accessory n., C2-3	Singly draw head toward shoulder; together flex head; raise thorax

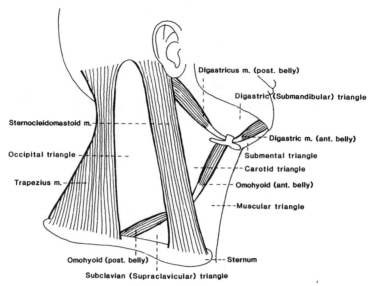

Figure 8.1. Subdivision of the cervical triangle.

Muscle	Origin	Insertion	Nerve	Action
Suprahyoid Muscles				
Digastric	Anterior belly from digastric fossa of mandible; posterior belly from mastoid notch	Intermediate tendon attached to hyoid bone	Posterior belly by facial n.; anterior belly by mylohyoid n. of trigeminal n.	Elevates hyoid and tongue; depresses mandible
Mylohyoid	Mylohoid line of mandible	Median raphe and hyoid bone	Mylohyoid n. of trigeminal n.	Elevates hyoid and tongue; depresses mandible
Stylohyoid	Styloid process	Body of hyoid	Facial n.	Elevates hyoid
Geniohyoid	Genial tubercle of mandible	Body of hyoid	C1 via hypoglossal n.	Elevates hyoid and tongue
Infrahyoid Muscles				
Sternohyoid	Manubrium sterni and medial end of clavicle	Body of hyoid	Ansa cervicalis	Depresses hyoid and larynx
Sternothyroid	Manubrium sterni; first costal cartilage	Oblique line of thyroid cartilage	Ansa cervicalis	Depresses thyroid cartilage and larynx
Thyrohyoid	Oblique line of thyroid cartilage	Body and greater horn of hyoid	C1 via hypoglossal n.	Depresses hyoid and larynx; elevates thyroid cartilage
Omohyoid	Inferior belly from medial lip of suprascapular notch and suprascapular ligament; superior belly from intermediate tendon	Inferior belly to intermediate tendon; superior belly to body of hyoid	Ansa Cervicalis	Depresses and retracts hyoid and larynx

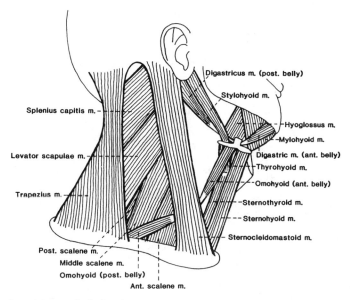

Figure 8.2. Muscles of the cervical triangle.

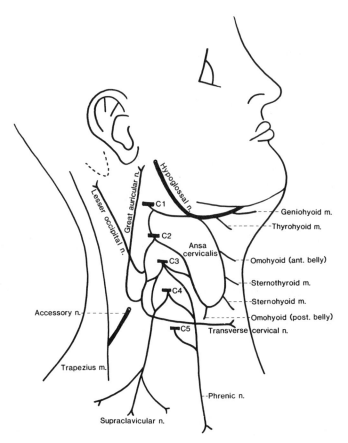

Figure 8.3. The cervical plexus.

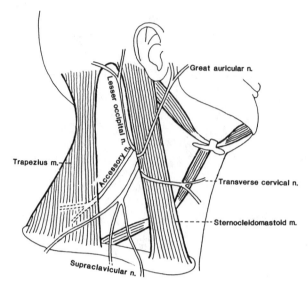

Figure 8.4. Cutaneous branches of the cervical plexus.

III. Nerves of Cervical Triangles

A. Accessory Nerve

–is formed by the union of cranial and spinal roots.

–its cranial roots arise from the medulla oblongata below the roots of the vagus.

–its spinal roots arise from the cervical segment of the spinal cord between C1 and C3 (C7). The spinal roots unite to form a trunk that extends between the dorsal and ventral roots of the spinal nerve in the vertebral canal and passes through the foramen magnum.

–both spinal and cranial portions traverse the jugular foramen, where they interchange fibers.

–its cranial portion contains motor fibers that join the vagus nerve and supply the soft palate, pharyngeal constrictors, and larynx.

–its spinal portion supplies the sternomastoid and trapezius muscles.

B. Cervical Plexus

–is formed by the ventral rami of the first four cervical nerves.

–gives rise to cutaneous branches, including the lesser occipital, greater auricular, transverse cervical, and supraclavicular nerves.

1. Lesser Occipital Nerve (C2)

–ascends along the posterior border of the sternomastoid to the scalp behind the auricle.

2. Greater Auricular Nerve (C2–C3)

–ascends on the sternomastoid to supply the skin behind the auricle and on the parotid gland.

3. **Transverse Cervical Nerve (C2-C3)**

  –turns around the posterior border of the sternomastoid and supplies the skin on the anterior cervical triangle.

4. **Supraclavicular Nerve (C3-C4)**

  –emerges as a common trunk from under the cover of the sternomastoid; then it divides into anterior, middle, and posterior branches to the skin over the clavicle and the shoulder.

–gives off motor nerves, including the ansa cervicalis to the infrahyoid muscles, the phrenic nerve to the diaphragm, and twigs to the sternomastoid, trapezius, levator scapulae, and scalenus muscles.

5. **Ansa Cervicalis**

  –is a nerve loop formed by the union of the superior root or descendens hypoglossi and the inferior root or descendens cervicalis.
  –its superior root is formed by nerve fibers from C1 or C1-2.
  –its inferior root is formed by nerve fibers from C2 and C3.
  –innervates the infrahyoid (or strap) muscles, such as omohyoid, sternohyoid, sternothyroid, and thyrohyoid muscles.

6. **Phrenic Nerve**

  –arises from the ventral rami of the cervial nerves C3,4,5.
  –runs in front of the anterior scalenus muscle.
  –passes into the thorax deep to the subclavian vein.
  –supplies the diaphragm, pericardium and pleura.
  –passes between the mediastinal pleura and fibrous pericardium.

C. **Brachial Plexus**

  –is formed by the union of the ventral primary rami of the lower four cervical and first thoracic nerves.
  –passes between the scalenus anterior and medius muscles.
  –its roots give rise to:

1. **Dorsal Scapular Nerve**

  –originates from C5 behind the scalenus anterior, runs through the scalenus medius and then deep to the trapezius.
  –passes deep to or through the levator scapulae and descends along with the dorsal scapular nerve on the deep surface of the rhomboids along the medial border of the scapula, supplying the levator scapulae and rhomboid muscles.

2. **Long Thoracic Nerve**

  –originates from C5, C6, and C7, pierces the scalenus medius muscle, descends behind the brachial plexus, and enters the axilla to supply the serratus anterior muscle.

–its upper trunk gives rise to:

3. **Suprascapular Nerve**

  –arises from C5 and C6, passes deep to the trapezius, and joins the suprascapular artery in a course toward the shoulder.
  –passes through the scapular notch under the transverse scapular ligament and supplies the supraspinatus and infraspinatus muscles.

4. Nerve to the Subclavius

–arises from C5 and descends in front of the plexus and behind the clavicle to supply the subclavius muscle.

–its middle and lower trunks give rise to no branches.

IV. Blood Vessels

A. Subclavian Artery

–is a branch of the brachiocephalic trunk on the right, but it arises directly from the arch of the aorta on the left.

–is divided into three parts by the scalenus anterior muscle: the first part passes from the origin of the vessel to the medial margin of the scalenus anterior, the second lies behind this muscle, and the third passes from the lateral margin of the muscle to the outer border of the first rib.

–its branches are the vertebral, thyrocervical, and internal thoracic from its first portion; the costocervical trunk from its second portion; and the dorsal scapular artery from its third portion.

1. Vertebral Artery

–arises from the first part of the subclavian and ascends between the scalenus anterior and the longus coli.

–ascends through the transverse foramina of the upper six cervical vertebrae, winds around the superior articular process of the atlas, and passes through the foramen magnum into the cranial cavity.

2. Thyrocervical Trunk

–is a short trunk from the first part of the subclavian artery that divides into the inferior thyroid, transverse cervical, and suprascapular arteries.

a. *Inferior Thyroid Artery*

–ascends in front of the scalenus anterior, turns medially behind the carotid sheath but in front of the vertebral vessels, and then arches downward to the lower pole of the thyroid gland.

–gives off an ascending cervical artery, which ascends on the scalenus anterior medial to the phrenic nerve.

b. *Transverse Cervical Artery*

–runs laterally across the scalenus anterior, phrenic nerve, and trunks of the brachial plexus, passing deep to the trapezius.

–divides into a superficial (or ascending) branch and a deep or descending branch, which is known as the dorsal or descending scapular artery.

c. *Suprascapular Artery*

–passes in front of the scalenus anterior and the brachial plexus parallel to but below the transverse cervical artery.

–passes superior to the transverse scapular ligament, whereas the suprascapular nerve passes inferior to it.

3. Costocervical Trunk

–arises from the posterior aspect of the subclavian artery behind the scalenus anterior and divides into the deep cervical and superior intercostal arteries.

    a. Deep Cervical Artery

        —passes between the transverse process of the seventh cervical vertebra and the neck of the first rib, ascends between the semispinalis capitis and cervicis, and anastomoses with the deep branch of the descending branch of the occipital artery.

    b. Superior Intercostal Artery

        —descends behind the cervical pleura, anterior to the necks of the first two ribs.

        —gives off the first two posterior intercostal arteries.

  4. Dorsal Scapular (or Descending Scapular) Artery

    —arises from either the third part of the subclavian artery or the deep or descending branch of the transverse cervical artery.

  5. Internal Thoracic Artery

    —arises from the first part of the subclavian artery, descends through thorax behind the upper six costal cartilages, and ends at the sixth intercostal space by dividing into the superior epigastric and musculophrenic arteries.

B. Common Carotid Artery

  —begins at the bifurcation of the brachiocephalic artery on the right and from the aortic arch on the left.

  —ascends within the carotid sheath and divides at the level of the upper border of the thyroid cartilage into the external and internal carotid arteries.

  —the carotid body at its bifurcation is sensitive to blood oxygenation (chemoreceptor).

  1. Carotid Body - *vagus nerve & Glanopharyngeal nerve*

    —lies at the bifurcation of the common carotid artery as an ovoid body.

    —functions as a **chemoreceptor** that is stimulated by chemical changes (such as oxygen tension) in the circulating blood.

    —is innervated by the nerve to the carotid body arising from the pharyngeal branch of the vagus nerve.

C. Internal Carotid Artery

  —has no branches in the neck.

  —ascends within the carotid sheath, in company with the vagus nerve and the internal jugular vein.

  —enters the cranium through the carotid canal in the petrous part of the temporal bone.

  —in the cranial fossa, gives off the ophthalmic artery and the anterior and middle cerebral arteries.

  1. Carotid Sinus — *Glanopharyngeal nerve*

    —is a spindle-shaped dilation located at the origin of the internal carotid artery.

    —functions as a **pressoreceptor** (baroreceptor), being stimulated by changes in blood pressure.

    —is innervated by the carotid branch of the glossopharyngeal nerve.

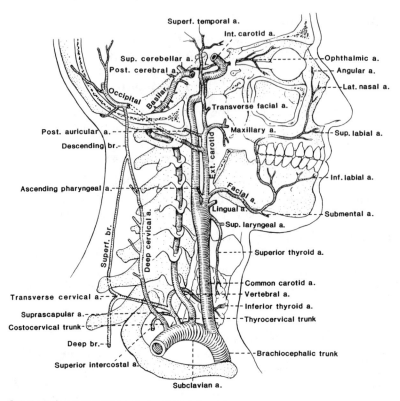

Figure 8.5. Subclavian and carotid arteries and their branches.

D. External Carotid Artery

–extends from the level of the upper border of the thyroid cartilage to the neck of the mandible, where it ends in the substance of the parotid gland by dividing into the maxillary and superficial temporal arteries.
–has eight named branches:

1. Superior Thyroid Artery

–arises below the level of the greater horn of the hyoid bone.
–descends obliquely forward in the carotid triangle and passes deep to the infrahyoid muscles to reach the superior pole of the thyroid gland.
–gives rise to an **infrahyoid** branch, a **sternomastoid** branch, a **superior laryngeal** branch, a **cricothyroid** branch, and several **glandular** branches.

2. Lingual Artery

–arises at the level of the tip of the greater horn of the hyoid bone.
–passes deep to the hyoglossus to reach the tongue.

3. Facial Artery

–arises just above the lingual artery and ascends forward deep to the posterior belly of the digastric and the stylohyoid muscles.

–hooks around the lower border of the mandible at the anterior margin of the masseter to enter the face.

4. Ascending Pharyngeal Artery

–arises from the deep surface of the external carotid artery in the carotid triangle and ascends between the internal carotid artery and the wall of the pharynx.

–gives rise to the pharyngeal, palatine, inferior tympanic, and meningeal branches.

5. Occipital Artery

–arises from the posterior surface of the external carotid artery, a little below the level of the hyoid bone.

–passes deep to the digastric posterior belly, occupies the groove on the mastoid process, and appears on the skin above the occipital triangle.

–gives off a branch to the sternocleidomastoid and the descending branch.

a. Descending Branch

–its superficial branch anastomes with the superficial (or ascending) branch of the transverse cervical artery.

–its deep branch anastomoses with the deep cervical artery of the costocervical trunk.

6. Posterior Auricular Artery

–arises from the posterior surface of the external carotid artery just above the digastric posterior belly.

–ascends superficial to the styloid process and deep to the parotid gland, and ends between the mastoid process and the external acoustic meatus.

–gives off the stylomastoid, auricular, and occipital branches.

7. Maxillary Artery

–arises behind the neck of the mandible as the larger terminal branch of the external carotid artery.

–runs deep to the neck of the mandible and enters the infratemporal fossa.

–its further course is described on page 285.

8. Superficial Temporal Artery

–arises behind the neck of the mandible as the smaller terminal branch of the external carotid artery.

–ascends in front of the external acoustic meatus into the scalp, accompanying the auriculotemporal nerve and the superficial temporal vein.

E. Retromandibular Vein

–is formed by the superficial temporal and maxillary veins.

–divides into an anterior branch, which joins the facial vein to form the common fascial vein, and a posterior branch, which joins the posterior auricular vein to form the external jugular vein.

F. External Jugular Vein

–is formed by the union of the posterior auricular vein and the posterior branch of the retromandibular vein.

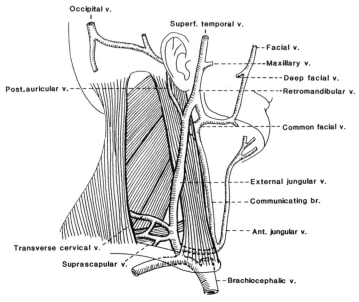

Figure 8.6. Veins in the cervical triangle.

–crosses the sternomastoid obliquely, under the platysma and ends in the subclavian (or sometimes the internal jugular) vein.

–receives the suprascapular, transverse cervical, and anterior jugular veins.

G. Internal Jugular Vein

–begins in the jugular foramen as a continuation of the sigmoid sinus and ends in the brachiocephalic vein.

–has the **superior bulb** at its beginning and the **inferior bulb** just above its termination.

–received blood from the brain, the face, and the neck.

–descends in the carotid sheath.

V. Deep Structures

A. Thyroid Gland

–develops as a diverticulum from the ventral wall of the pharynx.

–consists of right and left lobes connected by the isthmus. (A muscular band descending from the hyoid bone to the isthmus is called the levator glandulae thyroideae.)

–is supplied by the superior and inferior thyroid arteries (and the arteria thyroidea ima, which is an inconsistent branch from the brachiocephalic trunk).

–its venous drainage is by way of the superior and middle thyroid veins to the internal jugular vein, and by the inferior thyroid vein to the brachiocephalic vein.

B. Parathyroid Glands

–are endocrine glands that are essential to life. (Removal of all glandular tissue results in the development of tetany and death.)

–are four (two to six) small ovoid bodies that lie against the dorsum of the thyroid gland under its sheath but with their own capsule.

–their hormone maintains the normal relationship between blood and skeletal calcium.

–are supplied chiefly by the inferior thyroid artery.

C. Thyroid Cartilage

–is a hyaline cartilage.

–forms a laryngeal prominence (the "Adam's apple").

–its superior horn is joined to the tip of the greater horn of the hyoid bone by the lateral thyroid ligament.

D. Sympathetic Trunk

–runs behind the carotid sheath and in front of the longus colli and longus capitis muscles.

–contains postganglionic sympathetic fibers and visceral afferent fibers with cell bodies in the upper thoracic dorsal root ganglia.

–receives gray rami communicantes but no white rami communicantes.

–bears the following cervical ganglia:

1. Superior Cervical Ganglion

–lies in front of cervical vertebrae 1 and 2.

–lies posterior to the internal carotid artery and anterior to the longus capitis.

–gives rise to the **internal carotid, pharyngeal, external carotid,** and **superior cervical cardiac** nerves.

2. Middle Cervical Ganglion

–lies at the level of the cricoid cartilage (cervical vertebra 6).

–gives off a middle cervical cardiac nerve, which is the largest of the three cervical sympathetic cardiac nerves.

3. Inferior Cervical Ganglion

–is present as the **cervicothoracic** ganglion by its fusion with the first thoracic ganglion.

–lies in front of the neck of the first rib and the transverse process of the seventh cervical vertebra and behind the dome of the pleura.

–gives rise to the inferior cervical cardiac nerve.

E. Ansa Subclavia

–is the cord connecting the middle and inferior cervical sympathetic ganglia, forming a loop around the first part of the subclavian artery.

VI. Cervical Fasciae

A. Superficial Layer (Investing Fascia)

–surrounds all of the deeper parts of the neck.

–splits to enclose the sternocleidomastoid and trapezius muscles.

B. Prevertebral Layer

–is cylindrical in form and encloses the vertebral column and its associated muscles.

–covers the scalene muscles and attaches to the external occipital protuberance.

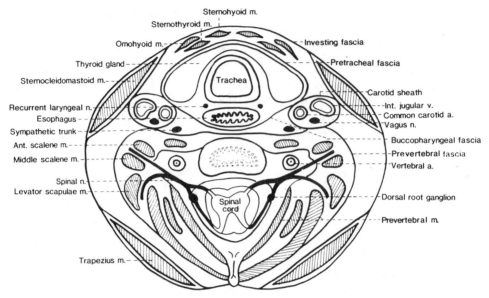

Figure 8.7. Cross-section of the neck.

C. Cervical Visceral Fascia

–consists of two fasciae, the **pretrachial fascia** anteriorly and the **buccopharyngeal fascia** posteriorly.

–encloses the pharynx, esophagus, trachea, thyroid gland, and parathyroid gland.

D. Carotid Sheath

–contains the common and internal carotid arteries, internal jugular vein, and vagus nerve.

–blends with the prevertebral, pretracheal, and investing fasciae.

–also attaches to the base of the skull.

–does not contain the sympathetic trunk, which lies posterior to the carotid sheath and anterior to the prevertebral fascia.

VII. Clinical Considerations

A. Injury of Upper Trunk of Brachial Plexus

–may be caused by a violent separation of the head from the shoulder, such as an incidence that occurs in a fall from a motorcycle. In this condition, the arm is in medial rotation due to the paralysis of the lateral rotators, resulting in a **"waiter's tip hand."**

–may be caused by hands of an obstetrician during a difficult delivery. This is referred to as **"birth palsy"** or **"obstetric paralysis."**

B. Neurovascular Compression Syndrome of Upper Limb

–is caused by an **abnormal insertion** of the scalenus anterior and posterior muscles and by the **cervical rib,** which is the cartilaginous accessory rib attached to the seventh cervical vertebra. Such cases can be corrected by cutting the cervical rib or the scalenus anterior muscle.

C. Fracture of Clavicle

–commonly occurs in a fall on the shoulder or hand, or by hands of an obstetrician during breech delivery.

–may damage the subclavian vein by bone fragments, resulting in a fatal hemorrhage and also thrombosis, leading to pulmonary embolism.

–may injure the lower trunk of the brachial plexus, causing paresthesias (abnormal sensations of burning, pricking, tickling, or tingling) in the area distributed by the lower trunk.

Face and Scalp

I. Skull

–is the skeleton of the head, composed of 8 cranial bones and 14 facial bones.

    a. The cranial bones are the frontal, occipital, two parietal, two temporal, ethmoid, and sphenoid.

    b. The facial bones are the two lacrimal, two nasal, two palates, two inferior turbinate, two superior maxillary, two malar, the vomer, and the maxilla.

–provides a case for accommodating the brain; cavities for housing the organs of special sense for sight, hearing, equilibration, taste, and smell; openings for passing food and air; and jaws with teeth for mastication.

A. Cranium

–means the skull without a mandible.

B. Calvaria

–represents the skullcap or vault of the skull without the facial bones.

C. Sutures

–are the immovable fibrous joints between the bones of the skull, such as the coronal, sagittal, squamous, and lambdoid sutures.

    1. Coronal Suture

       –lies between the frontal bone and the two parietal bones.

    2. Sagittal Suture

       –lies between the two pariental bones.

    3. Squamous Suture

       –lies between the parietal bone and the squamous part of the temporal bone.

    4. Lambdoid Suture

       –lies between the two parietal bones and the occipital bone.

D. Lambda

–is the point where the two parietal bones and the occipital bone come together.

E. Bregma

–is the intersection of the sagittal and coronal sutures.

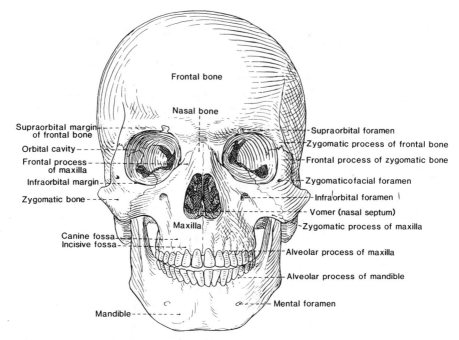

Figure 8.8. Anterior view of the skull.

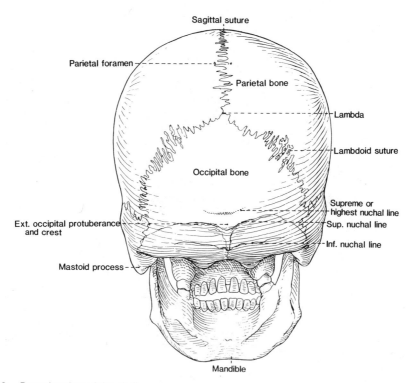

Figure 8.9. Posterior view of the skull.

F. Pterion

—is a craniometric point at the junction of the frontal, parietal, temporal, and great wing of the sphenoid bone.

II. Muscles of Facial Expression

Muscle	Origin	Insertion	Nerve	Action
Occipitofron-talis	Superior nuchal line; upper orbital margin	Epicranial apo-neurosis	Facial n.	Elevates eye-brows; wrinkles forehead
Corrugator supercilii	Medial supraorbital margin	Skin of medial eyebrow	Facial n.	Draws eyebrows downward medially
Orbicularis oculi	Medial orbital margin; medial palpebral ligament; lacrimal bone	Skin and rim of orbit; tarsal plate; lateral palpebral raphe	Facial n.	Sphincter of eye; closes eyelids
Procerus	Nasal bone and cartilage	Skin between eyebrows	Facial n.	Wrinkles skin over bones
Nasalis	Maxilla lateral to incisive fossa	Ala of nose	Facial n.	Draws ala of nose toward septum
Depressor septi	Incisive fossa of maxilla	Ala and nasal septum	Facial n.	Constricts nares
Orbicularis oris	Maxilla above incisor teeth	Skin of lip	Facial n.	Closes lips
Levator anguli oris	Canine fossa of maxilla	Angle of mouth	Facial n.	Elevates angle of mouth
Levator labii superioris	Maxilla above infraorbital foramen	Skin of upper lip	Facial n.	Elevates upper lip; dilates nares
Levator labii superioris alaeque nasi	Frontal process of maxilla	Skin of upper lip	Facial n.	Elevate ala of nose and upper lip
Zygomaticus major	Zygomatic arch	Angle of mouth	Facial n.	Draws angle of mouth backward and upward
Depressor labii inferioris	Mandible below mental foramen	Orbicularis oris and skin of lower lip	Facial n.	Depresses lower lip
Depressor anguli oris	Oblique line of mandible	Angle of mouth	Facial n.	Depresses angle of mouth
Risorius	Fascia over masseter	Angle of mouth	Facial n.	Retracts angle of mouth
Buccinator	Mandible; pterygomandibular raphe; alveolar processes	Angle of mouth	Facila n.	Presses cheek to keep it taut
Mentalis	Incisive fossa of mandible	Skin of chin	Facial n.	Elevates and protrudes lower lip
Auricularis anterior, superior, and posterior	Temporal fascia; epicranial aponeurosis; mastoid process	Anterior, superior, and posterior sides of auricle	Facial n.	Retract and elevate ear

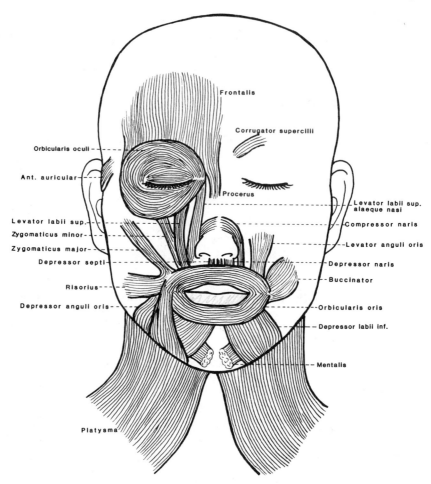

Figure 8.10. Muscles of facial expression.

III. Nerve Supply

A. Trigeminal Nerve

–is sensory to the skin of the face, whereas the facial nerve supplies the muscles of facial expression.

1. Ophthalmic Nerve

–supplies the area above the upper eyelid and dorsum of the nose.
–its branches are the supraorbital, supratrochlear, infratrochlear, external nasal, and lacrimal nerves.

2. Maxillary Nerve

–supplies the face below the level of the eyes and above the upper lip.
–its branches are the zygomaticofacil, zygomaticotemporal, and infraorbital nerves.

Herpetic lesion around opthalmic nerve

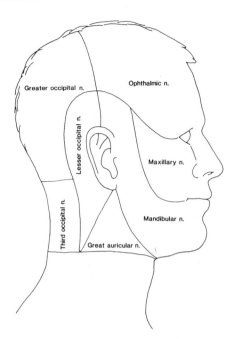

Figure 8.11. Cutaneous innervation of the face and scalp.

3. Mandibular Nerve
  –supplies the face below the level of the lower lip.
  –its branches are the auriculotermporal, buccal, and mental nerves.

* Trigeminal Neuralgia (Tic Douloureux)
  –marked by a paroxysmal pain along the course of the trigeminal nerve.
  –its pain may be alleviated by sectioning the sensory root of the trigeminal nerve in the trigeminal (Meckel's) cave in the middle cranial fossa. · *gt effech als Manllay and Mamdblar neue*

B. Facial Nerve
  –comes through the **stylomastoid foramen** of the skull and appears posterior to the parotid gland.
  –enters the parotid gland to give five terminal branches, which radiate forward in the face as **temporal, zygomatic, buccal, mandibular**, and **cervical** branches.
  –supplies the muscles of facial expression and sends the posterior auricular branch to muscles of the auricle and the occipitalis muscle.
  –also supplies the digastric posterior belly and stylohyoid muscles.

1. Bell's Palsy (Facial Paralysis)
  –is a unilateral paralysis of the facial muscles due to a lesion of the facial nerve.
  –is characterized by the presence of the characteristic distortion of the face such as (*a*) the sagging corner of the mouth and the inability to smile, whistle or blow, as well as (*b*) the drooping upper eyelid, the everting lower eyelid, and the inability to close or blink the eye.

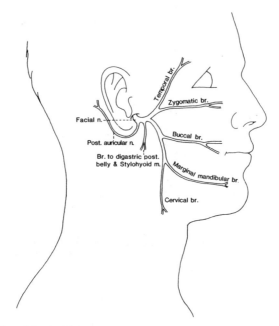

Figure 8.12. Distribution of the facial nerve.

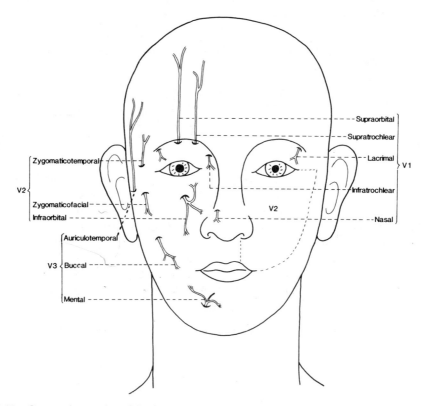

Figure 8.13. Sensory innervation of the face.

–causes decreased lacrimation (due to lesion of the greater petrosal nerve), a loss of taste for the anterior two-thirds of the tongue (chroda tympani), painful sensitivity to sounds (nerve to the stapedius), and deviation of the lower jaw and tongue (nerve to the digastric muscle).

2. Corneal Reflex

–is the closure of the eyes caused by blowing on the cornea or touching it with a wisp of cotton wool, due to bilteral contraction of the orbicularis oculi muscles.

–its efferent limb (of the reflex arc) is the facial nerve, whereas the afferent limb is the nasociliary nerve.

IV. Blood Vessels

A. Facial Artery

–arises from the external carotid artery just above the upper border of the hyoid bone.

–passes deep to the mandible, winds around the lower border of the mandible, and runs upward and forward on the face, giving off the **inferior labial, superior labial**, and **lateral nasal** branches, before ending as an **angular** artery.

–terminates as an angular artery that anastomoses with the palpebral and dorsal nasal branches of the ophthalmic artery and thus establishes a communication between the external and internal carotid arteries.

B. Superficial Temporal Artery

–arises behind the neck of the mandible as the smaller terminal branch of the external carotid artery.

–ascends anterior to the external acoustic meatus into the scalp.

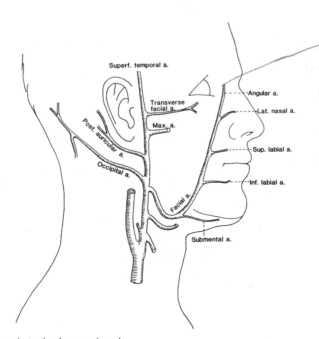

Figure 8.14. Blood supply to the face and scalp.

–accompanies the auriculotemporal nerve along its anterior surface.

–gives off the **transverse facial** artery, which passes forward across the masseter between the zygomatic arch above and the parotid duct below.

–also gives off the zygomatico-orbital, middle temporal, anterior auricular, frontal, and parietal branches.

C. Facial Vein

–begins as an angular vein by the confluence of the supraorbital and supratrochlear veins.

–communicates with the superior and inferior ophthalmic veins and thus with the cavernous sinus.

–receives tributaries corresponding to the branches of the artery and also receives the infraorbital and deep facial veins.

–drains either directly into the internal jugular vein or by joining the anterior branch of the retromandibular vein to form the common facial vein, which then enters the internal jugular vein.

D. Retromandibular Vein

–is formed by the union of the superficial temporal and maxillary veins behind the mandible.

–divides into an anterior branch, which joins the facial vein to form the common facial vein, and a posterior branch, which joins the posterior auricular vein to form the external jugular vein.

V. Scalp

–consists of five layers:

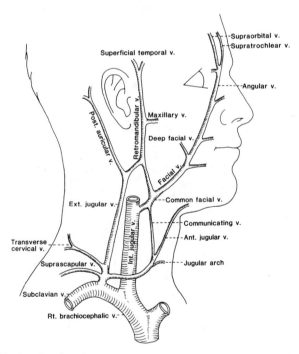

Figure 8.15. Veins of the head and neck.

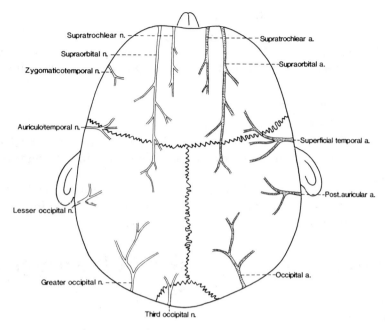

Figure 8.16. Nerves and arteries of the scalp.

1. **Skin**
2. **Connective Tissue (or Close Subcutaneous Tissue)**
   —contains the larger blood vessels and nerves. Because of its toughness, the scalp gapes when cut, and the blood vessels do not contract, leading to severe bleeding.
3. **Aponeurosis Epicranialis (Galea Aponeurotica)**
   —is a fibrous sheet that covers the vault of the skull and unites the occipitalis and frontalis muscles.

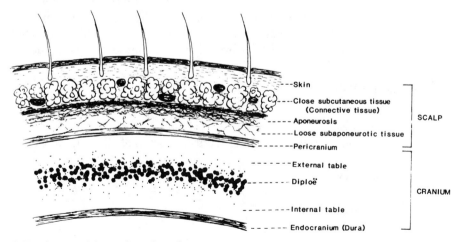

Figure 8.17. Layers of the scalp and cranium.

4. Loose Connective Tissue

–forms the subaponeurotic space and contains the emissary veins.

–is termed a "dangerous area" because infection (blood and pus) can spread easily in it or from the scalp to intracranial sinuses by way of the emissary veins.

5. Pericranium

–is the periosteum over the surface of the skull.

–is innervated by the **supratrochlear, supraorbital, zygomaticotemporal, auriculotemporal, lesser occipital, greater occipital**, and **third occipital** nerves.

–is supplied by the **supratrochlear** and **supraorbital** branches of the internal carotid and by the **superficial temporal, posterior auricular**, and **occipital** branches of the external carotid arteries.

Temporal, Infratemporal, and Pterygopalatine Fossae

I. Boundaries of Fossae

A. Infratemporal Fossa

–its boundaries

a. *Anterior*

–posterior surface of the maxilla.

b. *Posterior*

–styloid process.

c. *Medial*

–lateral pterygoid plate of the sphenoid bone.

d. *Lateral*

–ramus and coronoid process of the mandible.

e. *Roof*

–infratemporal surface of the greater wing of the sphenoid bone.

–contains the lower portion of the temporalis, the lateral and medial pterygoids, the pterygoid plexus of veins, the mandibular nerve and its branches, the maxillary artery and its branches, the chorda tympani, the otic ganglion, etc.

B. Temporal Fossa

–its boundaries

a. *Anterior*

–zygomatic process of the frontal process of the zygomatic.

b. *Posterior*

–temporal line.

c. *Superior*

–temporal line.

d. *Inferior*

–zygomatic arch.

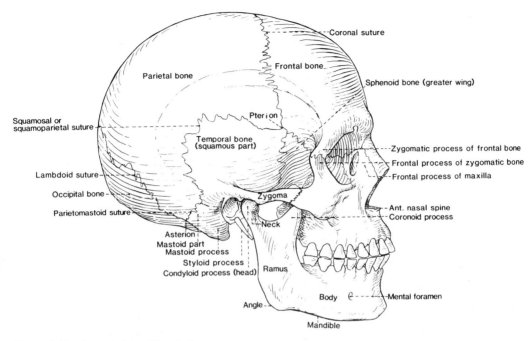

Figure 8.18. Lateral view of the skull.

e. Floor

—parts of the frontal, parietal, temporal, and greater wing of the sphenoid.

—contains the temporalis muscle.

II. Muscles of Mastication

Muscle	Origin	Insertion	Nerve	Action
Temporalis	Temporal fossa	Coronoid process and ramus of mandible	Mandibular n. (CN V3)	Elevates and retracts mandible
Masseter	Lower border and medial surface of zygomatic arch	Lateral surface of coronoid process, ramus and angle of mandible	Mandibular n. (CN V3)	Elevates mandible
Lateral ptery-goid	Upper head from infratemporal surface of sphenoid: lateral head from lateral surface of lateral pterygoid plate	Neck of mandible; capsule of temporomandibular joint	Mandibular n. (CN V3)	Protracts and depresses mandible
Medical ptery-goid	Tuber of maxilla; medial surface of lateral pterygoid plate; pyramidal process of palatine bone	Medial surface of angle and ramus of mandible	Mandibular n. (CN V3)	Protrudes and elevates mandible

→ Lateral pterygoid got 2 heads. Upper head is active during Jaw closing while Lower head is active during Jaw opening.

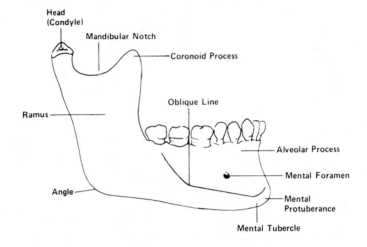

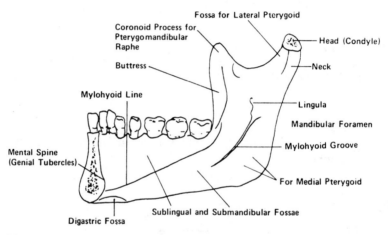

Figure 8.19. External and internal surfaces of the mandible.

III. Nerves

A. Mandibular Nerve

–passes through the foramen ovale.
–supplies the tensor veli palatini, tensor tympani, muscles of mastication (temporalis, masseter, lateral and medial pterygoid), anterior belly of digastric, and mylohyoid muscles.
–is sensory to the lower part of the face below the lower lip and mouth as well as to lower teeth.

1. Meningeal Branch

–accompanies the middle meningeal artery and enters the cranium through the foramen spinosum.

2. Masseteric, Deep Temporal, Medial Pterygoid, and Lateral Pterygoid Nerves

–supply the corresponding muscles of mastication.

3. **Buccal Nerve**

   –descends between the two heads of the lateral pterygoid muscles.
   –supplies skin and fascia on the buccinator and penetrates the muscle to supply the mucous membrane of the cheek and gums.

4. **Auriculotemporal Nerve**

   –arises by two roots that encircle the middle meningeal artery.
   –supplies sensory branches to the temporomandibular joint.
   –carries postganglionic parasympathetic and sympathetic fibers to the parotid gland.
   –its terminal branches supply the skin of the auricle and the scalp.

5. **Lingual Nerve**

   –descends deep to the lateral pterygoid muscle, where it joins the chorda tympani, which conveys the preganglionic parasympathetic (secretary) fibers to the submandibular ganglion and taste fibers from the anterior two-thirds of the tongue.
   –lies anterior to the inferior alveolar nerve on the medial pterygoid, deep to the ramus of the mandible.
   –crosses the lateral to the styloglossus and hyoglossus, passes deep to the mylohyoid, and descends across the submandibular duct.
   –supplies the anterior two-thirds of the tongue for general sensation.

6. **Inferior Alveolar Nerve**

   –passes deep to the lateral pterygoid and then between the spheno-mandibular ligament and the ramus of the mandible.
   –enters the mandibular canal through the foramen.
   –gives off the following branches:

   a. The **mylohyoid nerve** to the mylohyoid and the anterior belly of the digastric muscle.
   b. The **inferior dental** branch to the lower teeth.
   c. The **mental** nerve to the skin over the chin.
   d. The **incisive** branch to the canine and incisor teeth.

B. Otic Ganglion

–lies in the infratemporal fossa, just below the foramen ovale, between the mandibular nerve and the tensor veli palatini.
–receives preganglionic parasympathetic fibers that run in the glosso-pharyngeal nerve, tympanic plexus, and lesser petrosal nerve and synapse in this ganglion.
–sends postganglionic fibers that run in the auriculotemporal nerve and supply the parotid gland.

IV. Blood Vessels

A. Maxillary Artery

–arises from the external carotid artery at the posterior border of the ramus of the mandible.
–divides into three parts:

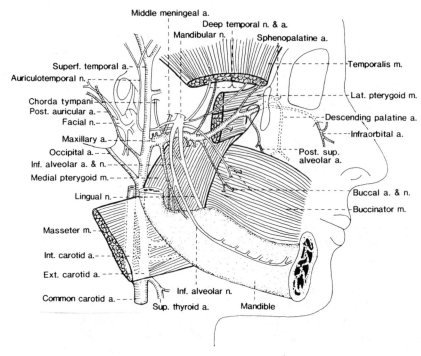

Figure 8.20. The infratemporal region.

1. Mandibular Part
  —runs anteriorly between the neck of the mandible and the spheno-mandibular ligament.

  a. Deep auricular artery
    —supplies the external acoustic meatus.

  b. Anterior Tympanic Artery
    —supplies the tympanic cavity and membrane.

  c. Middle Meningeal Artery
    —arises from the maxillary artery.
    —is embraced by two roots of the auriculotemporal nerve.
    —enters the middle cranial fossa through the foramen spinosum.
    —runs between the dura mater and the periosteum.
    —its damage results in epidural hematoma.

  d. Accessory Meningeal Artery
    —passes through the foramen ovale.

  e. Inferior Alveolar Artery
    —follows the inferior alveolar nerve between the sphenomandibular ligament and the ramus of the mandible.
    —enters the mandibular canal through the mandibular foramen.
    —supplies the tissues of the chin and lower teeth.

2. Pterygoid Part

   —runs anteriorly deep to the temporalis and lies superficial or deep to the lateral pterygoid muscle.

   —its branches include the anterior and posterior **deep temporal, pterygoid, masseteric**, and **buccal** arteries, which supply the muscles of mastication.

3. Pterygopalatine Part

   —runs between the two heads of the lateral pterygoid and then through the pterygomaxillary fissure into the pterygopalatine fossa.

   —its branches include the posterior superior alveolar, infraorbital, descending palatine, artery of the pterygoid canal, pharyngeal, and sphenopalatine.

   a. *Posterior Superior Alveolar Artery*

      —runs downward on the posterior surface of the maxilla and supplies the molar and premolar teeth and the maxillary sinus.

   b. *Infraorbital Artery*

      —runs upward and forward to enter the orbit through the inferior orbital fissure.

      —traverses the infraorbital groove and canal and emerges on the face through the infraorbital foramen.

      —divides into branches to supply the lower eyelid, the lacrimal sac, the upper lip, and the cheek.

      —gives off the anterior superior alveolar branch to the anterior upper teeth and the maxillary sinus.

   c. *Descending Palatine Artery*

      —descends in the pterygopalatine fossa and the palatine canal.

      —gives off the greater and lesser palatine arteries, which pass through the greater and lesser palatine foramina, respectively, and supplies the soft palate.

   d. *Artery of Pterygoid Canal*

      —passes through the pterygoid canal and supplies the upper part of the pharynx, the auditory tube, and the tympanic cavity.

   e. *Pharyngeal Artery*

      —supplies the roof of the nose and pharynx, the sphenoid sinus, and the auditory tube.

   f. *Sphenopalatine Artery*

      —is the terminal branch of the maxillary artery.

      —enters the nasal cavity through the sphenopalatine foramen in company with the nasopalatine branch of the maxillary nerve.

      —is the principal artery to the nasal cavity, supplying the conchae, meatus, and paranasal sinuses.

      —results in bleeding from the nose (epistaxis) by its damage.

Bleeds during Epistaxis

B. Pterygoid Plexus of Veins

   —lies in the infratemporal fossa, on the lateral surface of the medial pterygoid.

—communicates with the cavernous sinus via:

    a. *Emissary veins*

    b. *Inferior Ophthalmic Vein*

—communicates with the facial vein via the deep facial vein.

C. Retromandibular Vein

—is formed by the superficial temporal vein and the maxillary vein.

—divides into an anterior branch, which joins the facial vein to form the common facial vein, and a posterior branch, which joins the posterior auricular vein to form the external jugular vein.

V. Parotid Gland

—is separated from the submandibular gland by the stylomandibular ligament (which extends from the styloid process to the angle of the mandible); thus, pus does not readily exchange between these two glands.

—its complete surgical removal may damage the facial nerve.

—is innervated by parasympathetic (secretomotor) fibers of the glossopharyngeal nerve by way of the lesser petrosal nerve, the otic ganglion, and the auriculotemporal nerve.

—mumps (a viral infection) irritates the auriculotemporal nerve, causing severe pain.

—its duct crosses the masseter, pierces the buccinator muscle and opens into the oral cavity opposite the second upper molar tooth.

VI. Joint and Ligaments

A. Temporomandibular Joint

—is a synovial joint between the mandibular fossa and articular tubercle of the temporal bone and the head of the mandible.

—has **two synovial cavities**, divided by an articular disc.

—combines a hinge and a gliding joint.

—has an articular capsule that extends from the articular tubercle and the margins of the mandibular fossa to the neck of the mandible.

—is reinforced by the **lateral (temporomandibular) ligament**, which extends from the tubercle on the zygoma to the neck of the mandible, and the **sphenomandibular ligament**, which extends from the spine of the sphenoid bone to the lingula of the mandible.

—is innervated by the auriculotemporal, masseteric and deep temporal branches of the mandibular division of the trigeminal nerve.

—is supplied by the superficial temporal, maxillary (middle meningeal and anterior tympanic branches), and ascending pharyngeal arteries.

B. Pterygomandibular Raphe

—is a ligamentous band that separates the buccinator from the superior pharyngeal constrictor.

—extends between the pterygoid hamulus superiorly and the posterior end of the mylohyoid line of the mandible inferiorly.

C. Stylomandibular Ligament

—extends from the styloid process to the posterior border of the ramus of the mandible near its angle.

Cranial Fossa

I. Some Characteristic Features

A. Foramen Cecum

–is a small pit in front of the crista galli between the ethmoid and frontal bones.

–transmits a small emissary vein from the nasal mucosa to the superior sagittal sinus.

B. Crista Galli

–is the triangular midline process of the ethmoid bone extending upward from the cribriform plate.

–gives attachment to the falx cerebri.

C. Cribriform Plate of Ethmoid Bone

–supports the olfactory bulb.

–transmits olfactory nerve fibers from the olfactory mucosa to the olfactory bulb.

D. Anterior Clinoid Processes

–are two anterior processes of the lesser wing of the sphenoid bone.

–give attachment to the free border of the tentorium cerebelli.

E. Posterior Clinoid Processes

–are two tubercles from each side of the dorsum sellae.

–give attachment to the attached border of the tentorium cerebelli.

F. Hypophyseal Fossa

–contains the hypophysis (pituitary gland).

–is located in the sella turcica of the sphenoid bone.

–is bounded anteriorly by the middle clinoid process, posteriorly by the dorsum sellae, and laterally by the cavernous dural venous sinus.

–its floor is formed by the roof of the sphenoid sinus.

G. Sella Turcica (Turk's Saddle) of Sphenoid Bone

–is bounded anteriorly by the **tuberculum sellae** and posteriorly by the **dorsum sellae**.

–lies directly above the sphenoid sinus located within the body of the sphenoid bone.

–is an important landmark for locating the pituitary gland or the hypophysis.

–its dural roof is formed by the **diaphragma sellae**.

H. Jugum Sphenoidale

–forms the roof for the sphenoidal air sinus.

I. Lesser Wing of Sphenoid Bone

–forms the anterior boundary of the middle cranial fossa, whereas the greater wing forms the floor of the middle cranial fossa.

II. Meninges of Brain

A. Pia Mater

—is a delicate investment that is closely applied to the brain and dips into fissures and sulci.

—enmeshes blood vessels on the surfaces of the brain.

B. Arachnoid

—is a filmy, transparent, spidery layer and is connected to the pia mater by web-like trabeculations.

—is separated from the pia mater by the subarachnoid space, which is filled with **cerebrospinal fluid** and also contains blood on hemorrhage of a cerebral artery.

—may have **arachnoid granulations**, which are tuft-like collections of highly folded arachnoid that project through the dura mater.

1. Cerebrospinal Fluid

—is contained in the subarachnoid space between the arachnoid and pia mater.

—is formed by vascular choroid plexuses in the ventricles of the brain.

—circulates through the ventricles, enters the subarachnoid space, and eventually filters into the venous system.

2. Arachnoid Granulations

—are aggregations of nonvascular villous processes of arachnoid tissue.

C. Dura Mater

—is the tough, fibrous, outermost layer of the meninges.

—has the subdural space internal to it (between the arachnoid and the dura).

—has the epidural space external to it, which contains the middle meningeal arteries in the cranial cavity.

—forms the dural venous sinuses, which are spaces between the periosteal and meningeal layers or between duplications of the meningeal layers.

1. Innervation of Cranial Dura

a. Anterior Cranial Fossa

—by the anterior and posterior ethmoidal branches of the ophthalmic nerve.

b. Middle Cranial Fossa

—by the meningeal branches of the maxillary and mandibular nerves.

c. Posterior Cranial Fossa

—by the meningeal branches of the vagus and hypoglossal nerves, both of which contain spinal nerve fibers.

III. Projections of Dura Mater

A. Falx Cerebri

—is a sickle-shaped double layer of the dura mater, lying between the two cerebral hemispheres.

—is attached anteriorly to the crista galli and posteriorly to the tentorium cerebelli.

—its inferior free concave border contains the inferior sagittal sinus.

—its upper convex margin encloses the superior sagittal sinus.

B. Falx Cerebelli

—is a small sickle-shaped projection between the two cerebellar hemispheres.

—is attached to the posterior and inferior part of the tentorium.

—contains the occipital sinus in its posterior border.

C. Tentorium Cerebelli

—is a crescentic fold of dura mater that supports the occipital lobes of the cerebral hemispheres and covers the cerebellum.

—its internal concave border is free and bounds the tentorial notch.

—its external convex border encloses the transverse sinus posteriorly and the superior petrosal sinus anteriorly.

—the free border is anchored to the anterior clinoid process, whereas the attached border is attached to the posterior clinoid process.

D. Diaphragma Sellae

—is a circular, horizontal fold of dura that forms a roof of the sella turcica, covering the pituitary gland or the hypophysis.

—has a central aperture for the hypophysial stalk or infundibulum.

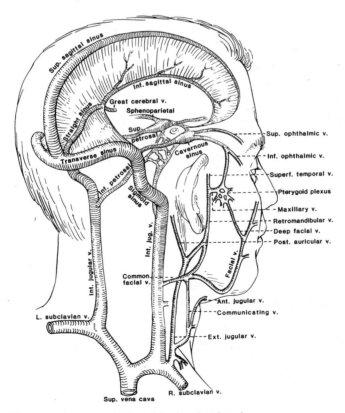

Figure 8.21. Cranial venous sinuses and veins of the head and neck.

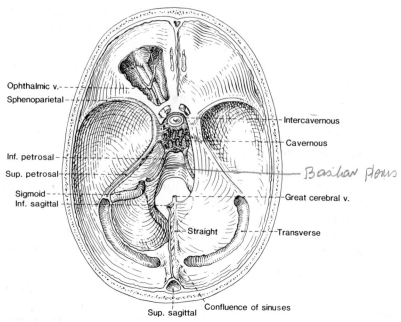

Ophthalmic v.
Sphenoparietal
Intercavernous
Cavernous
Inf. petrosal
Sup. petrosal
Basilar plexus
Sigmoid
Inf. sagittal
Great cerebral v.
Straight
Transverse
Sup. sagittal
Confluence of sinuses

Figure 8.22. Cranial venous sinuses.

IV. Cranial Venous Sinuses of Dura Mater

A. Superior Sagittal Sinus

—lies in the midline along the convex border of the falx cerebri.
—receives the cerebral, diploic, meningeal, and parietal emissary veins.
—begins at the crista galli.

B. Inferior Sagittal Sinus

—lies in the free edge of the falx cerebri.
—is joined by the great cerebral vein (the great vein of Galen) to form the straight sinus.

C. Straight Sinus

—runs along the line of attachment of the falx cerebri to the tentorium cerebelli.

D. Transverse Sinus

—runs laterally from the confluence along the edge of the tentorium cerebelli.

E. Sigmoid Sinus

—is a continuation of the transverse sinus and arches downward and medially in an S-shaped groove on the mastoid part of the temporal bone.
—enters the superior bulb of the internal jugular vein.

F. Cavernous Dural Venous Sinuses

—are located on each side of the sella turcica and the body of the sphenoid bone.

–lie between the meningeal and periosteal layers of the dura mater.

–the internal carotid artery and the abducens nerve pass through these sinuses.

–the oculomotor, trochlear, ophthalmic, and maxillary nerves pass forward in the lateral wall of these sinuses.

–communicate with the pterygoid plexus of veins by emissary veins.

–receive the superior orbital vein.

G. Superior Petrosal Sinus — *separate middle and posterior cranial fossa*

–lies in the margin of the tentorium cerebelli.

–runs from the posterior end of the cavernous sinus to the transverse sinus.

H. Inferior Petrosal Sinus

–drains the cavernous sinus into the bulb of the internal jugular vein.

–runs in a groove between the petrous part of the temporal bone and the basilar part of the occipital bone.

I. Sphenoparietal Sinus — *separate anterior and middle cranial fossa*

–lies along the posterior edge of the lesser wing of the sphenoid bone.

–drains into the cavernous sinus.

J. Occipital Sinus

–lies in the falx cerebelli.

–drains into the confluence of sinuses.

K. Marginal Sinus

–runs around the foramen magnum.

L. Basilar Plexus

–consists of interconnecting venous channels on the basilar part of the occipital bone.

–connects the two inferior petrosal sinuses.

–communicates with the internal vertebral venous plexus.

M. Diploic Veins

–lie in the diploë of the skull.

–are connected with the cranial dural sinuses by the emissary veins.

N. Emissary Veins

–are small veins connecting the venous sinuses of the dura with the diploic veins and the veins of the scalp.

V. Blood Supply of Brain

A. Internal Carotid Artery

–gives no branches to the neck.

–enters the carotid canal in the petrous portion of the temporal bone.

–is separated from the tympanic cavity by a thin bony structure.

–lies within the cavernous sinus and gives rise to small twigs to the wall of the cavernous sinus, to the hypothesis, and to the semilunar ganglion of the trigeminal nerve.

–pierces the dural roof of the cavernous sinus between the anterior and middle clinoid processes.

–gives off the **superior hypophyseal, ophthalmic, posterior commu-**

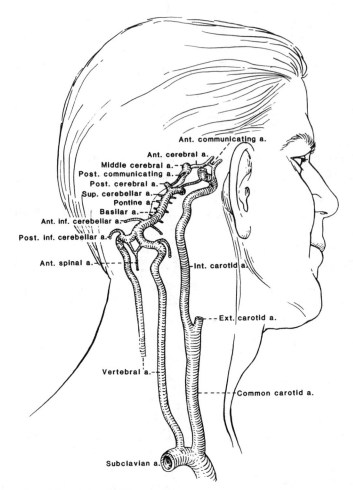

Figure 8.23. Formation of the circle of Willis.

nicating, **anterior choroid, anterior cerebral,** and **middle cerebral** arteries.

B. Vertebral Artery

–is the first branch of the first part of the subclavian artery.

–ascends through the transverse foramina of the upper six cervical vertebrae.

–curves posteriorly behind the lateral mass of the atlas.

–pierces the dura mater into the vertebral canal and then enters the cranial cavity through the foramen magnum.

–on each side joins to form the basilar artery.

–gives rise to the posterior inferior cerebellar artery and the anterior and posterior spinal arteries.

1. Anterior Spinal Artery

–arises as two roots from the vertebral arteries shortly before two vertebrals join in the basilar artery.

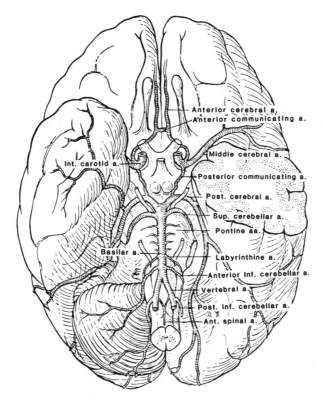

Figure 8.24. Arterial circle on the inferior surface of the brain.

–descend in front of the medulla and unite to form a single median trunk at the level of the foramen magnum.

2. **Posterior Spinal Artery.**

–arises from the vertebral or the posterior inferior cerebellar artery, descends on the side of the medulla, and is united at the lower cervical region.

3. **Posterior Inferior Cerebellar Artery**

–is the largest branch of the vertebral artery and distributes to the posterior inferior surface of the cerebellum.
–gives rise to the posterior spinal artery.

C. **Basilar Artery**

–is formed by the union of the two vertebral arteries at the lower border of the pons.
–gives rise to the **pontine, anterior inferior cerebellar, labyrinthine, superior cerebellar** arteries, and end at the upper border of the pons by dividing into the two **posterior cerebral** arteries.

D. **Circle of Willis (Circulus Arteriosus)**

–is formed by the **posterior cerebral, posterior communicating, internal carotid, anterior cerebral**, and **anterior communicating** arteries.
–forms an important means of collateral circulation in the event of obstruction.

VI. Intracranial Hemorrhage

A. Epidural Hemorrhage
–is due to the rupture of the middle meningeal artery.

B. Subdural Hemorrhage
–results from the rupture of cerebral veins as they pass from the brain surface into one of the venous sinuses.

C. Subarachnoid Hemorrhage
–is due to rupture of cerebral arteries.

D. Pial Hemorrhage
–occurs upon damage to the small vessels of the pia and brain tissue.

Cranial Nerves

I. Olfactory Nerves
–pass through the foramina in the cribriform plate of the ethmoid bone.
–supply the olfactory area which lies in the upper one-third of the nasal mucosa.

II. Optic Nerve
–is formed by the axons of ganglion cells of the retina, which converge at the optic disc.
–leaves the orbit through the optic canal and ends in the optic chiasma.
–carries afferent fibers of vision from the retina to the brain.
–from one eye joins the optic nerve from the other eye to form the optic chiasma (chiasma means "cross"), at which point fibers from the nasal side of either retina cross over to the opposite side of the brain.

III. Oculomotor Nerve
–leaves the cranium through the superior orbital fissure.
–supplies the muscles of eye movement, including the medial, superior, and inferior recti; inferior oblique; and levator palpebrae superioris.
–contains preganglionic parasympathetic fibers whose cell bodies are located in the Edinger-Westphal nucleus and postganglionic fibers derived from the ciliary ganglion supply the sphincter pupillae and the ciliary muscle.

[handwritten margin note: Located between superior cerebellar and posterior cerebellar arteries]

IV. Trochlear Nerve
–passes through the lateral wall of the cavernous sinus during its course.
–enters the orbit by passing through the superior orbital fissure.
–is the smallest cranial nerve.
–is the only cranial nerve that emerges from the dorsal aspect of the brain stem.
–supplies the superior oblique muscle.

V. Trigeminal Nerve
–is sensory to the face, mucous membranes of the nose and mouth, and deep structures of the head.
–divides into the ophthalmic, maxillary, and mandibular divisions.
–has ganglion (semilunar or trigeminal) that consists of cell bodies of afferent fibers and occupies the trigeminal impression on the petrous portion of the temporal bone.

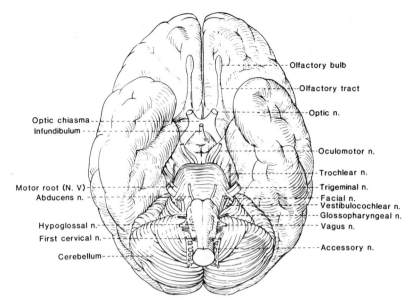

Figure 8.25. Cranial nerves on the base of the brain.

A. Ophthalmic Nerve

—runs in the dura of the lateral wall of the cavernous sinus.
—enters the orbit through the superior orbital fissure.
—is sensory to the skin of the face above the eye.

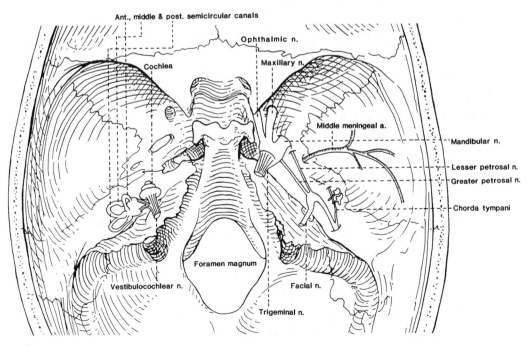

Figure 8.26. Temporal bone in the interior of the base of the skull.

B. Maxillary Nerve

–passes through the lateral wall of the cavernous sinus.
–passes through the foramen rotundum.
–is sensory to the skin of the face below the eye but above the upper lip.

C. Mandibular Nerve

–passes through the foramen ovale.
–supplies the tensor veli palati, tensor tympani, muscles of mastication (temporalis, masseter, lateral and medial pterygoid), anterior belly of the digastric, and mylohyoid muscles.
–is sensory to the lower part of the face below the lower lip and mouth as well as lower teeth.

VI. Abducens Nerve

–pierces the dura on the dorsum sellae of the sphenoid bone.
–passes through the cavernous sinus.
–enters the orbit through the superior orbital fissure.
–supplies the lateral rectus muscle.

VII. Facial Nerve

–enters the internal acoustic meatus.
–its motor portion passes through the stylomastoid foramen and enters the parotid gland, where it gives off its terminal branches such as the temporal, zygomatic, buccal, marginal mandibular, and cervical branches.
–supplies all muscles of facial expression, as well as the stylohyoid, digastric posterior belly, and stapedius muscles.
–has no cutaneous branches of the face.
–has the nervus intermedius branch, which exits the skull through the petrotympanic fissure as the chorda tympani carrying taste fibers from the anterior two-thirds of the tongue and parasympathetic preganglionic (secretormotor) fibers to the submandibular ganglion (for the submandibular glands) and to the pterygopalatine ganglion (for the lacrimal gland).
–has a sensory ganglion, called the geniculate ganglion, that lies at the knee-shaped bend or genu (L. "knee").

VIII. Vestibulocochlear (Acoustic) Nerve

–enters the internal acoustic meatus and remains within the temporal bone to supply the cochlea and semicircular canals.
–is split into a cochlear portion for hearing and a vestibular portion for equilibrium.

IX. Glossopharyngeal Nerve

–passes through the jugular foramen.
–gives rise to the lesser petrosal nerve, which transmits preganglionic parasympathetic fibers to the otic ganglion.
–supplies the stylopharyngeal muscle.
–supplies the muscles of the pharynx that are involved in swallowing.
–supplies the posterior third of the tongue for general and special (taste) sensation, including the vallate papillae.
–also supplies the dorsum of the soft palate, auditory tube, tympanum, eardrum, mastoid antrum, and mastoid air cells.
–provides innervation to the carotid sinus (the pressure receptors).

X. Vagus Nerve

–passes through the jugular foramen.

–is motor to smooth muscle and cardiac muscle, secretory to all glands, and afferent from all mucous membranes in the thoracic and abdominal visceral organs (except for the descending colon and pelvic organs).

–is motor to all muscles of the larynx, the pharynx (except stylopharyngeus), and palate (except tensor veli palatini).

–supplies the taste buds on the root of the tongue near the epiglottis.

–gives rise to the pharyngeal, superior laryngeal, recurrent laryngeal, cardiac, and other branches.

–has superior laryngeal branch that divides into an internal laryngeal nerve, which is sensory to the larynx above the vocal cord, and an external laryngeal nerve, which supplies the cricothyroid and inferior pharyngeal constrictor muscles.

–gives off the recurrent laryngeal nerve, which is sensory to the larynx below the vocal cord and is motor to all muscles of the larynx except the cricothyroid muscle.

XI. Accessory Nerve

–passes through the jugular foramen.

–its spinal roots unite to form the trunk that ascends between dorsal and ventral roots of the spinal nerves and passes through the foramen magnum.

–supplies the sternomastoid and trapezius muscles.

–its cranial portion contains motor fibers that join the vagus nerve and supply the pharynx, larynx, and palate.

XII. Hypoglossal Nerve → *panei (etue patermai Caidio auo internal Jugulau vessels*

–passes through the hypoglossal canal.

–loops around the occipital artery and passes between the external carotid and internal jugular vessels.

–passes above the hyoid bone on the lateral surface of the hyoglossus muscle and deep to the mylohyoid muscle.

–supplies all of the intrinsic and extrinsic muscles of the tongue except the palatoglossus muscle, which is supplied by the vagus nerve.

XIII. Cranial Nerves

Nerves	Cranial Exit	Cell Bodies	Components	Chief Functions
1. Olfactory	Cribriform plate	Nasal mucosa	SVA	Smell
2. Optic	Optic canal	Ganglion cells of retina	SSA	Vision
3. Oculomotor	Superior orbital fissure	Nucleus III (midbrain)	GSE	Eye movements
		Edinger-Westphal Nucleus (midbrain)	GVE	Contraction of pupil and accommodation
4. Trochlear	Superior orbital fissure	Nucleus IV (midbrain)	GSE	Eye movements
5. Trigeminal	Superior orbital fissure; formen rotundum and foramen ovale	Pons Motor V nucleus	SVE	Mastication
		Trigeminal ganglion	GSA	Sensation in head

Nerves	Cranial Exit	Cell Bodies	Components	Chief Functions
6. Abducens	Superior orbital fissure	Nucleus VI (pons)	GSE	Eye movements
7. Facial	Stylomastoid foramen	Motor VII nucleus (pons)	SVE	Facial expression
		Salivatory nucleus (pons)	GVE	Lacrimal and salivary secretion
		Geniculate ganglion	SVA	Taste
8. Vestibulo-cochlear	Does not leave skull	Vestibular ganglion	SSA	Equilibrium
		Spiral ganglion	SSA	Hearing
9. Glosso-pharyngeal	Jugular foramen	Nucleus ambiguus (medulla)	SVE	Elevation of pharynx
		Dorsal nucleus (medulla)	GVE	Secretion of saliva
		Inferior ganglion	GVA	Sensation in tongue and pharynx
		Inferior ganglion	SVA	Taste
		Inferior ganglion	GSA	Sensation in middle ear
10. Vagus	Jugular foramen	Nucleus ambiguus (medulla)	SVE	Movements of pharynx and larynx
		Dorsal nucleus (medulla)	GVE	Involuntary muscle and gland control
		Inferior ganglion	GVA	Sensation in pharynx, larynx and other viscerae
		Inferior ganglion	SVA	Taste
		Superior ganglion	GVA	Sensation in external ear
11. Accessory	Jugular foramen	Nucleus ambiguus (medulla)	SVE	Movements of pharynx and larynx
		Spinal cord (cervical)	SVE	Movements of head and shoulder
12. Hypoglossal	Hypoglossal canal	Nucleus XII (medulla)	GSE	Movements of tongue

[a]SVA, special visceral afferent; GVA, general visceral afferent; SSA, special somatic afferent; GSE, general somatic efferent; GVE, general visceral efferent; SVE, special visceral efferent; GSA, general somatic afferent.

Foramina of Skull and Their Contents

I. Interior of Skull

A. Anterior Cranial Fossa

1. Cribriform Plate
—olfactory nerve.

   2. **Foramen Cecum**
      —occasional small emissary vein from nasal mucosa to superior sagittal sinus.

B. **Middle Cranial Fossa**

   1. **Optic Canal**
      —optic nerve, ophthalmic artery.

   2. **Superior Orbital Fissure**
      —oculomotor, trochlear, ophthalmic division of trigeminal nerve, abducens, ophthalmic vein.

   3. **Foramen Rotundum**
      —maxillary division of trigeminal nerve.

   4. **Foramen Ovale**
      —mandibular division of trigeminal nerve, accessory meningeal artery, emissary vein(s), occasionally lesser petrosal nerve.

   5. **Foramen Spinosum**
      —middle meningeal artery.

   6. **Foramen Lacerum**
      —(nothing?) upper part traversed by internal carotid artery.

   7. **Carotid Canal**
      —internal carotid artery, sympathetic nerves (carotid plexus).

C. **Posterior Cranial Fossa**

   1. **Internal Auditory Meatus**
      —facial and statoacoustic nerves.

   2. **Jugular Foramen**
      —glossopharyngeal nerve, vagus nerve, spinal accessory nerve, beginning of internal jugular vein.

   3. **Hypoglossal Canal**
      —hypoglossal nerve, a meningeal artery.

   4. **Foramen Magnum**
      —spinal cord, spinal accessory nerve, vertebral arteries, venous plexus of vertebral canal, anterior and posterior spinal arteries.

   5. **Condyloid foramen**
      —vein from transverse sinus.

   6. **Mastoid Foramen**
      —branch of occipital artery to dura mater, vein to transverse sinus.

II. Front of Skull

A. **Inferior Orbital Fissure and Infraorbital Groove**
   —maxillary division of trigeminal nerve.

B. **Supraorbital Notch**
   —supraorbital nerve and vessels.

C. Infraorbital Foramen
–infraorbital nerve and vessels.

D. Mental Foramen
–mental nerve and vessels.

III. Base of Skull

A. Foramen Ovale
–mandibular nerve.

B. Foramen Spinosum
–middle meningeal artery.

C. Foramen Lacerum
–upper part traversed by internal carotid artery.

D. Carotid Canal
–internal carotid artery and sympathetic nerve.

E. Jugular Foramen
–cranial nerves IX, X, XI and jugular vein.

F. Hypoglossal Canal
–hypoglossal nerve, meningeal artery.

G. Foramen Magnum
–spinal cord, spinal accessory nerve, vertebral artery, and venous plexus.

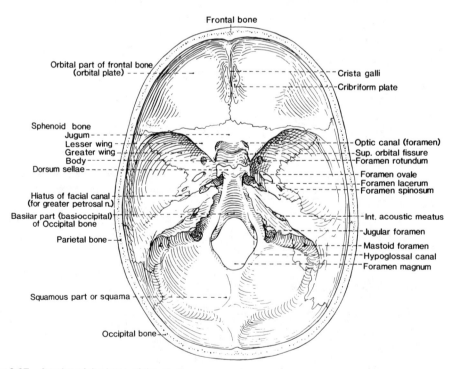

Figure 8.27. Interior of the base of the skull.

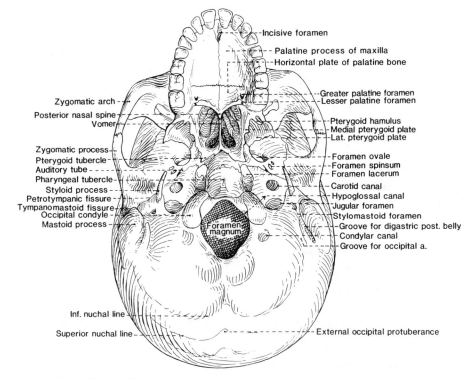

Figure 8.28. Base of the skull.

H. Petrotympanic Fissure
–chorda tympani.

I. Stylomastoid Foramen
–facial nerve.

J. Incisive Canal
–nasopalatine nerve.

K. Greater Palatine Canal
–greater palatine nerve and vessels.

L. Lesser Palatine Canal
–lesser palatine nerve and vessels.

IV. Nasal Cavity

A. Incisive Foramen
–nasopalatine nerve.

B. Lateral Wall

1. Sphenoethmoidal Recess
–opening of sphenoid sinus into posterior part.

2. Superior Meatus
–opening of posterior ethmoidal air cells.

3. Middle Meatus

—opening of frontal sinus into infundibulum; openings of middle ethmoidal air cells on ethmoidal bulla; openings of anterior ethmoidal air cells and maxillary sinus in hiatus semilunaris.

4. Inferior Meatus

—opening of nasolacrimal duct.

5. Sphenopalatine Foramen

—opening into pterygopalatine fossa.

6. Choanae

—communication of nose with nasopharynx.

V. Pterygopalatine Fossa

A. Posterior Openings

1. Foramen Rotundum

—maxillary nerve.

2. Pterygoid Canal

—nerve of pterygoid canal (postganglionic sympathetics and preganglionic parasympathetic from seventh cranial nerve), artery of canal.

B. Lateral Openings

1. Pterygomaxillary Fissure

—to infratemporal fossa.

C. Medial Openings

1. Sphenopalatine Foramen

—to nasal cavity (sphenopalatine artery).

D. Superior Opening

1. Inferior Orbital Fissure

—maxillary nerve.

E. Inferior Opening

1. Pterygopalatine Canal

—greater and lesser palatine canals.

VI. Mandible

A. Mandibular Foramen

—medial surface of ramus (inferior alveolar nerve and vessels).

B. Mental Foramen

—mental nerve.

Orbit

I. Bony Orbit

A. Orbital Margin

—is formed by the frontal, the maxilla, and the zygomatic.

B. Walls of Orbit

1. **Superior Wall or Roof**

   —orbital part of frontal bone and lesser wing of sphenoid bone.

2. **Lateral Wall**

   —zygomatic bone (frontal process) and greater wing of sphenoid bone.

3. **Inferior Wall or Floor**

   —maxilla (orbital surface), zygomatic, and palatine bones.

4. **Medial Wall**

   —ethmoid (orbital plate), frontal, lacrimal, and sphenoid bones.

C. Fissures and Canals

1. **Superior Orbital Fissure**

   —communicates with the middle cranial fossa.
   —is bounded by the greater and lesser wings of the sphenoid.
   —transmits the oculomotor, trochlear, abducens, and ophthalmic nerves (all three branches) as well as the ophthalmic veins.

2. **Inferior Orbital Fissure**

   —communicates with the infratemporal and pterygopalatine fossae.
   —is bounded by the greater wing of the sphenoid (above) and the maxillary and palatine bone (below).
   —transmits the maxillary nerve and its zygomatic branch and the infraorbital vessels.

3. **Optic Canal**

   —connects the orbit with the middle cranial fossa.
   —is situated in the posterior part of the roof of the orbit.
   —is formed by the two roots of the lesser wing of the sphenoid.
   —transmits the optic nerve and ophthalmic artery.

4. **Infraorbital Groove and Foramen**

   —transmits the infraorbital nerve and vessels.

5. **Supraorbital Notch or Foramen**

   —transmits the supraorbital nerve and vessels.

II. Nerves

A. Ophthalmic Nerve

—enters the orbit through the superior orbital fissure and divides into three branches.

1. **Lacrimal Nerve**

   —enters the orbit through the superior orbital fissure.
   —enters the lacrimal gland, giving off branches to the lacrimal gland, the conjunctiva, and the skin of the upper eyelid.

2. **Frontal Nerve**

   —enters the orbit through the superior orbital fissure.
   —divides into the supraorbital (which supplies the scalp, forehead, fron-

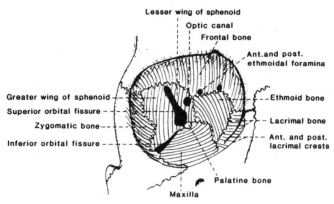

Figure 8.29. The bony orbit.

tal sinus and upper eyelid) and the supratrochlear (which supplies the scalp, forehead and upper eyelid) nerves.

3. **Nasociliary Nerve**
   –is the sensory nerve to the eye.
   –enters the orbit through the superior orbital fissure, within the common tendinous ring.
   –gives off:

   a. A communicating branch to the ciliary ganglion.
   b. Short ciliary nerves that carry postganglionic parasympathetic and sympathetic fibers to the ciliary body and iris.
   c. Long ciliary nerves that transmit postganglionic sympathetic fibers to the dilator pupillae and afferent fibers from the iris and cornea.
   d. The infratrochlear nerve to the eyelids, conjunctiva skin of the nose, and lacrimal sac.
   e. The posterior ethmoidal nerve that passes through the posterior ethmoidal foramen to the sphenoidal and posterior ethmoidal sinuses.
   f. The anterior ethmoidal nerve, which passes through the anterior ethmoidal foramen. It divides into internal nasal branches (which supply the septum and lateral walls of the nasal cavity) and external nasal branches (which supply the skin of the nose).

B. **Optic Nerve**
   –leaves the orbit passing through the optic canal.
   –carries afferent fibers of vision from the retina to the brain.
   –joins the optic nerve from the other eye to form the optic chiasma. (Chiasma means "cross," so the fibers from the nasal side of the retina cross and go to the opposite—i.e., temporal—side of the brain.)

C. **Oculomotor Nerve**
   –leaves the cranium through the superior orbital fissure.
   –supplies the muscles of eye movement, including the medial, superior, and inferior recti; the inferior oblique; and the levator palpebrae superioris.

–contains preganglionic parasympathetic fibers whose cell bodies are located in the Edinger-Westphal nucleus.

D. Trochlear Nerve

–passes through the lateral wall of the cavernous sinus during its course.
–enters the orbit by passing through the superior orbital fissure.
–is the smallest cranial nerve.
–is the only cranial nerve that emerges from the dorsal aspect of the brain stem.
–supplies the superior oblique muscle.

E. Abducens Nerve

–pierces the dura on the dorsum sellae of the sphenoid bone.
–passes through the cavernous sinus.
–enters orbit through the superior orbital fissure.
–supplies the lateral rectus muscle.

F. Ciliary Ganglion

–is a parasympathetic ganglion.
–receives preganglionic parasympathetic fibers (with cell bodies in the Edinger-Westphal nucleus of cranial nerve III in the mesencephalon), which run in the inferior division of the oculomotor nerve.
–its postganglionic parasympathetic fibers pass to the sphincter pupillae (iris) and the ciliary muscle (ciliary body) via the short ciliary nerves.
–is formed by the cell bodies of the postganglionic parasympathetic fibers.
–receives postganglionic sympathetic fibers arising from the superior cervical ganglion that reach the dilator pupillae muscle by way of the ciliary ganglion (without synapsing) and short ciliary nerves.
–is situated behind the eyeball, between the optic nerve and the lateral rectus muscle.
–its sensory root is connected to the nasociliary nerve.

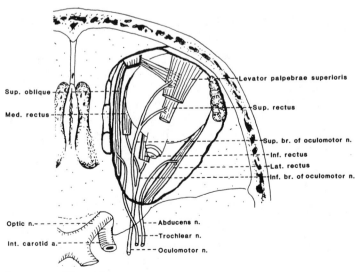

Figure 8.30. Motor nerves of the orbit.

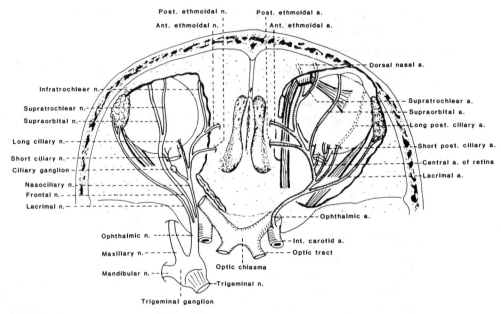

Figure 8.31. Branches of the ophthalmic nerve and artery.

III. Blood Vessels

A. Ophthalmic Artery

–is a branch of the internal carotid artery and enters the orbit through the optic canal beneath the optic nerve.

–gives off the **ocular** vessels, such as the artery of the retina, the short and long posterior ciliary and anterior ciliary arteries, and the **orbital** vessels, such as the lacrimal, muscular, supraorbital, anterior and posterior ethmoidal, medial palpebral, supratrochlear, and dorsal nasal arteries.

–ends by dividing into the dorsal nasal and supratrochlear arteries.

1. Central Artery of Retina

–is the most important branch of the ophthalmic artery.

–travels in the optic nerve; it divides into superior and inferior branches at the optic disc, each of which further divide into temporal and nasal branches.

–is an end-artery in the sense that no direct communications occur between arterioles and venules, the junction being by way of capillary networks only.

–occlusion results in blindness.

B. Ophthalmic Vein

1. Superior Ophthalmic Vein

–is formed by the union of the supraorbital and angular veins.

–receives branches corresponding to most of those of the ophthalmic artery and, in addition, it receives the inferior ophthalmic vein, before draining into the cavernous sinus.

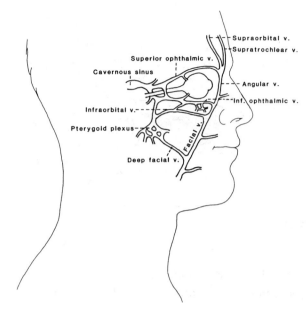

Figure 8.32. Ophthalmic veins.

2. Inferior Ophthalmic Vein

—begins by the union of small veins in the floor of the orbit.

—communicates with the pterygoid venous plexus and often with the infraorbital vein.

—terminates directly or indirectly in the cavernous sinus.

IV. Muscles of Eye Movement

Muscle	Origin	Insertion	Nerve	Actions
Superior rectus	Common tendinous ring	Sclera just behind cornea	Oculomotor n.	Elevates eyeball
Inferior rectus	Common tendinous ring	Sclera just behind cornea	Oculomotor n.	Depresses eyeball
Medial rectus	Common tendinous ring	Sclera just behind cornea	Oculomotor n.	Adducts eyeball
Lateral rectus	Common tendinous ring	Sclera just behind cornea	Abducens n.	Abducts eyeball
Levator palpebrae superioris	Lesser wing of sphenoid above and anterior to optic canal	Tarsal plate and skin of upper eyelid	Oculomotor n.	Elevates upper eyelid
Superior oblique	Sphenoid bone above optic canal	Sclera beneath superior rectus	Trochlear n.	Rotates downward and medially; depresses adducted eye
Inferior oblique	Floor of orbit lateral to lacrimal groove	Sclera beneath lateral rectus	Oculomotor n.	Rotates upward and laterally; elevates adducted eye

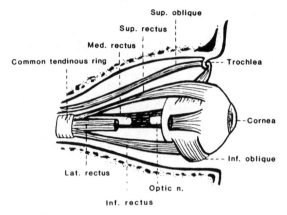

Figure 8.33. Muscles of the orbit.

A. Innervation of Muscles of Eyeball
–can be summarized as follows: SO_4, LR_6, Remainder$_3$.

B. Intorsion
–is an inward rotation of the vertical corneal meridians.
–is caused by the superior oblique and superior rectus muscles.

C. Extorsion
–is an outward rotation of the vertical corneal meridians.
–is caused by the inferior oblique and inferior rectus muscles.

V. Lacrimal Apparatus

A. Lacrimal Gland
–lies in the upper lateral region of the orbit, on the lateral rectus and the levator palpebrae superioris.
–is drained by a dozen lacrimal ducts that open into the superior conjunctival fornix.

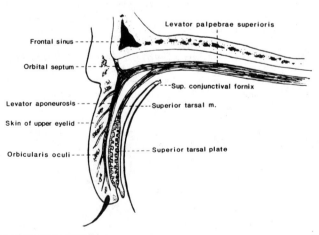

Figure 8.34. Structure of the upper eyelid.

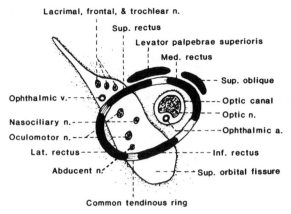

Figure 8.35. The common tendinous ring.

B. Lacrimal Canaliculi

—are two curved canals, which begin as a **lacrimal punctum** or pore in the margin of the eyelid and open into the lacrimal sac.

C. Lacrimal Sac

—is the upper dilated end of the **nasolacrimal duct**, which opens into the inferior meatus of the nasal cavity.

D. Tears

—are produced by the lacrimal gland.
—pass through excretory ductules into the superior conjunctival fornix.
—are spread evenly over the eyeball by blinking movements.
—accumulate in the area of the lacrimal lake.
—enters the lacrimal canaliculi through their lacrimal puncta before draining into the lacrimal sac, nasolacrimal duct, and finally the inferior nasal meatus.

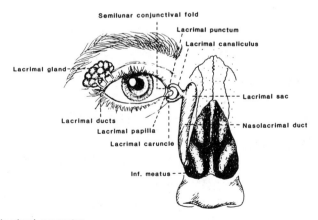

Figure 8.36. The lacrimal apparatus.

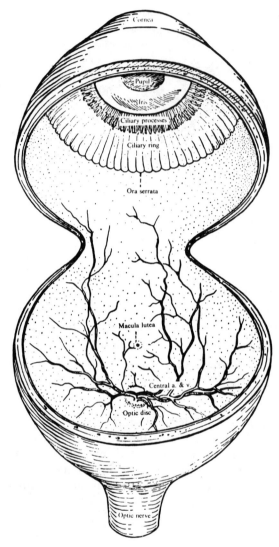

Figure 8.37. Vessels of the retina.

VI. Features in Eyeball

A. Optic Disc or Blind Spot

–has no receptors and is insensitive to light.

–consists merely of optic nerve fibers and marks their exist.

–is located nasal (or medial) to the fovea centralis and the posterior pole of the eye.

–has a depression in its center, termed the "physiological cup."

B. Macula or Yellow Spot (Macula Lutea)

–is a yellowish area of the retina on the temporal side of the optic disc.

–contains a pit called the fovea centralis.

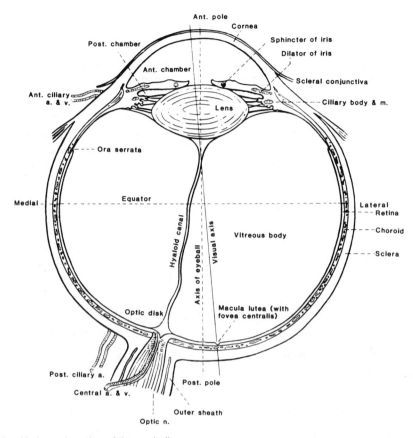

Figure 8.38. Horizontal section of the eyeball.

C. Fovea Centralis

–is a central depression or foveola in the macula.
–is avascular and is nourished by the choriocapillary lamina of the choroid.
–has cones only (no rods), each of which is connected with only one ganglion cell.
–functions in detailed vision.

D. Rods

–are 100–120 million in number.
–are most numerous about 0.5cm from the fovea centralis.
–contain a visual purple pigment called rhodopsin.
–are associated with dim vision as in the night or twilight.

E. Cones

–are 7 million in number.
–are most numerous in the foveal region.
–are associated with visual acuity (sharpest vision) and color vision.

VII. Other Features

A. Structures Passing through the Common Tendinous Ring

1. The oculomotor, nasociliary, and abducens nerves enter the orbit through the superior orbital fissure and the common tendinous ring.
2. The optic nerve, the ophthalmic artery, and the central artery of the retina enter the orbit through the optic canal and the tendinous ring.
3. The superior ophthalmic vein and the trochlear, frontal, and lacrimal nerves enter the orbit through the superior orbital fissure but outside of the tendinous ring.

B. Horner's Syndrome

—is caused by injury to cervical sympathetic fibers.
—is characterized by:

1. **Miosis**

   —constriction of a pupil due to paralysis of the associated dilator pupillae muscle.

2. **Ptosis**

   —drooping of an upper eyelid due to paralysis of the smooth muscle component of the levator palpebrae superioris muscle.

3. **Enophthalmos**

   —retraction of an eyeball due to paralysis of the tarsal muscle.

4. **Anhidrosis**

   —absence of sweating.

5. **Vasodilation**

   —in the facial and cervical regions.

Oral Cavity and Salivary Glands

I. Palate

—forms the **roof** of the mouth and the **floor** of the nasal cavity.
—consists of the hard palate (anterior two-thirds) and the soft palate (posterior third).

A. Hard Palate

—forms a bony partition between the nasal and oral cavities.
—consists of the palatine processes of the **maxillae** and horizontal parts of the **palatine bones.**
—contains the incisive foramen in its median plane anteriorly, and the greater and lesser palatine foramina posteriorly.

B. Soft Palate

—is a fibromuscular fold, extended from the posterior border of the hard palate.
—moves posteriorly against the pharyngeal wall to close the oropharyngeal (faucial) isthmus in swallowing and during speech.
—is continuous with the palatoglossal and palatopharyngeal folds.
—receives blood from the greater and lesser palatine arteries of the **de-**

scending palatine artery, the ascending palatine artery of the **facial** artery, and the palatine branch of the **ascending pharyngeal** artery.
—receives sensory innervation through the greater and lesser palatine nerves.
—has five muscles: the palatoglossus, palatopharyngeus, musculus uvulae, levator veli palatini, and tensor veli palatini.

C. Muscles

Muscle	Origin	Insertion	Nerve	Action
Tensor veli palatini	Scaphoid fossa; spine of sphenoid; cartilage of auditory tube	Tendon hooks around hamulus of ptery-goid to insert into aponeurosis of soft palate	Mandibular branch of trigeminal n.	Tenses soft palate
Levator veli palatini	Petrous part of temporal bone; cartilage of auditory tube	Aponeurosis of soft palate	Vagus n. via pharyngeal plexus	Elevates soft palate
Palatoglossus	Aponeurosis of soft palate	Dorsolateral side of tongue	Vagus n. via pharyngeal plexus	Elevates tongue
Palatopharyngeus	Aponeurosis of soft palate	Thyroid cartilage and side of pharynx	Vagus n. via pharyngeal plexus	Elevates pharynx; closes nasopharynx
Musculus uvulae	Posterior nasal spine; palatine aponeurosis	Mucous membrane of uvula	Vagus n. via pharyngeal plexus	Elevates uvula

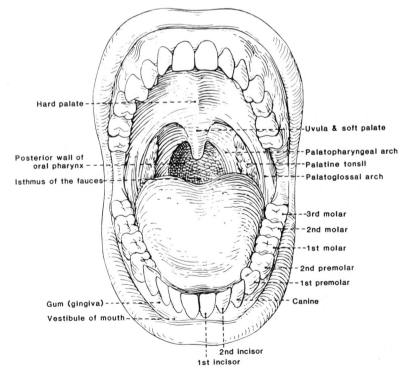

Figure 8.39. The oral cavity.

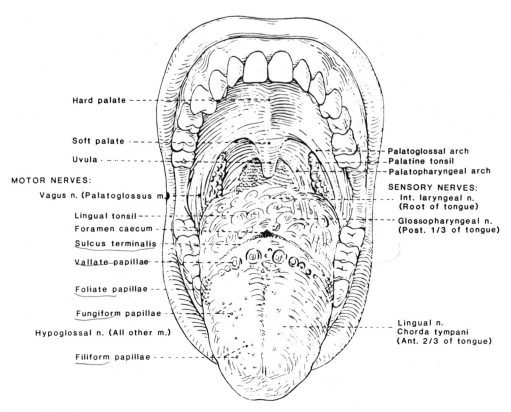

Hard palate

Soft palate

Uvula

MOTOR NERVES:

Vagus n. (Palatoglossus m.)

Lingual tonsil

Foramen caecum

Sulcus terminalis

Vallate papillae

Foliate papillae

Fungiform papillae

Hypoglossal n. (All other m.)

Filiform papillae

Palatoglossal arch
Palatine tonsil
Palatopharyngeal arch

SENSORY NERVES:
Int. laryngeal n.
(Root of tongue)

Glossopharyngeal n.
(Post. 1/3 of tongue)

Lingual n.
Chorda tympani
(Ant. 2/3 of tongue)

Figure 8.40. The tongue.

II. Tongue

—is attached by muscles to the hyoid bone, mandible, styloid process, and pharynx.

—is divided by a V-shaped **sulcus terminalis**, into two parts, an anterior two-thirds and a posterior one-third, which differ developmentally, structurally, and in innervation.

—has the **foramen cecum** at the apex of the V, which inciates the site of origin of the thyroglossal duct in the embryo.

A. Lingual Papillae

—are small, nipple-shaped projections on the anterior two-thirds of the dorsum of the tongue.

—include the **vallate, fungiform**, and **filiform** papillae. Foliate papillae are found in certain animals but are rudimentary in man.

1. Vallate Papillae

—are arranged in the form of a V in front of the sulcus terminalis.

—are studded with numerous taste buds.

—are innervated by the glossopharyngeal nerve.

B. Lingual Tonsil

—is the collection of nodular masses of lymphoid follicles on the posterior third of the dorsum of the tongue.

C. Innervation

–its extrinsic and intrinsic muscles are innervated by the hypoglossal nerve except for the palatoglossus muscle, which is supplied by the vagus nerve.

–its anterior two-thirds is innervated by the lingual nerve for general sensation and by the chorda tympani for special sensation (taste).

–its posterior one-third and the vallate papillae are innervated by the glossopharyngeal nerve for both general and special sensation.

–its root near the epiglottis is innervated by the internal laryngeal nerve of the vagus nerve for both general and special sensation.

D. Lingual Artery

–arises from the external carotid artery at the level of the tip of the greater horn of the hyoid bone in the carotid triangle.

–passes deep to the hyoglossus and lies on the middle pharyngeal constrictor.

–gives off the suprahyoid, dorsal lingual, and sublingual arteries and terminates as the deep lingual artery, which ascends between the genioglossus and inferior pharyngeal constrictor.

E. Muscles

Muscle	Origin	Insertion	Nerve	Action
Styloglossus	Styloid process	Side and inferior aspect of tongue	Hypoglossal n.	Retracts and elevates tongue
Hyoglossus	Body and greater horn of hyoid bone	Side and inferior aspect of tongue	Hypoglossal n.	Depresses and retracts tongue
Genioglossus	Genial tubercle of mandible	Inferior aspect of tongue; body of hyoid bone	Hypoglossal n.	Protrudes and depresses tongue
Palatolglossus	Aponeurosis of soft palate	Dorsolateral side of tongue	Vagus n. via pharyngeal plexus	Elevates tongue

III. Teeth and Gum (Gingiva)

A. Structure of Teeth

1. Enamel

–is the hardest substance that covers the crown.

2. Dentine

–is a hard substance that is nurtured through the fine dental tubules of odontoblasts lining the central pulp space.

3. Pulp

–fills the central cavity, which is continuous with the root canal.

–contains numerous blood vessels, nerves, and lymphatics, which enter the pulp through an apical foramen at the apex of the root.

B. Parts of Teeth

1. Crown

–projects above the gingival surface and is covered by enamel.

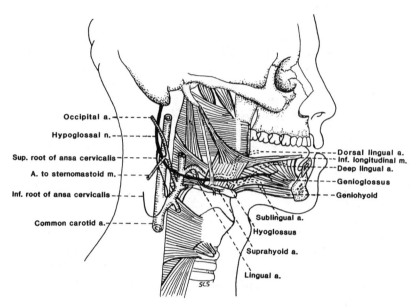

Occipital a.
Hypoglossal n.
Sup. root of ansa cervicalis
A. to sternomastoid m.
Inf. root of ansa cervicalis
Common carotid a.
Dorsal lingual a.
Inf. longitudinal m.
Deep lingual a.
Genioglossus
Geniohyoid
Sublingual a.
Hyoglossus
Suprahyoid a.
Lingual a.

Figure 8.41. Muscles of the tongue.

2. Neck
−is the constricted area of junction of crown and root.

3. Root
−is embedded in the alveolar part of the maxilla or mandible.
−is covered with cement, which is connected to the bone of the alveolus by a layer of modified periosteum, the periodontal ligament.

C. Basic Types of Teeth

1. Incisors
−are chisel-shaped and are for cutting or biting.

2. Canines
−have a single prominent cone and are for tearing.

3. Premolars
−usually have two cusps and are for grinding.

4. Molars
−usually have three cusps and are for grinding.

D. Two Sets of Teeth

1. Deciduous Teeth
−have two incisors, one canine, and two molars in each quadrant.

2. Permanent Teeth
−have two incisors, one canine, two premolars, and three molars in each quadrant.

E. Innervation of Teeth

1. Maxillary Teeth

—are innervated by the anterior, middle, and posterior alveolar branches of the maxillary nerve.

2. Mandibular Teeth

—are innervated by the inferior alveolar branch of the mandibular nerve.

F. Innervation of Gingiva (Gum)

1. Outer Aspect

a. Maxillary Gingiva

—posterior, middle, and anterior superior alveolar and infraorbital nerves.

b. Mandibular Gingiva

—buccal and mental nerves.

2. Inner Aspect

a. Maxillary Gingiva

—greater palatine and nasopalatine nerves.

b. Mandibular Gingiva

—lingual nerve.

IV. Salivary Glands

A. Submandibular Gland

—is ensheathed by the investing layer of the deep cervical fascia.
—is located between the hyoglossus and styloglossus medially and the mylohyoid laterally, and between the lingual nerve above and the hypoglossal nerve below.
—its duct (Wharton's) runs forward between the mylohyoid, genioglossus and hyoglossus muscles. It is crossed laterally by the lingual nerve.
—its duct further runs between the sublingual gland and the genioglossus and empties into the mouth on the summit of the sublingual papilla (caruncle) at the side of the frenulum of the tongue.
—is innervated by parasympathetic secretomotor fibers from the facial nerve, which run in the chorda tympani.

B. Sublingual Gland

—is located in the floor of the mouth between the mucous membrane above and the mylohyoid muscle below.
—surrounds the terminal portion of the submandibular duct.
—empties into the floor of the mouth by a dozen short ducts, of which some enter the submandibular duct.
—is supplied by postganglionic parasympathetic fibers from the submandibular ganglion either directly or through the lingual nerve.

V. Autonomic Nerve

A. Submandibular Ganglion

—lies on the hyoglossus muscles, deep to the mylohyoid.

–is a parasympathetic ganglion that is attached to the lingual nerve by a few short connecting branches.

–receives preganglionic parasympathetic (secretomotor) fibers through the chorda tympani.

–its postganglionic fibers join the lingual nerve to innervate the submandibular and sublingual glands.

Pharynx

I. Subdivisions

A. Nasopharynx

–is situated behind the oral cavity above the soft palate and communicates with the nasal cavities through the choanae.

–has the pharyngeal tonsils in its posterior wall.

–is connected with the tympanic cavity through the auditory tube.

B. Oropharynx

–extends between the soft palate above and the superior border of the epiglottis below.

–communicates with the mouth through the faucial (oropharyngeal) isthmus.

–contains the palatine tonsils, which are lodged in the tonsilar fossae bounded by the palatoglossal and palatopharyngeal folds.

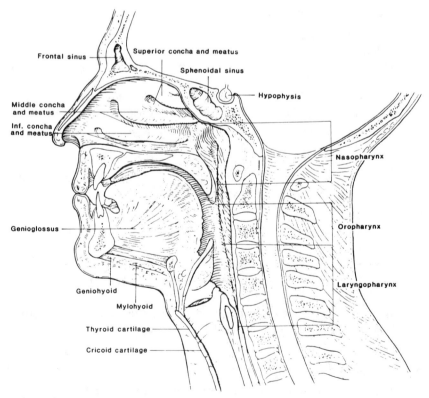

Figure 8.42. The pharynx.

C. Laryngopharynx

—extends from the upper border of the epiglottis to the lower border of the cricoid cartilage.

—contains the piriform recesses, one on each side of the opening of the larynx, into which swallowed foreign bodies may be lodged.

II. Muscles

Muscle	Origin	Insertion	Nerve	Action
Circular Muscles				
Superior constrictor	Medial pterygoid plate; pterygoid hamulus; pterygomandibular raphe; mylohyoid line of mandible; side of tongue	Medial raphe and pharyngeal tubercle of skull	Vagus n. via pharyngeal plexus	Constricts upper pharynx
Middle constrictor	Greater and lesser horns of hyoid; stylohyoid ligament	Median raphe	Vagus n. via pharyngeal plexus	Constricts middle pharynx
Inferior constrictor	Arch of cricoid and oblique line of thyroid cartilages	Median raphe of pharynx	Vagus n. via pharyngeal plexus, recurrent and external laryngeal n.	Constricts lower pharynx
Longitudinal muscles				
Stylopharyngeus	Styloid process	Thyroid cartilage and muscles of pharynx	Glossopharyngeal n.	Elevates pharynx and larynx
Palatopharyngeus	Hard palate; aponeurosis of soft palate	Thyroid cartilage and muscles of pharynx	Vagus n. via pharyngeal plexus	Elevates pharynx and closes nasopharynx
Salpingopharyngeus	Caritlage of auditory tube	Muscles of pharynx	Vagus n. via pharyngeal plexus	Elevates nasopharynx; opens auditory tube

III. Innervation and Blood Supply

A. Pharyngeal Plexus

—is formed by the pharyngeal branches of the glossopharyngeal and vagus nerves and sympathetic branches from the superior cervical ganglion.

—innervates all of the muscles of the pharynx with the exception of the **stylopharyngeus**, which is supplied by the glossopharyngeal nerve.

—lies on the middle pharyngeal constrictor.

B. Arteries

—are the ascending pharyngeal, the ascending palatine, and the descending palatine arteries.

IV. Tonsils

A. Pharyngeal Tonsil

—is found in the posterior wall and roof of the nasopharynx.

—is called the **adenoid** when enlarged.

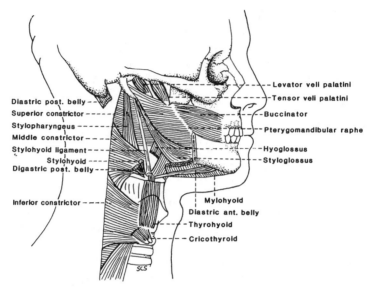

Figure 8.43. Muscles of the pharynx.

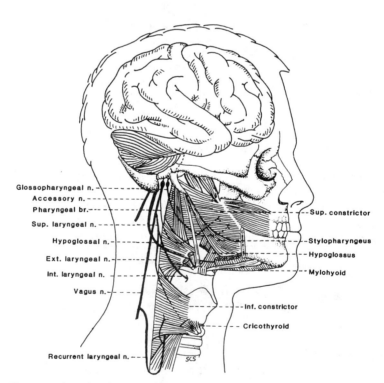

Figure 8.44. Nerve supply to the pharynx.

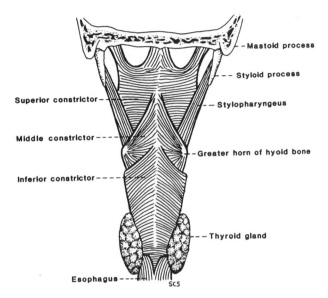

Figure 8.45. Pharyngeal constrictors.

B. Palatine Tonsil

–lies on each side of the oropharynx in an interval between the palato-glossal and palatopharyngeal folds.

–receives blood from the ascending palatine, descending palatine, ascending pharyngeal, and dorsal lingual arteries.

C. Waldeyer's Ring

–is a sort of tonsillar ring at the oropharyngeal isthmus, formed of the lingual, palatine, and pharyngeal tonsils.

V. Fascia and Space

A. Retropharyngeal Space

–lies posterior to the buccopharyngeal fascia and anterior to the prevertebral fascia.

–is closed laterally by the carotid sheath.

B. Pharyngobasilar Fascia

–blends with the periosteum of the base of the skull.

–forms the submucosa of the pharynx.

–lies internal to the muscular coat of the pharynx; these muscles are covered externally by the buccopharyngeal fascia.

Nasal Cavity and Pterygopalatine Fossa

I. Nasal Cavity

–opens on the face through the anterior nasal apertures (nares or nostrils) and communicates with the nasopharynx through a posterior opening, the **choana**.

—has a slight dilatation inside the aperture of each nostril called the **vestibule** which is lined largely by skin containing hair, sebaceous glands, and sweat glands.

A. Roof

—is formed by the nasal, frontal, ethmoid (cribriform plate), and sphenoid (body) bones.

B. Floor

—is formed by the palatine process of the **Maxilla** and the horizontal part of the **palatine bone**.

C. Medial Wall or Nasal Septum

—is formed primarily by the perpendicular plate of the ethmoid bone, vomer(bone), and septal cartilage.

—is also formed by the processes of the palatine, maxillary, frontal, sphenoid, and nasal bones.

D. Lateral Wall

—is formed by the superior and middle conchae of the ethmoid bone; inferior concha (a bone itself); nasal bone; frontal process and nasal surface of the

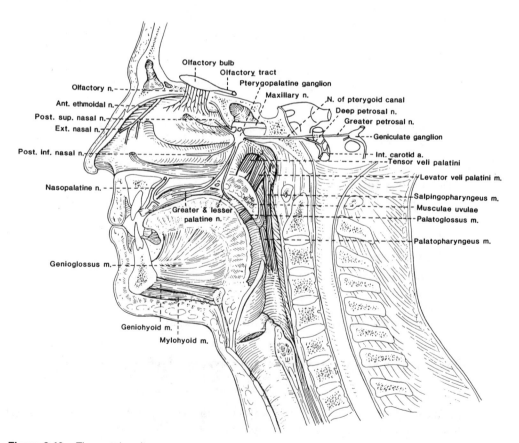

Figure 8.46. The nasal cavity.

maxilla; lacrimal bone; perpendicular plate of the palatine bone; and medial pterygoid plate of the sphenoid bone.

II. Mucous Membrane

A. Respiratory Region

–consists of the lower two-thirds of the nasal cavity.

–is covered by mucous membrane with pseudostratified, ciliated columnar epithelium.

B. Olfactory Region

–consists of the superior nasal concha and the upper third of the nasal septum.

–is innervated by the olfactory nerve, which enters the cranial cavity through the cribriform plate of the ethmoid bone to end in the olfactory bulb.

III. Blood Supply

A. Anterior and Posterior Ethmoidal Branches of Ophthalmic Artery

–supply the anterior portion of the superior and middle conchae and meatuses and an adjacent area of septum.

B. Sphenopalatine Branch of Maxillary Artery — *Bleeds during Epistani.*

–enters the nasal cavity through the sphenopalatine foramen.

–supplies the conchae, meatuses, and paranasal sinuses and ends on the nasal septum.

C. Greater Palatine Branch of Maxillary Artery

–sends a terminal branch through the incisive canal to reach the lower part of the nasal septum.

D. Septal Branch of Superior Labial Artery of Face

–supplies the lower anterior part of the nasal septum.

IV. Nerve Supply

A. Anterior and Posterior Ethmoidal Branches of Ophthalmic Nerve

–supply the anterior half of the nasal cavity.

B. Posterior Nasal Branch of Maxillary Nerve

–passes through the sphenopalatine foramen and supplies the posterior half of the nasal cavity.

C. Anterior Superior Alveolar Branch of Maxillary Nerve

–supplies the anterior end of the inferior concha.

V. Paranasal Sinuses

A. Ethmoidal Sinus

–consists of ethmoidal air cells, which are numerous small cavities within the ethmoidal labyrinth between the orbit and the nasal cavity.

–can be subdivided into three groups: posterior, middle, and anterior air cells:

    a. Posterior Ethmoidal Air Cells

      –drain into the **superior nasal meatus**.

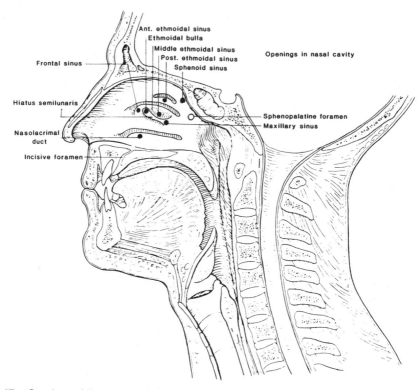

Figure 8.47. Openings of the paranasal sinuses.

   b. Middle Ethmoidal Air Cells
    —drain into the summit of the ethmoidal bulla of the **middle nasal meatus**.
   c. Anterior Ethmoidal Air Cells
    —drain into the anterior aspect of the hiatus semilunaris in the **middle nasal meatus**.

B. Frontal Sinus

  —lies in the frontal bone.
  —opens into the anterior part of the **middle nasal meatus** by way of the frontonasal duct.
  —is innervated by the supraorbital branch of the ophthalmic nerve.

C. Maxillary Air Sinus

  —is the largest of the paranasal air sinuses and is the only paranasal sinus that may be present at birth.
  —lies in the maxilla on each side, lateral to the lateral wall of the nasal cavity and inferior to the floor of the orbit.
  —drains into the posterior aspect of the hiatus semilunaris in the **middle meatus**.

D. Sphenoidal Sinus

–is contained within the body of the sphenoid bone.

–opens into the **sphenoethmoidal recess** of the nasal cavity.

–is supplied by branches from the maxillary nerve.

* Nasolacrimal Duct

–lies in the nasolacrimal canal, formed by the maxilla, the lacrimal bone, and the inferior nasal concha.

–opens into the **inferior nasal meatus** about 1 cm behind the anterior end of the inferior concha.

VI. Pterygopalatine Fossa

–is located between the pterygoid process of the sphenoid bone and the palatine bone.

–contains the terminal branches of the maxillary artery, the maxillary nerve and the pterygopalatine ganglion.

–its boundaries:

   a. Anterior

   –posterior surface of the maxilla.

   b. Posterior

   –lateral pterygoid plate and greater wing of the sphenoid.

   c. Medial

   –perpendicular plate of the palatine.

   d. Lateral

   –open.

   e. Roof

   –orbital process of the palatine and body of the sphenoid.

A. Maxillary Nerve

–passes through the lateral wall of the cavernous sinus.

–enters the pterygopalatine fossa through the foramen rotundum.

–is sensory to the skin of the face below the eye but above the upper lip.

–gives off the following branches:

1. **Meningeal Branch**

   –innervates the dura mater of the middle cranial fossa.

2. **Communicating Branches**

   –are connected to the pterygopalatine ganglion.

3. **Posterior Superior Alveolar Nerve**

   –descends through the pterygopalatine fissure and enters the posterior superior alveolar canals.

   –innervates the cheek, gums, molar teeth, and maxillary sinus.

4. **Zygomatic Nerve**

   –enters the orbit through the inferior orbital fissure, divides into the zygomaticotemporal and zygomaticofacial branches and supplies the skin of the temple and face. It joins the lacrimal nerve in the orbit.

5. Infraorbital Nerve

–enters the orbit through the inferior orbital fissure and runs through the infraorbital groove and canal.

–emerges through the infraorbital foramen and divides on the face into the inferior palpebral, nasal, and superior labial branches.

–gives off the middle and anterior superior alveolar nerves, which supply the maxillary sinus, teeth, and gums.

6. Branches of Pterygopalatine Ganglion

a. Orbital Branches

–supply the periosteum of the orbit and the mucous membrane of the posterior ethmoidal and sphenoidal sinuses.

b. Pharyngeal Branch

–runs in the pharyngeal canal and supplies the roof of the pharynx and the sphenoidal sinus.

c. Posterior Superior Lateral Nasal Branches

–enter the nasal cavity through the sphenopalatine foramen and supply the posterior part of the septum, the posterior ethmoidal air cells, and the superior and middle conchae.

d. Greater Palatine Nerve

–descends through the palatine canal and emerges through the greater palatine foramen to supply the palate.

–gives off the inferior lateral nasal branches.

e. Lesser Palatine Nerve

–descends through the palatine canal and emerges through the lesser palatine foramen to supply the soft palate and the palatine tonsil.

f. Nasopalatine Nerve

–runs obliquely downward and forward on the septum, supplying the septum, and passes through the incisive canal.

B. Pterygopalatine Ganglion

–lies in the pterygopalatine fossa just below the maxillary nerve, lateral to the sphenopalatine foramen and anterior to the pterygoid canal.

–receives its preganglionic parasympathetic fibers from the facial nerve by way of the greater petrosal nerve and the nerve of the pterygoid canal.

–sends its postganglionic parasympathetic fibers to the nasal and palatine glands and to the lacrimal gland by way of the maxillary, zygomatic, and lacrimal nerves.

–also receives postganglionic sympathetic fibers (by way of the deep petrosal nerve and the nerve of the pterygoid canal) which are distributed with the postganglionic parasympathetic fibers.

Larynx and Prevertebral Region

I. Larynx

–extends from the lower part of the pharynx to the trachea.

–acts as a valve, to prevent the passage of foods into the airway.

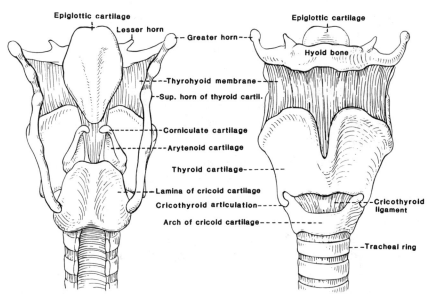

Figure 8.48. Cartilages of the larynx.

—controls the airway during swallowing and vocalization (or phonation).
—regulates the flow of air to and from the lungs for sound production.
—forms a framework of cartilage for the attachment of ligaments and muscles.

II. Cartilages of Larynx

A. Thyroid Cartilage
   —is a **single** cartilage and composed of **hyaline** cartilage.
   —forms a median elevation, called the laryngeal prominence ("Adam's apple").
   —its superior horn is attached to the tip of the greater horn of the hyoid bone.
   —its inferior horn articulates with the cricoid cartilage.
   —has an oblique line on the lateral surface of its lamina, which gives attachment for the inferior pharyngeal constrictor, sternothyroid, and thyrohyoid muscles.

B. Cricoid Cartilage
   —is a **single** cartilage and composed of **hyaline** cartilage.
   —is signet ring shaped.
   —marks the end of the pharynx and larynx at its lower border.

C. Epiglottis
   —is a **single** cartilage and composed of **elastic** cartilage.
   —is a spoon-shaped plate that lies behind the root of the tongue.
   —its lower end is attached to the back of the thyroid cartilage.

D. Arytenoid Cartilages
   —are **paired** cartilages and composed of **elastic** and **hyaline** cartilages.
   —are shaped like pyramids.

–have vocal processes that give attachment to the vocal ligament and muscular processes that give attachment to the thyroarytenoid, lateral and posterior cricoarytenoid muscles.

E. Corniculate Cartilages

–are **paired** cartilages and composed of **elastic** cartilage.
–lie on the apices of the arytenoid cartilages.
–are enclosed within the aryepiglottic folds of mucous membrane.

F. Cuneiform Cartilages

–are **paired** cartilages and composed of **elastic** cartilage.
–lie in the aryepiglottic folds anterior to the corniculate cartilages.

III. Ligaments of Larynx

A. Thyrohyoid Membrane

–extends from the thyroid cartilage to the medial surface of the hyoid bone.
–its median part (the median thyrohyoid ligament) is pierced by the internal laryngeal nerve and the superior laryngeal vessels.

B. Cricothyroid Ligament

–extends from the arch of the cricoid cartilage to the thyroid cartilage and the vocal processes of the arytenoid cartilages.

C. Vocal Ligament

–extends from the posterior surface of the thyroid cartilage to the vocal process of the arytenoid cartilage.
–is considered as the upper border of the conus elasticus.

D. Vestibular (Ventricular) Ligament

–extends from the thyroid cartilage to the anterior lateral surface of the arytenoid cartilage.

E. Conus Elasticus (or Cricovocal Ligament)

–is a fibroelastic membrane that extends upward from the entire arch of the cricoid cartilage to the vocal ligaments (and the thyroid cartilage and the vocal process of the arytenoid cartilage).
–is formed by the cricothyroid, median cricothyroid and vocal ligaments.

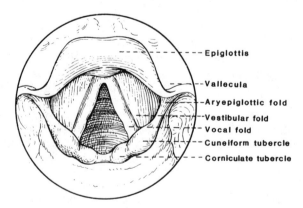

Figure 8.49. Interior view of the larynx from above.

IV. Cavities and Folds of Larynx

—The larynx is divided into three portions by the vestibular and the vocal folds: the vestibule, ventricle, and infraglottic cavity.

A. Vestibule

—extends from the laryngeal inlet to the vestibular (ventricular) folds.

B. Ventricles

—extend between the ventricular fold and the vocal fold.

C. Infraglottic Cavity

—extends from the rima glottis to the lower border of the cricoid cartilage.

D. Rima Glottis

—is the space between the vocal folds and arytenoid cartilages.
—is the narrowest part of the laryngeal cavity.

E. Vestibular (Ventricular) Folds or False Vocal Cords

—extend from the thyroid cartilage above the vocal ligament to the arytenoid cartilage.

F. Vocal Folds or True Vocal Cords

—extend from the angle of the thyroid cartilage to the vocal processes of the arytenoid cartilages.
—contain the vocal ligament near their free margin and the vocalis muscle, which forms the bulk of the vocal fold.
—are important in voice production because they control the stream of air passing thorugh the rima glottis.
—alter the shape and size of the rima by movements of the arytenoids to facilitate respiration and phonation. (The rima glottis is wide during inspiration and narrow and wedge-shaped during expiration and sound production.)

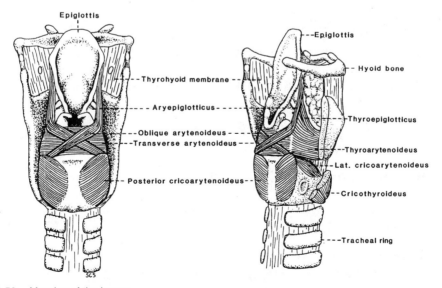

Figure 8.50. Muscles of the larynx.

V. Muscles of Larynx

Muscle	Origin	Insertion	Nerve	Action on Vocal Cords
Cricothyroid	Arch of cricoid cartilage	Inferior horn and lower lamina of thyroid cartilage	External laryngeal n.	Tenses
Posterior cricoarytenoid	Posterior surface of lamina of cricoid cartilage	Muscular process of arytenoid cartilage	Recurrent laryngeal n.	Abducts
Lateral cricoarytenoid	Arch of cricoid cartilage	Muscular process of arytenoid cartilage	Recurrent laryngeal n.	Adducts
Transverse artytenoideus	Posterior surface of arytenoid cartilage	Opposite arytenoid cartilage	Recurrent laryngeal n.	Adducts
Oblique artytenoideus	Muscular process of arytenoid cartilage	Apex of opposite arytenoid	Recurrent laryngeal n.	Adducts
Aryepiglotticus	Apex of arytenoid cartilage	Side of epiglottic cartilage	Recurrent laryngeal n.	Adducts
Thyroarytenoid	Inner surface of thyroid lamina	Anterolateral surface of arytenoid cartilage	Recurrent laryngal n.	Adducts
Thyroepi-glotticus	Anteromedial surface of lamina of thyroid cartilage	Lateral margin of epiglottic cartilage	Recurrent laryngeal n.	Adducts
Vocalis	Anteromedial surface of lamina of thyroid cartilage	Vocal process	Recurrent laryngeal n.	Adducts and tenses

VI. Innervation of Larynx

A. Recurrent (Inferior) Laryngeal Nerve

–supplies all of the intrinsic muscles of the larynx except the cricothyroid, which is innervated by the external laryngeal branch of the superior laryngeal nerve of the vagus nerve.

–supplies the sensory innervation below the vocal cord.

–its terminal portion above the cricoid cartilage is called the **inferior laryngeal nerve.**

B. Internal Laryngeal Nerve

–innervates the mucous membrane above the vocal cord.

–is accompanied by the superior laryngeal artery and pierces the thyrohyoid membrane.

C. External Laryngeal Nerve

–innervates the cricothyroid and inferior pharyngeal constrictor muscles.

–is accompanied by the superior thyroid artery.

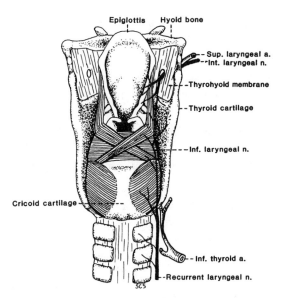

Figure 8.51. Nerve supply to the larynx.

VII. Prevertebral Muscles[a]

Muscle	Origin	Insertion	Nerve	Action
Lateral Vertebral				
Scalenus anterior	Transverse processes of CV3-6	Scalene tubercle on first rib	Lower cervical (C5-C8)	Elevates first rib; bends neck
Scalenus medius	Transverse processes of CV1-7	Upper surface of first rib	Lower cervical (C5-C8)	Elevates first rib; bends neck
Scalenus posterior	Transverse processes of CV4-6	Outer surface of second rib	Lower cervical (C6-C8)	Elevates second rib; bends neck
Anterior Vertebral				
Longus capitus	Transverse processes of CV3-6	Basilar part of occipital bone	C1-C4	Flexes and rotates head
Longus colli (L. cervicis)	Transverse processes and bodies of CV3-TV3	Anterior tubercle of atlas; bodies of CV2-4; transverse process of CV5-6	C2-C6	Flexes and rotates head
Rectus capitis anterior	Lateral mass of atlas	Basilar part of occipital bone	C1-C2	Flexes and rotates head
Retus capitis lateralis	Transverse process of atlas	Jugular process of occipital bone	C1-C2	Flexes head laterally

[a]CV, cervical vertebra; TV, thoracic vertebra.

VIII. Fasciae

A. Preverterbral Fascia

—is a part of the cervical fascia that encloses the cervical vertebral column and its associated musculature.

–covers the scalene muscles and attaches to the external occipital protuberance.

B. Pretracheal Fascia

–is the layer of the cervical fascia investing the larynx and trachea, enclosing the thyroid gland, and contributing to the formation of the carotid sheath.

C. Buccophyaryngeal Fascia

–covers the buccinator muscles and the pharynx.
–is attached to the pharyngeal tubercle and the pterygomandibular raphe.

D. Pharyngobasilar Fascia

–is the fibrous coat in the wall of the pharynx, situated between the mucous membrane and the pharyngeal constrictor muscles.

Ear

I. Tympanic (or Middle Ear) Cavity

–its boundaries

   a. Roof

   –tegmen tympani.

   b. Floor

   –jugular fossa.

   c. Lateral

   –tympanic membrane.

   d. Medial

   –medial wall of the inner ear.

   e. Anterior

   –carotid canal.

   f. Posterior

   –mastoid air cells and mastoid antrum through the *aditus ad antrum*.

–communicates anteriorly with the nasopharynx via the auditory tube and posteriorly with the mastoid air cells and the mastoid antrum through the *aditus ad antrum*.
–is traversed by the chorda tympani and lesser petrosal nerve.

A. Tympanic Membrane

–its most depressed center point of the concavity is called the umbo.
–its lateral concave surface is covered by epidermis and supplied by cranial nerves V and X.
–its medial surface is covered by the mucous membrane, innervated by cranial nerve IX, and gives attachment for the handle of the malleus.

B. Promontory of Middle Ear

–is the rounded prominence on the inner wall of the middle ear, formed by the first coil of the cochlea.

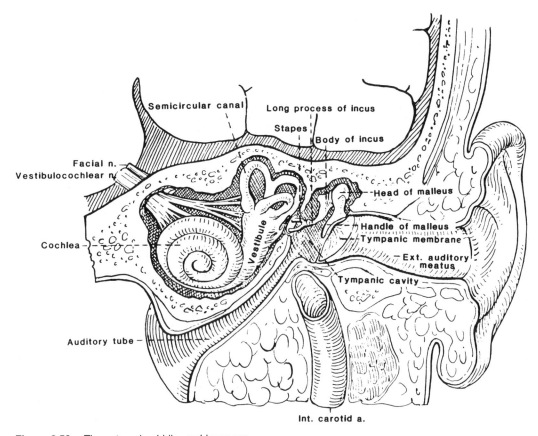

Figure 8.52. The external, middle, and inner ear.

II. Muscles of Middle Ear

A. Stapedius Muscle

—is the smallest of the skeletal muscles in the human body.

—arises from the pyramidal eminence on the posterior wall of the tympanic cavity.

—inserts on the neck of the stapes.

—is innervated by a branch of the facial nerve.

—pulls the head of the stapes posteriorly, thereby tilting the base of the stapes in the vestibular window.

—prevents excessive oscillation of the stapes.

B. Tensor Tympani Muscle

—arises from the cartilaginous portion of the auditory tube.

—inserts on the handle (manubrium) of the malleus.

—is innervated by the mandibular branch of the trigeminal nerve.

—draws the manubrium medially, thereby making the tympanic membrane taut.

III. Auditory Ossicles

A. Malleus (Hammer)

–consists of a head, a neck, a handle (or manubrium), and anterior and posterior processes.

–its rounded head articulates with the incus in the epitympanic recess.

–its **handle** (or **Manubrium**) is fused to the medial surface of the tympanic membrane and gives an attachment for the **tensor tympani** muscle.

B. Incus (Anvil)

–consists of a body and two processes (or crura).

–its long process descends vertically, parallel to the handle of the malleus, and articulates with the stapes.

C. Stapes (Stirrup)

–consists of a head and neck, two processes (or crura), and a base (or foot plate).

–its neck provides insertion of the stapedius muscle.

–has a hole through which the stapedial artery is transmitted in the embryo but which is closed by an obturation in the adult.

IV. Nerves

A. Facial Nerve

–enters the internal acoustic meatus, and then the facial canal.

–its motor portion passes through the stylomastoid foramen and enters the parotid gland, where it gives off its terminal branches, such as the temporal, zygomatic, buccal, marginal mandibular, and cervical branches.

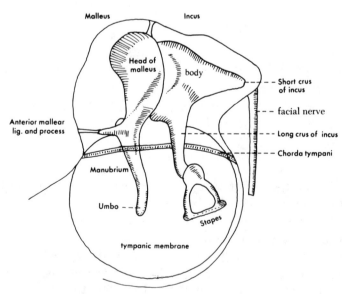

Figure 8.53. Ossicles of the middle ear.

–supplies all muscles of facial expression as well as the stylohyoid, digastric belly, and stapedius muscles.

–has no cutaneous branches of the face.

–its nervus intermedius branch exits the skull through the petrotympanic fissure as the **chorda tympani**, carrying taste fibers from the anterior two-thirds of the tongue and parasympathetic preganglionic (secretomotor) fibers to the submandibular ganglion (for the submandibular glands) and to the pterygopalatine ganglion (for the lacrimal gland).

1. **Chorda Tympani**

    –arises from the facial nerve, just above the stylomastoid foramen.

    –crosses the tympanic cavity between the handle of the malleus and the long process of the incus.

    –leaves the skull through the petrotympanic fissure and joins the lingual nerve in the infratemporal fossa.

    –contains special sensory fibers for taste from the anterior two-thirds of the tongue and the soft palate, with the cell bodies being in the geniculate ganglion.

    –also contains parasympathetic preganglionic (secretomotor) fibers that synapse in the submandibular ganglion and go on to supply the submandibular, sublingual, and lingual glands.

    –communicates with the otic ganglion below the base of the skull.

2. **Greater Petrosal Nerve**

    –arises from the facial nerve adjacent to the geniculate ganglion.

    –emerges at the hiatus of the canal for the greater petrosal nerve in the middle cranial fossa.

    –is joined by the deep petrosal nerve to form the nerve of the pterygoid canal.

    –contains secretomotor (preganglionic parasympathetic) fibers for the lacrimal and nasal glands, that synapse in the pterygopalatine ganglion.

    –also contains taste fibers, with cell stations in the geniculate ganglion, which pass from the palate through the pterygopalatine ganglion and nerve of the pterygoid canal.

B. **Lesser Petrosal Nerve**

    –is a continuation of the tympanic nerve beyond the tympanic plexus.

    –passes forward through the petrous portion of the temporal bone and joins a branch from the geniculate ganglion of the facial nerve.

    –runs just lateral to the greater petrosal nerve and leaves the middle cranial fossa through either the foramen ovale or the fissure between the petrous bone and the great wing of the sphenoid to enter the otic ganglion.

    –contains preganglionic parasympathetic secretomotor fibers that run in the glossopharyngeal and tympanic nerves before synapsing in the otic ganglion. (The postganglionic fibers arising from this ganglion are passed to the parotid gland by the auriculotemporal nerve.)

    –also transmits postganglionic sympathetic fibers to the parotid gland.

C. Tympanic Plexus

–is formed by the tympanic nerve of the glossopharyngeal nerve, an an-
astomotic branch from the geniculate ganglion of the facial, and the sympathetic (caroticotympanic) branches of the internal carotid plexus.

–lies in grooves on the promontory of the medial wall of the middle ear.

–supplies the mucosa of the middle ear, the auditory tube, and the mastoid
air cells, and gives rise to the lesser petrosal nerve to the otic ganglion.

D. Vestibulocochlear (Acoustic) Nerve

–enters the internal acoustic meatus and remains within the temporal bone
to supply the cochlea and semicircular canals.

–is split into a cochlear portion for hearing and a vestibular portion for
equilibrium.

V. Blood Supply of Middle Ear

A. Chief Arteries

–are the **anterior tympanic** artery from the maxillary artery to the tympanic membrane and the **stylomastoid** artery from the posterior auricular artery to the tympanic antrum and mastoid air cells.

Autonomics of the Head and Neck

I. Parasympathetic Ganglia and Associated Nerves

A. Ciliary Ganglion

–is situated behind the eyeball, between the optic nerve and the lateral
rectus muscle.

–receives preganglionic parasympathetic fibers (with cell bodies in the
Edinger-Westphal nucleus of cranial nerve III in the mesencephalon),
which run in the inferior division of the oculomotor nerve.

–sends its postganglionic parasympathetic fibers to the sphincter pupillae
(iris) and the ciliary muscle (ciliary body) via the short ciliary nerves.

–receives postganglionic sympathetic fibers (derived from the superior cervical ganglion) that reach the dilator pupillae muscle by way of the sympathetic plexus on the internal carotid artery, ciliary ganglion (without
synapsing), and short ciliary nerves.

B. Pterygopalatine Ganglion

–lies in the pterygopalatine fossa just below the maxillary nerve, lateral
to the sphenopalatine foramen and anterior to the pterygoid canal.

–receives its preganglionic parasympathetic fibers from the facial nerve
by way of the greater petrosal nerve and the nerve of the pterygoid canal.

–sends its postganglionic parasympathetic fibers to the nasal and palatine
glands and to the lacrimal gland by way of the maxillary, zygomatic, and
lacrimal nerves.

–also receives postganglionic sympathetic fibers (derived from the superior
cervical ganglion) by way of the plexus on the internal carotid artery, the
deep petrosal nerve, and the nerve of the pterygoid canal. The fibers
merely pass through the ganglion and are distributed with the postganglionic parasympathetic fibers.

1. **Greater Petrosal Nerve**
   —contains preganglionic parasympathetic fibers and joins the deep petrosal nerve (containing postganglionic sympathetic fibers) to form the nerve of the pterygoid canal (or Vidian nerve).
   —also contains taste fibers, which pass from the palate nonstop through the pterygopalatine ganglion, nerve of the pterygoid canal, and greater petrosal nerve to the geniculate ganglion (where the bodies are found).

2. **Deep Petrosal Nerve**
   —arises from the plexus on the internal carotid artery.
   —contains postganglionic sympathetic fibers whose cell bodies are located in the superior cervical ganglion. These fibers run in the nerve of the pterygoid canal, merely pass through the pterygopalatine ganglion without synapsing, and then join the postganglionic parasympathetic fibers in supplying the lacrimal gland and the nasal and oral mucosa.

3. **Nerve of Pterygoid Canal (Vidian Nerve)**
   —consists of preganglionic parasympathetic fibers from the greater petrosal nerve and postganglionic sympathetic fibers from the deep petrosal nerve.
   —passes through the pterygoid canal and ends in the pterygopalatine ganglion, which is slung from the maxillary nerve. The postganglionic parasympathetic fibers with cell bodies in the pterygopalatine ganglion, along with some postganglionic sympathetic fibers, are distributed to the lacrimal glands and the nasal and palatine glands.
   —also contains taste fibers from the palate.

C. Submandibular Ganglion
   —lies on the lateral surface of the hyoglossus muscle but medial to the mylohyoid muscle and is suspended from the lingual nerve.
   —receives preganglionic parasympathetic secretomotor fibers that run in the facial nerve, chorda tympani, and lingual nerve.
   —sends its postganglionic fibers to supply the submandibular gland mostly, although some of the fibers join the lingual nerve to reach the sublingual gland.

1. **Chorda Tympani**
   —contains preganglionic parasympathetic fibers that synapse on the postganglionic neuron cell bodies in the submandibular ganglion. Their postganglionic fibers innervate the submandibular and sublingual glands.
   —passes through the petrotympanic fissure, runs in the infratemporal fossa, and joins the lingual nerve.
   —also contains taste fibers from the anterior two-thirds of the tongue whose cell bodies are located in the geniculate ganglion.

D. Otic Ganglion
   —lies in the infratemporal fossa, just below the foramen ovale, between the mandibular nerve and the tensor veli palatini.
   —receives preganglionic parasympathetic fibers that run in the glosso-

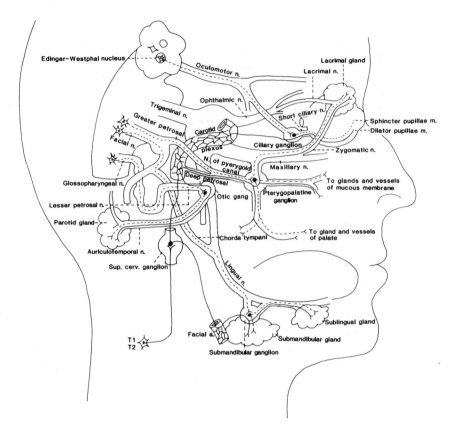

Figure 8.54. Autonomics of the head and neck.

pharyngeal nerve, tympanic plexus, and lesser petrosal nerve and synapse in this ganglion.

—sends postganglionic fibers that run in the auriculotemporal nerve and supply the parotid gland.

1. **Tympanic Nerve**

   —contains preganglionic parasympathetic secretomotor fibers for the parotid gland.

   —arises from the inferior ganglion of the glossopharyngeal nerve.

   —passes through a small canal between the jugular foramen and the carotid canal into the tympanic cavity.

   —enters the tympanic plexus on the promontory of the medial wall of the tympanic cavity.

2. **Lesser Petrosal Nerve**

   —is a continuation of the tympanic nerve beyond the tympanic plexus.

   —passes forward through the petrous portion of the temporal bone and joins a branch from the geniculate ganglion of the facial nerve.

   —runs just lateral to the greater petrosal nerve, and leaves the middle cranial fossa through either the foramen ovale or the fissure between the petrous bone and the great wing of the sphenoid to enter the otic ganglion.

—contains preganglionic parasympathetic secretomotor fibers that run in the glossopharyngeal and tympanic nerves before synapsing in this otic ganglion. (The postganglionic fibers arising from the ganglion are passed to the parotid gland by the auriculotemporal nerve.)
—also transmits postganglionic sympathetic fibers to the parotid gland.

II. Summary of Parasympathetic Ganglia

Ganglion	Location	Parasympathetic Fibers	Sympathetic Fibers	Chief Distribution
Ciliary	Lateral to optic n.	Oculomotor n. and its inferior division	Internal carotid plexus	Ciliary muscle, and sphincter pupillae (parasympathetic; dilator pupillae and tarsal muscles (sympathetic)
Pterygotopalatine	In pterygopalatine fossa	Facial, greater petrosal, and n. of pterygoid canal	Internal carotid plexus	Lacrimal gland, and glands in nose and palate
Submandibular	On hyoglossus	Facial n., chorda tympani, and lingula n.	Plexus on facial a.	Submandibular and sublingual glands
Otic	Below foramen ovale	Glossopharyngeal n., its tympanic branch and lesser petrosal	Plexus on middle meningeal a.	Parotid gland

Structure Passing through Cavernous Sinus → Abducent nerve

Review Test

HEAD AND NECK

DIRECTIONS: For each of the questions or incomplete statements in this section, *one* or *more* of the answers or completions given is correct. Choose answer:

A. if only **1, 2,** and **3** are correct.
B. if only **1** and **3** are correct.
C. if only **2** and **4** are correct.
D. if only **4** is correct.
E. if all are correct.

8.1. Which of the following cavities are separated from the middle cranial fossa by a thin layer of bone?

1. cochlea.
2. middle ear cavity.
3. sigmoid sinus.
4. sphenoid sinus.

8.2. The palatine tonsil

1. is bounded by the palatoglossal and palatopharyngeal folds.
2. receives sensory innervation from the glossopharyngeal nerve.
3. is supplied by branches of the facial artery.
4. is located on each side of the nasopharynx.

8.3. Nerves that pass through the jugular foramen include the

1. vagus.
2. spinal accessory.
3. glossopharyngeal.
4. hypoglossal.

8.4. Concerning the orbicularis oculi muscle

1. it is supplied by temporal and zygomatic branches of the facial nerve.
2. it functions to close the eyelids.
3. its paralysis results in spilling of tears.
4. it is not branchiomeric in origin.

8.5. The innervation of the cranial dura includes

1. vagus nerve.
2. trigeminal nerves.
3. upper cervical spinal nerves.
4. facial nerves.

8.6. The carotid sinus is

1. located at the origin of the external carotid artery.
2. innervated mainly by the glossopharyngeal nerve.
3. stimulated by changes in pH of blood.
4. stimulated by changes in blood pressure.

8.7. Which of the following structures pass(es) through the optic canal?

1. optic nerve.
2. ophthalmic vein.
3. ophthalmic artery.
4. ophthalmic nerve.

8.8. A cancer of the maxillary sinus may

1. cause cutaneous pain superficial to the maxilla.
2. cause pain in the soft palate and the palatine tonsil.
3. accompany toothache in the upper molars.
4. block the nasolacrimal duct.

8.9. Severance of the greater petrosal nerve results in

1. decreased lacrimal gland secretion.
2. decreased diameter of the pupil.
3. dryness in the nose and palate.
4. decreased parotid gland secretion.

8.10. The nerve of the pterygoid canal (Vidian nerve)

1. contains preganglionic parasympathetic fibers whose cell bodies are in the geniculate ganglion.
2. contains taste fibers from the palate.
3. contains postganglionic parasympathetic fibers.
4. contains postganglionic sympathetic fibers.

8.11. Preganglionic fibers connecting the central nervous system with autonomic ganglia include:

1. thoracolumbar outflow by ventral roots of the thoracic (T1–T12) and the upper two lumbar (L1–L2) cord segments.
2. sacral outflow via the ventral roots of S1–S5.
3. cranial outflow by visceral motor fibers in the oculomotor (III), facial (VII), glossopharyngeal (IX), and vagus (X) nerves.
4. cranial outflow by visceral motor fibers in the trochlear (VI), trigeminal (V), and abducens (VI) nerves.

8.12. The digastric muscle is innervated by the

1. spinal accessory nerve.
2. trigeminal nerve.
3. ansa cervicalis.
4. facial nerve.

8.13. The following structures are located within the carotid sheath:

1. vagus (X) nerve.
2. common carotid artery.
3. internal jugular vein.
4. sympathetic trunk.

8.14. The following muscles are innervated by the facial nerve:

1. buccinator.
2. stylohyoid.
3. posterior belly of the digastric.
4. tensor tympani.

8.15. The middle meatus of the nasal cavity communicates with the

1. sphenoidal sinus.
2. frontal sinus.
3. posterior ethmoidal air cells.
4. middle ethmoidal air cells.

8.16. The internal laryngeal nerve

1. is a branch of the superior laryngeal nerve.
2. is an indirect branch of the vagus nerve.
3. is sensory to the mucosa of the larynx.
4. is motor to the cricothyroideus muscle.

8.17. which of the following muscles are innervated by the trigeminal nerve?

1. tensor veli palatini.
2. platysma.
3. masseter.
4. frontalis.

8.18. Damage to the eardrum and middle ear ossicles is avoided by contraction of two muscles located in the middle ear. These are innervated by

1. chorda tympani.
2. trigeminal nerve.
3. auditory nerve.
4. facial nerve.

8.19. Which of the following, if cut, would eliminate the pupillary light reflex?

1. short ciliary nerves.
2. oculomotor nerve.
3. optic nerve.
4. long ciliary nerves before they join the short ciliary nerves.

8.20. If the pupil remains small even in a room with subdued lighting, which of the following nervous structure(s) could be damaged?

1. trochlear nerve.
2. superior cervical ganglion.
3. oculomotor nerve.
4. cervical sympathetic trunk.

8.21. Which nerve(s) could be damaged if the corneal surface is dry due to lack of fluid for keeping it moist?

1. terminal portion of lacrimal nerve.
2. zygomatic branch of maxillary nerve.
3. greater petrosal nerve.
4. lesser petrosal nerve.

8.22. The frontal sinus

1. extends into the parietal bone.
2. communicates with the middle nasal meatus.
3. receives sensory innervation via the maxillary nerve.
4. receives blood supply via branches of the ophthalmic artery.

8.23. The tongue

1. has intrinsic and extrinsic muscle attachments.
2. contains lymphoid tissue.
3. receives fibers from cranial nerves V, VII, IX, and XII.
4. receives blood from a direct branch of the internal carotid artery.

8.24. The foramen magnum

1. is surrounded by dura, periosteum, and ligaments.
2. contains a medulla-cord junction and cerebrospinal fluid.
3. is traversed by vertebral and anterior spinal arteries.
4. contains the accessory nerve (spinal accessory nerve).

8.25. which of the following nervous structure(s) could be damaged if the patient moves the eyeball entirely normally and sees distant objects clearly but cannot focus on near objects?

1. ciliary ganglion.
2. oculomotor nerve.
3. short ciliary nerves.
4. superior cervical ganglion.

8.26. Veins of the brain are direct tributaries of the

1. emissary veins.
2. pterygoid venous plexus.
3. diploid veins.
4. dural sinuses.

8.27. Stimulation of the parasympathetic fibers to the eyeball result in which of the following?

1. enhanced vision for distance objects.
2. dilation of the pupil.
3. contraction of capillaries in the iris.
4. contraction of the ciliary muscle (accommodation).

8.28. The pituitary gland (hypophysis)

1. lies in a depression in the ethmoid bone.
2. is bordered on either side by the left and right carotid sinuses.
3. lies nearer the posterior cerebral arteries than it does the internal carotid arteries.
4. is situated in the hypophyseal fossa of the sella turcica.

8.29. Which of the following structures throughout part of their course do *not* lie embedded in the walls of the cavernous sinus?

1. oculomotor nerves.
2. optic nerves.
3. trochlear nerves.
4. mandibular division of the trigeminal nerves.

8.30. Which of the following structures enter(s) the orbit through both the superior orbital fissure and the common tendinous ring?

1. nasociliary nerve.
2. oculomotor nerve.
3. abducent nerve.
4. trochlear nerve.

8.31. Of the following ganglia in the head and neck, which ones form a synaptic point for preganglionic secretory fibers from the facial nerve?

1. pterygopalatine (sphenopalatine).
2. geniculate.
3. submandibular.
4. ciliary.

8.32. Muscles that are attached to the styloid process are innervated by the following nerves.

1. facial nerve.
2. hypoglossal nerve.
3. glossopharyngeal nerve.
4. vagus nerve.

8.33. Of the following, which would most likely result in a functional defect to the act of swallowing? Damage to the

1. vagus nerve.
2. maxillary division of the trigeminal nerve.
3. mandibular division of the trigeminal nerve.
4. buccal branch of the facial nerve.

8.34. A nerve that carries preganglionic parasympathetic fibers to the otic ganglion (Jacobson's nerve):

1. is a branch of the facial.
2. is the deep petrosal nerve.
3. synapses with fibers of the lesser superficial petrosal nerve.
4. is a branch of the glossopharyngeal.

8.35. Of the following arteries, which are usually *not* direct branches of the subclavian artery?

1. highest thoracic.
2. vertebral.
3. inferior thyroid.
4. internal thoracic.

DIRECTIONS: For each numbered item, select the *one* lettered heading that is most closely associated with it. Each lettered heading may be selected once, more than once, or not at all.

A. Cavernous sinus
B. Sigmoid sinus
C. Superior sagittal sinus
D. Transverse sinus
E. Straight sinus

8.36. Lies at the junction of the falx cerebri with tentorium cerebelli.

8.37. This sinus curves laterally and forward in the convex outer border of the tentorium cerebelli.

8.38. Lies in the superior convex border of the falx cerebri.

8.39. Communicates directly with the ophthalmic veins.

8.40. At the jugular foramen it becomes continuous with the internal jugular vein.

A. hypoglossal nerve
B. Vagus nerve
C. Chorda tympani nerve
D. Lingual nerve
E. Glossopharyngeal nerve

8.41. provides motor innervation to the intrinsic muscles of the larynx.

8.42. Carries general sensation from the anterior two-thirds of the tongue.

8.43. Is the source of parasympathetic innervation for the parotid gland.

8.44. Provides motor innervation to the intrinsic muscles of the tongue.

8.45. Carries sensory information from pressure receptors in the carotid sinus.

A. Foramen ovale
B. Foramen spinosum
C. Foramen rotundum
D. Foramen lacerum
E. Superior orbital fissure

8.46. Transmits the ophthalmic nerve.

8.47. Related to the internal carotid artery.

8.48. Transmits the middle meningeal artery.

8.49. Injury to the nerve that passes through this structure leads to a general loss of sensation of the maxillary teeth.

8.50. Injury to the nerve that passes through this structure leads to a loss of sensation of the temporomandibular joints.

A. Stylomastoid foramen
B. Pterygoid canal
C. Pterygomaxillary fissure
D. Sphenopalatine foramen
E. Jugular foramen

8.51. Transmits the nerve that innervates the muscles of facial expression.

8.52. Is traversed by sensory fibers from the posterior one-third of the tongue.

8.53. Is traversed by sensory fibers from the mucosa of the nasal septum, posterior lateral nasal wall, and anterior portion of the hard palate.

8.54. Is the passageway between the infratemporal fossa and the pterygopalatine fossa for the terminal part of the maxillary artery.

8.55. Is traversed by preganglionic parasympathetic fibers to the lacrimal gland.

DIRECTIONS: Each of the questions or incomplete statements below is followed by five suggested answers or completions. Choose the *one* that is *best* in each case.

8.56. When a descending (dorsal) scapular artery is present off the third part of the subclavian, it usually replaces functionally which of the following?

1. superficial branch of transverse cervical artery.
2. deep branch of transverse cervical artery.
3. subscapular artery.
4. suprascapular artery.
5. internal thoracic artery.

8.57. In a low tracheotomy (i.e., performed in the interval between the isthmus of the thyroid gland and the suprasternal notch) a vessel or vessels that probably would never be encountered in a clean operation is (are) the

1. inferior thyroid vein or its tributaries.
2. jugular arch.
3. costocervical trunk.
4. thyroidea ima artery.
5. brachiocephalic (left) vein.

8.58. During thyroid surgery, a nerve that is closely associated with the superior thyroid artery may be damaged, in inability to:

A. relax the vocal cords.
B. rotate the arytenoid cartilages.
C. tense the vocal cords.
D. adduct the vocal cords.
E. abduct the vocal cords.

8.59. One of the following branches of the cervical plexus contains no cutaneous branches:

A. phrenic nerve.
B. greater auricular nerve.
C. transverse nerve of neck.
D. supraclavicular nerve.
E. lesser occipital nerve.

8.60. Which one of the following structures does not empty or open into the middle nasal meatus?

A. middle ethmoidal air cells.
B. maxillary sinus.
C. sphenoid sinus.
D. anterior ethmoidal air cells.
E. frontal sinus.

8.61. The superior laryngeal artery is accompanied by the

A. external laryngeal nerve.
B. internal laryngeal nerve.
C. superior laryngeal nerve.
D. hypoglossal nerve.
E. vagus nerve.

8.62. Which of the following nerves is responsible for the sensory innervation of the mucosa of the pharynx?

A. transverse cervical nerves.
B. phrenic nerves.
C. vagus nerves.
D. glossopharyngeal nerves.
E. ansa cervicalis (hypoglossi).

8.63. Select the incorrect statement.

A. All cutaneous (sensory) nerves of the neck are branches of the cervical plexus.
B. The cutaneous nerve supplying most of the skin of the neck is the transversus colli (transverse cervical) nerve.
C. The supraclavicular nerves innervate the platysma muscle.
D. Motor nerves to most of the infrahyoid muscles are branches of the ansa cervicalis.
E. Anterior primary rami from cervical nerves 2, 3, and 4 contribute to the cervical plexus.

8.64. A named artery that is never a branch of the thyrocervical trunk is the

A. inferior thyroid.
B. transverse cervical.
C. Suprascapular.
D. deep cervical
E. none of the above.

8.65. Normally, on either side of the body, the phrenic nerve in the neck passes

A. across the anterior surface of the subclavian vein.
B. across the posterior surface of the subclavian artery.
C. across the deep surface of the scalenus anterior muscle.
D. medial to the common carotid artery.
E. across the superficial surface of the scalenus anterior muscle.

8.66. A muscle that is a "landmark" for finding the glossopharyngeal nerve in the neck is the: (Note: This muscle is also innervated by the glossopharyngeal nerve.)

A. inferior pharyngeal constrictor.
B. stylopharyngeus muscle.
C. posterior belly of the digastric.
D. longus colli.
E. rectus capitis anterior.

8.67. The nerve that innervates the cricothyroid muscle also sends some fibers to the

A. inferior constrictor muscle.
B. thyrohyoid.
C. sternohyoid.
D. stylohyoid.
E. sternothyroid.

8.68. Taste cells associated with the fungiform papillae on the tongue are innervated by fibers that originate in cranial nerve:

A. XII.
B. VII.
C. V.
D. X.
E. IX.

8.69. Identify the correct statement.

A. The inlet to the larynx is formed by the aryepiglottic folds.
B. The true vocal folds are found inferior to the ventricle of the larynx.
C. The afferent nerve fibers from the larynx are carried by the vagus nerve.
D. The larynx extends inferiorly to the level of the sixth cervical vertebra.
E. All of the above are correct.

8.70. The superior orbital fissure provides a passageway in the floor of the cranial cavity for all but one of the following. Which one does *not* pass through it?

A. abducens nerve.
B. ophthalmic nerve.
C. oculomotor nerve.
D. trochlear nerve.
E. optic nerve.

8.71. Concerning the anterior and posterior ethmoidal nerves

A. both have terminal branches called external nasal nerves.
B. are branches of the infraorbital nerve.
C. both leave the orbit by way of the posterior ethmoidal foramina.
D. both send branches to the ethmoidal air sinuses.
E. one leaves the orbit with the zygomatico-temporal nerve.

8.72. Most of the postganglionic parasympathetic fibers to the gland in the palate originate in the following ganglion:

A. nodose.
B. otic.
C. pterygopalatine (sphenopalatine).
D. submandibular.
E. ciliary.

8.73. Select the incorrect statement.

A. The duct of the submandibular gland opens into the sublingual region of the mouth.
B. The duct of the submandibular gland pierces the mylohyoid muscle.
C. The duct of the parotid gland pierces the buccinator muscle.
D. The duct of the parotid gland opens into the vestibule of the mouth.
E. Along part of its course, the parotid duct parallels the transverse facial artery.

8.74. Select the incorrect statement.

A. The attachments of the conchae are limited to the lateral wall of the nasal cavity.
B. The ethmoid bone contributes to the roof, medial, and lateral borders of the nasal cavity.
C. The septum of the nasal cavity is partially cartilaginous.
D. The major portion of the floor of the nasal cavity is formed by the palatine bone.
E. The vomer bone forms part of the floor of the nasal cavity.

8.75. In Bell's palsy (or facial paralysis), a possible inflammation of the cornea leads to corneal ulceration, resulting from the following:

A. sensory loss of the cornea and conjunctiva.
B. lack of secretion of the salivary glands.
C. absence of the blinking reflex due to paralysis of the closing muscle(s) of the eyelid.
D. absence of the blinking due to paralysis of the opening muscle(s) of the eyelids.
E. constriction of the pupil due to paralysis of the dilator pupillae.

8.76. Of the following, which are direct tributaries to the straight dural sinus in the cranial cavity?

A. transverse and sigmoid sinuses.
B. inferior sagittal sinus and greater cerebral vein.
C. superior sagittal sinus and confluence of sinuses.
D. superior and inferior petrosal sinuses.
E. cavernous sinus and basilar plexus.

8.77. The abducens (VI) nerve is severed proximal to its entrance into the orbit. Which of the following is a correct result?

A. ptosis of the upper eyelid.
B. loss of ability to dilate the pupil.
C. external strabismus (lateral deviation).
D. loss of visual accommodation.
E. loss of adduction of the eye.

8.78. The bilateral severance of the following cranial nerves at the base of the skull may result in death of the subject

A. trigeminal.
B. facial.
C. vagus.
D. accessory.
E. hypoglossal.

8.79. If the middle meningeal artery is ruptured but the meninges remain intact, blood enters the

A. subarachnoid space.
B. subdural space.
C. epidural space.
D. subpial space.
E. dural sinuses.

8.80 Preganglionic neurons of the parasympathetic nervous system are located in the

A. cervical and sacral spinal cord.
B. cervical and thoracic spinal cord.
C. brain stem and cervical spinal cord.
D. thoracic and lumbar spinal cord.
E. brain stem and sacral spinal cord.

8.81. The taste buds in the anterior two-thirds of the tongue are innervated by branches of the

A. glossopharyngeal nerve.
B. trigeminal nerve.
C. vagus nerve.
D. facial nerve.
E. spinal accessory nerve.

8.82. The pituitary gland lies in the sella turcica immediately posterior and adjacent to the

A. frontal sinus.
B. maxillary sinus.
C. ethmoid cells.
D. mastoid cells.
E. sphenoidal sinus.

8.83. Choose the incorrect answer. The carotid sheath

A. is partially reinforced by cervical visceral fascia.
B. contains the vagus nerve.
C. is continued into the mediastinum as adventitia of the great vessels.
D. encloses a portion of the ansa cervicalis.
E. contains the sympathetic chain trunk ganglia.

8.84. The sella turcica is part of the

A. frontal bone.
B. ethmoid bone.
C. temporal bone.
D. basioccipital bone.
E. sphenoid bone.

8.85. Choose the correct answer.

A. When the ciliary muscle contracts, the lens of the eye becomes thinner.
B. The ciliary muscle contracts if its parasympathetic fibers are stimulated.
C. During accommodation for seeing objects close to the eye, the lens become thinner.
D. Accommodation for seeing objects close to the eye is mediated by sympathetic nerve action.
E. The lens does not change in shape during accommodation, but simply moves forward or backward.

8.86. A characteristic of an open scalp wound is excessive bleeding. This happens because:

A. the skin of the scalp has a richer blood supply than does the skin of other parts of the body.
B. the connective tissue fibers of the scalp are unique in that they tend to hold the cut walls of scalp arteries open, whereas in other parts of the body they permit them to collapse.
C. venous return from the scalp is less than from the skin of other parts of the body.
D. most of the arteries in the scalp lie deep to the galea aponeurotica.
E. blood in vessels of the scalp does not clot as fast as it does in skin of other parts of the body.

8.87. A horizontal cut through the neck that would sever the inferior thyroid arteries would *not* sever the

A. recurrent laryngeal nerves.
B. external carotid arteries.
C. inferior thyroid veins.
D. vagus nerves.
E. trachea.

8.88. The dural venous sinus nearest the pituitary gland would be the

A. straight.
B. cavernous.
C. superior petrosal.
D. sigmoid.
E. confluence of sinuses.

8.89. The chorda tympani

A. carries taste fibers from the vallate papillae.
B. usually joins the inferior alveolar division of the mandibular nerve.
C. brings parasympathetic fibers to the submandibular ganglion.
D. mediates taste from the posterior one-third of the tongue.
E. carries preganglionic fibers that synapse in the pterygopalatine ganglion.

8.90. Concerning the pterygopalatine fossa, it

A. is located in the petrous portion of the temporal bone.
B. contains the otic ganglion.
C. communicates with the middle cranial cavity through the foramen rotundum.
D. is located directly inferior to the maxillary sinus.
E. communicates with the infratemporal fossa through the sphenopalatine foramen.

8.91. Which of the following statements on the tensor tympani muscle is incorrect? It

A. inserts on the handle of the malleus and functions to tighten the tympanic membrane.
B. is innervated by a branch of the facial nerve.
C. runs parallel to the auditory tube.
D. arises chiefly from the cartilaginous portion of the auditory tube.
E. is innervated by the branch of the trigeminal nerve.

8.92. Which of the following muscles causes abduction of the vocal cords during quiet breathing?

A. vocalis muscle
B. cricothyroid muscles.
C. oblique arytenoid muscles.
D. posterior cricoarytenoid muscles.
E. thyroarytenoid muscle.

8.93. Severance of the occulomotor nerve may *not* cause one of the following:

A. partial ptosis.
B. abduction of the eyeball.
C. a dilated pupil.
D. impaired lacrimal secretion.
E. paralysis of the ciliary muscle.

8.94. Choose one of the following nerves that supplies striated muscles not of branchiomeric origin.

A. vagus.
B. glossopharyngeal.
C. oculomotor.
D. facial.
E. trigeminal.

8.95. Which of the following pairs of muscles probably would be most necessary in preventing food from getting into the larynx and trachea during the process of swallowing?

A. sternohyoids and sternothyroids.
B. oblique arytenoids and aryepiglotticus.
C. inferior pharyngeal constrictors and thyrohyoids.
D. levator veli palatini and tensor veli palatinis.
E. musculus uvulae and geniohyoids.

DIRECTIONS: Each set of lettered headings below is followed by a list of numbered words or phrases. Choose answer:

A. if the item is associated with **A** only.
B. if the item is associated with **B** only.
C. if the item is associated with both **A** and **B**.
D. if the item is associated with neither **A** nor **B**.

A. Greater (superficial) petrosal nerve
B. Deep petrosal nerve
C. Both
D. Neither

8.96. Contains postganglionic sympathetic nerve fibers.

8.97. Contains preganglionic parasympathetic nerve fibers to the pterygopalatine ganglion.

8.98. Contributes fibers to form the nerve of the pterygoid canal.

8.99. Contains taste fibers from the palate.

8.100. Some of the motor fibers found in this nerve have their cell bodies in the geniculate ganglion.

A. Buccinator muscle
B. Masseter muscle
C. Both
D. Neither

8.101. Is an important muscle used in elevating the mandible.

8.102. Is innervated by a branch of the same cranial nerve that innervates the digastric muscle.

8.103. Is crossed superficially by the parotid duct.

8.104. Is pierced by the parotid duct.

8.105. Has no attachment to the mandible.

A. Costocervical trunk
B. Thyrocervical trunk
C. Both
D. Neither

8.106. Arises from the subclavian artery.

8.107. Gives rise to the superior intercostal artery, which supplies the first two posterior intercostal spaces.

8.108. The deep cervical artery is a direct branch of this trunk.

8.109. Its branch (direct or indirect) anastomoses with the descending branch of the occipital artery.

8.110. Typically has three branches.

A. Trigeminal nerve
B. Facial nerve
C. Both
D. Neither

8.111. Contains nerve fibers whose major functional components convey general sensation (touch, pain, and temperature) from the face and scalp.

8.112. Contains nerve fibers that pass through the greater palatine foramen.

8.113. Has preganglionic parasympathetic fibers that synapse in the pterygopalatine ganglion.

8.114. Has nerve fibers that stimulate secretion of the mucous glands in the nasal cavity.

8.115. Gives off the buccal nerve (directly or indirectly).

A. Tensor tympani muscle
B. Tensor veli palatini muscle.
C. Both
D. Neither

8.116. Arises from the cartilaginous portion of the auditory tube.

8.117. Inserts on the handle (manubrium) of the malleus.

8.118. Is innervated by the nerve that passes through the foramen ovale.

8.119. Receives blood from the branch of the maxillary artery.

8.120. Its tendon winds around pterygoid hamulus.

Answers and Explanations

HEAD AND NECK

8.1. C. The middle ear cavity and the sphenoid sinus are separated from the middle cranial fossa by a thin layer of bone.

8.2. A. The palatine tonsil is located on each side of the oropharynx between the palatoglossal and palatopharyngeal folds. It receives sensory innervation from the glossopharyngeal nerve and blood from branches of the facial artery.

8.3. A. The jugular foramen transmits the glossopharyngeal, accessory, and vagus nerves as well as the internal jugular vein.

8.4. A. The obicularis oculi muscle, derived from the second pharyngeal (or hyoid) arch, is innervated by the facial nerve and is active in eye closure. Its paralysis results in drooping of the lower eyelid and spilling of tears.

8.5. A. The cranial dura is innervated by the ophthalmic nerve in the anterior cranial fossa, by the maxillary and mandibular nerves in the middle cranial fossa, and by the vagus and hypoglossal nerves in the posterior cranial fossa.

8.6. C. The carotid sinus is a spindle-shaped dilation at the origin of the internal carotid artery, functions as a pressoreceptor that is stimulated by changes in blood pressure, and is innervated by the glossopharyngeal nerve.

8.7. B. The optic canal transmits the optic nerve and ophthalmic artery. The ophthalmic nerve and vein pass through the superior orbital fissure.

8.8. E. The medial wall of the maxillary sinus is formed by the lateral wall of the nasal cavity and the roof is formed by the floor of the orbit. The maxillary sinus is supplied by the anterior, middle, and posterior superior alveolar and infraorbital nerves. The cancer of the maxillary sinus may damage (a) the anterior, middle, and posterior alveolar nerves that run in the wall of the maxillary sinus and supply the sinus and the upper gums and teeth; (b) the infraorbital nerve that traverses the floor of the orbit and supplies the skin of the face superficial to the maxilla and lateral to the nose; and (c) the greater and lesser palatine nerves that traverse through the palatine canal situated in the posteromedial wall of the sinus and supply the soft palate and the palatine tonsil.

8.9. B. The greater petrosal nerve transmits parasympathetic (preganglionic) fibers, which are secretomotor fibers, to the lacrimal glands and mucous glands in the nasal cavity and palate.

8.10. C. The nerve of the pterygoid canal (vidian nerve) contains taste fibers from the palate, postganglionic sympathetic fibers and preganglionic parasympathetic fibers.

8.11. A. The preganglionic autonomic fibers connecting the central nervous system with autonomic ganglia include the efferent fibers of the thoracolumbar outflow (T1–L2), sacral outflow (S2–4), and cranial outflow (cranial nerves, III, VII, IX, X).

8.12. C. The digastric anterior belly is innervated by the trigeminal nerve, whereas the digastric posterior belly is innervated by the facial nerve.

8.13. A. The carotid sheath contains the vagus nerve, the common carotid artery, and the internal jugular vein.

8.14. A. the tensor tympani is innervated by the mandibular division of the trigeminal nerve.

8.15. C. The sphenoidal sinus opens into the sphenoethmoidal recess of the nasal cavity. The frontal sinus opens into the anterior part of the middle nasal meatus via the front nasal duct. The posterior ethmoidal air cells drain into the superior nasal meatus and the middle ethmoidal air cells drain into the summit of the ethmoidal bulla of the middle nasal meatus.

8.16. A. The internal laryngeal nerve is a branch of the superior laryngeal nerve of the vagus nerve and is sensory to the mucosa of the larynx above the vocal cord. The external laryngeal nerve supplies the cricothyroid and inferior pharyngeal constrictor muscles.

8.17. B. The platysma and frontalis muscles are innervated by the facial nerve.

8.18. C. The tensor tympani muscle is innervated by the trigeminal nerve and the stapedius muscle by the facial nerve.

8.19. A. The efferent limbs of the reflex arc concerned in the pupillary light reflex (such as constriction of the pupil in response to illumination of the retina) are composed of parasympathetic preganglionic fibers in the oculomotor nerve and parasympathetic postganglionic fibers in the short ciliary nerves. The afferent limbs of this reflex are optic nerve fibers.

8.20. C. The pupil remains small even in a dimly lit room, indicating that sympathetic fibers innervating the dilator pupillae (radial muscles of the iris) are damaged.

8.21. A. The secretomotor fibers to the lacrimal gland are parasympathetic fibers that run in the facial, greater petrosal, Vidian, maxillary, zygomatic and lacrimal nerves.

8.22. C. The frontal sinus communicates with the middle nasal meatus and receives blood from branches of the ophthalmic artery.

8.23. A. The tongue has nodular masses of lymphoid follicles that are collectively called the lingual tonsil on the dorsum of its posterior one-third. The tongue is innervated by (a) the trigeminal nerve via lingual nerve for general sensation on its anterior two-thirds, (b) the facial nerve via chorda tympani for taste sensation from its anterior two-thirds, (c) the glossopharyngeal nerve for general and taste sensations from its posterior one-third, (d) the vagus nerve via internal laryngeal nerve for taste sensation from its root near the epiglottis, and (e) the hypoglossal nerve for motor fibers to its intrinsic and extrinsic muscles.

8.24. E. The foramen magnum is the large opening at the center of the base of the skull, surrounded by the dura and periosteum. It transmits the medulla-spinal cord junction, the meninges, the spinal roots of the accessory nerves, the vertebral arteries, the anterior and posterior spinal arteries, the ligaments passing between the occipital bone and the axis, etc. The cerebrospinal fluid is located in the subarachnoid space between the pia and arachnoid maters.

8.25. B. The patient cannot focus on close objects (accommodation) because of damage to the parasympathetic fibers in the ciliary ganglion or in the short ciliary nerves. The patient sees distant objects clearly because the long ciliary nerve carries sympathetic fibers to the dilator pupillae. The patient moves his eyeball normally, indicating that the oculomotor, trochlear, and abducens nerves are intact.

8.26. D. Veins of the brain are direct tributaries of the dural venous sinuses. The emissary veins connect the dural venous sinuses with the veins of the scalp, whereas the diploic veins lie in channels in the diploë of the skull and communicate with the dural sinuses, the veins of the scalp, and the meningeal veins. The pterygoid venous plexus communicates with the cavernous sinus by an emissary vein.

8.27. D. If the parasympathetic fibers to the eyeball are stimulated, the pupil is constricted and the ciliary muscle is contracted, resulting in a thicker lens and enhanced vision for near objects (accommodation). Contraction of capillaries in the iris and enhanced ability to see distant objects (lens becomes flattened) are actions of the sympathetic nerve.

8.28. D. The pituitary gland is situated in the hypophyseal fossa of the sella turcica of the sphenoid bone.

8.29. C. The optic nerve and the mandibular division of the trigeminal nerve do not lie in the wall of the cavernous sinus.

8.30. A. The trochlear, lacrimal, and frontal nerves and the ophthalmic vein enter the orbit through the superior orbital fissure but outside the common tendinous ring.

8.31. B. Some preganglionic parasympathetic fibers from the facial nerve run in the greater petrosal nerve and the nerve of the pterygoid canal and synapse in the pterygopalatine ganglion, and others run in the chorda tympani and synapse in the submandibular ganglion.

8.32. A. The stylohyoid muscle is innervated by the facial nerve; the styloglossus muscle by the hypoglossal nerve; and the stylopharyngeus muscle by the glossopharyngeal nerve.

8.33. B. Swallowing involves movements of the tongue to push the food into the oropharynx, elevation of the soft palate to close the entrance of the nasopharynx, elevation of the hyoid bone and the larynx to close the opening into the larynx, and contraction of the pharyngeal constrictors to move the food through the pharynx. The mandibular division of the trigeminal nerve supplies the suprahyoid muscles such as the digastric anterior belly and mylohyoid muscles. The vagus nerve innervates the muscles of the palate, the larynx, and the pharynx.

8.34. D. The preganglionic parasympathetic fibers run in the tympanic (Jacobson's) nerve, which is a branch of the glossopharyngeal nerve, and then in the lesser petrosal nerve to reach the otic ganglion where they synapse with postganglionic neurons.

8.35. B. The supreme (highest) thoracic artery is a branch of the costocervical trunk, whereas the inferior thyroid artery is a branch of the thyrocervical trunk.

8.36. E. The straight sinus runs along the line of attachment of the falx cerebri with the tentorium cerebelli.

8.37. D. The transverse sinus runs laterally and forward in the convex outer border of the tentorium cerebelli.

8.38. C. The superior sagittal sinus lies in the superior convex border of the falx cerebri.

8.39. A. The cavernous sinus communicates directly with the ophthalmic veins.

8.40. B. The sigmoid sinus becomes continuous with the internal jugular vein.

8.41. B. The vagus nerve provides motor innervation to the intrinsic muscles of the larynx through the recurrent and external laryngeal nerves.

8.42. D. The lingual nerve carries general sensation from the anterior two-thirds of the tongue.

8.43. E. The glossopharyngeal nerve carries the preganglionic parasympathetic fibers that run in the tympanic and lesser petrosal nerves and synapse in the otic ganglion. The postganglionic parasympathetic fibers run in the auriculotemporal nerve and innervate the parotid gland.

8.44. A. The hyoglossal nerve provides motor innervation to the intrinsic and extrinsic muscles of the tongue except for the palatoglossus muscle, which is innervated by the vagus nerve.

8.45. E. The glossopharyngeal nerve carries sensory information from pressure receptors in the carotid sinus.

8.46. E. The superior orbital fissure transmits the ophthalmic nerve.

8.47. D. The foramen lacerum transmits nothing, but its superior portion is occupied by the internal carotid artery.

8.48. B. The foramen spinosum transmits the middle meningeal artery.

8.49. C. The foramen rotundum transmits the maxillary division of the trigeminal nerve, and its injury leads to a loss of general sensation of the maxillary teeth.

8.50. A. The foramen ovale transmits the mandibular division of the trigeminal nerve, and its injury leads to a loss of sensation of the temporomandibular joint.

8.51. A. The stylomastoid foramen transmits the facial nerve, which innervates the muscles of facial expression.

8.52. E. The jugular foramen transmits the glossopharyngeal nerve, which carries sensory fibers from the posterior one-third of the tongue.

8.53. D. The sphenopalatine foramen transmits the sphenopalatine nerve, which carries sensory fibers from the mucosa of the nasal septum, the posterior lateral nasal wall, and the anterior portion of the hard palate.

8.54. C. The pterygomaxillary fissure is the passageway between the infratemporal fossa and the pterygopalatine fossa for the terminal part of the maxillary artery.

8.55. B. The pterygoid canal transmits the nerve of the pterygoid canal, which contains preganglionic parasympathetic fibers to the lacrimal gland.

8.56. B. When the dorsal scapular artery arises from the third part of the subclavian artery, it replaces a deep branch of the transverse cervical artery.

8.57. C. The costocervical trunk is a snort trunk from the subclavian artery, which arches to the neck of the first rib, where it divides into the deep cervical and supreme intercostal arteries. Thus it is not closely associated with the isthmus of the thyroid gland.

8.58. C. The superior thyroid artery is accompanied by the external laryngeal nerve, which supplies the cricothyroid muscle. Damage to this nerve results in inability to tense the vocal cords.

8.59. A. The phrenic nerve contains motor and sensory fibers but no cutaneous nerve fibers.

8.60. C. The sphenoid sinus opens into the sphenoethmoidal recess in the nasal cavity.

8.61. B. The superior laryngeal artery is accompanied by the internal laryngeal nerve.

8.62. D. The glossopharyngeal nerve supplies sensory innervation of the mucosa of the pharynx.

8.63. C. The supraclavicular nerve is a cutaneous branch of the cervical plexus and supplies skin over the pectoralis major and deltoid muscles.

8.64. D. The deep cervical artery is a branch of the costocervical trunk.

8.65. E. The phrenic nerve descends on the superficial surface of the scalenus anterior muscle and enters the thorax by passing between the subclavian artery and vein.

8.66. B. The stylopharyngeus is a "landmark" for finding the glossopharyngeal nerve, because this nerve curves posteriorly around the lateral margin of the stylopharyngeus muscle to enter the pharyngeal wall.

8.67. A. The external laryngeal branch of the superior laryngeal nerve supplies the cricothyroid and inferior pharyngeal constrictor muscles.

8.68. B. Taste cells associated with the fungiform papillae on the anterior two-thirds of the tongue are innervated by the chorda tympani, which originates in the facial nerve.

8.69. E. The afferent nerve fibers from the larynx are carried by the internal laryngeal branch of the superior laryngeal nerve and the recurrent laryngeal nerve.

8.70. E. The optic nerve passes through the optic canal in company with the ophthalmic artery.

8.71. D. Both the anterior and posterior ethmoidal nerves are branches of the nasociliary nerve and send branches to the ethmoidal air cells.

8.72. C. The postganglionic parasympathetic fibers originating in the pterygopalatine ganglion innervate the glands in the palate.

8.73. B. The duct of the submandibular gland passes between the mylohyoid and hyoglossus muscles, where it is crossed laterally by the lingual nerve.

8.74. E. The vomer bone forms part of the nasal septum.

8.75. C. In Bell's palsy (or facial paralysis), a possible inflammation of the cornea leads to corneal ulceration, which is most likely attributable to absence of the blinking reflex due to paralysis of the closing muscle(s) of the eyelid.

8.76. B. The inferior sagittal sinus and the greater cerebral vein are direct tributaries to the straight sinus in the cranial cavity.

8.77. E. The abducens (VI) nerve innervates the lateral rectus muscle, which abducts the eyeball.

8.78. C. The bilateral severance of the vagus nerves may result in death.

8.79. C. Rupture of the middle meningeal artery in the cranial cavity causes an epidural hemorrhage.

8.80. E. Preganglionic neurons of the parasympathetic nervous system are located in the brain stem (cranial outflow) and sacral spinal cord segments S2–4 (sacral outflow).

8.81. D. The taste buds in the anterior two-thirds of the tongue are innervated by the chorda tympani of the facial nerve.

8.82. E. The pituitary gland lies in the hypophysial fossa of the sella turcica of the sphenoid bone, which lies immediately posterior and superior to the sphenoid sinus and medial to the cavernous sinus., It is roofed by the diaphragma sellae.

8.83. E. The carotid sheath contains the vagus nerve, the common carotid artery, and the internal jugular vein. The sympathetic trunk lies posterior to the carotid sheath.

8.84. E. The sella turcica is part of the sphenoid bone.

8.85. B. If parasympathetic fibers are stimulated, the ciliary muscle contracts and thus the lens of the eye becomes thicker. Accommodation for seeing objects close to the eye is mediated by the parasympathetic nerve action, and the lens becomes thicker during accommodation.

8.86. B. A characteristic of an open scalp wound is excessive bleeding. This happens because the connective tissue fibers of the scalp are unique in that they tend to hold the cut walls of scalp arteries open, whereas in other parts of the body they permit them to collapse.

8.87. B. A horizontal cut through the neck would sever the inferior thyroid arteries and the common carotid arteries but not the external carotid arteries.

8.88. B. The dural venous sinus nearest the pituitary gland is the cavernous sinus.

8.89. C. The chorda tympani carries parasympathetic fibers to the submandibular ganglion and taste fibers from the anterior two-thirds of the tongue.

8.90. C. The pterygopalatine fossa lies between the pterygoid plates of the sphenoid and palatine bone, below the apex of the orbit. It contains the pterygopalatine ganglion and communicates with the middle cranial cavity through the foramen rotundum and with the infratemporal fossa through the pterygomaxillary fissure.

8.91. B. The tensor tympani is innervated by the mandibular branch of the trigeminal nerve.

8.92. D. The posterior cricoarytenoid muscle is the only muscle that abducts the vocal cords during quiet breathing.

8.93. D. The oculomotor nerve carries parasympathetic fibers to the constrictor pupillae and the ciliary muscle. The secretomotor fibers for lacrimal secretion come through the pterygopalatine ganglion.

8.94. C. Nerves that supply the muscles of the tongue and the eyeball are not of branchiomeric origin.

8.95. B. The oblique arytenoids and aryepiglotticus can prevent food from getting into the larynx and trachea during the process of swallowing.

8.96. B. The deep petrosal nerve contains postganglionic sympathetic fibers whose cell bodies are located in the superior cervical ganglion.

8.97. A. The greater petrosal nerve contains preganglionic parasympathetic fibers that synapse in the pterygopalatine ganglion.

8.98. C. The nerve of the pterygoid canal is formed by the greater petrosal and deep petrosal nerves.

8.99. A. The taste fibers, with cell bodies in the geniculate ganglion, pass from the palate through the palatine nerve, pterygopalatine ganglion, nerve of the pterygoid canal, and greater petrosal nerve to the geniculate ganglion.

8.100. D. The geniculate ganglion is composed of cell bodies of sensory nerves.

8.101. B. The masseter muscle elevates the mandible.

8.102. C. The buccinator muscle is innervated by the facial nerve, which also innervates the posterior belly of the digastric muscle. However, the masseter muscle is innervated by the trigeminal nerve, which also innervates the anterior belly of the digastric muscle.

8.103. B. The parotid duct superficially crosses the masseter muscle, pierces the buccinator muscle, and empties into the vestibule of the mouth opposite the upper second molar tooth.

8.104. A. See 8.103.

8.105. D. The buccinator originates from the alveolar process of the maxilla and mandible, whereas the masseter inserts on the coronoid process and the ramus and angle of the mandible.

8.106. C. Both the costocervical and thyrocervical trunks arise from the subclavian artery.

8.107. A. The costocervical trunk gives rise to the superior intercostal artery, which supplies the first two posterior intercostal spaces.

8.108. A. The deep cervical artery is a direct branch of the costocervical trunk.

8.109. C. The deep cervical branch of the costocervical trunk anastomoses with the deep branch of the descending branch of the occipital artery. The ascending (superficial) branch of the transverse cervical artery of the thyrocervical trunk anastomoses with the superficial branch of the descending branch of the occipital artery.

8.110. B. The thyrocervical trunk typically has three branches, including the inferior thyroid, transverse cervical, and suprascapular branches, whereas the costocervical trunk typically has two branches, including the deep cervical and superior intercostal branches

8.111. A. The trigeminal nerve contains nerve fibers whose major functional components convey general sensation from the face and scalp.

8.112. A. The trigeminal (maxillary division) contains sensory nerve fibers that pass through the greater palatine foramen and reach the palate.

8.113. B. The facial nerve contains preganglionic parasympathetic fibers that run through the greater petrosal nerve and the nerve of the pterygoid canal to synapse in the pterygopalatine ganglion.

8.114. B. The trigeminal nerve (maxillary division) contains sensory nerve fibers that stimulate secretion of the mucous glands in the nasal cavity.

8.115. C. The buccal nerve from the trigeminal nerve is sensory, whereas the buccal nerve from the facial nerve is motor.

8.116. C. Both the tensor tympani and tensor veli palatini muscles arise from the cartilaginous portion of the auditory tube, receive blood from a branch of the maxillary artery, and are innervated by the mandibular division of the trigeminal nerve, which passes through the foramen ovale.

8.117. A. The tensor tympani inserts on the handle of the malleus.

8.118. B. See 8.116.

8.119. C. See 8.116.

8.120. B. The tendon of the tensor veli palatini muscle winds around the pterygoid hamulus of the medial pterygoid plate and inserts into the soft palate (palatine aponeurosis).

SUGGESTED READINGS

Anderson JE. (1983) *Grant's Atlas of Anatomy*, Eighth Edition. Williams & Wilkins Company, Baltimore.

Hollinshead WH, Rosse C. (1985) *Textbook of Anatomy*, Fourth Edition. Harper & Row, Philadelphia.

Lachman E, Faulkner KK (1981) Case Studies in Anatomy, Third Edition. Oxford University Press, New York.

Moore KL (1980) *Clinically Oriented Anatomy*. Williams & Wilkins, Baltimore.

O'Rahilly R. (1986) *Gardner-Gray-O'Rahilly's Anatomy, A Regional Study of Human Structure*, Fifth Edition. WB Saunders, Philadelphia.

Woodburne RT. (1983) *Essentials of Human Anatomy*, Seventh Edition. Oxford University Press, New York.

INDEX